# FIRST AID FOR THE

*FIRST EDITION*

# WARDS

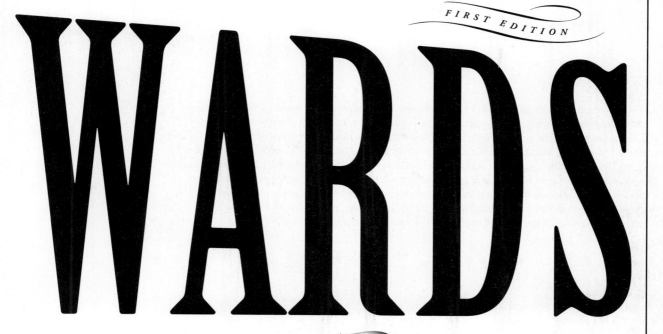

INSIDER **FOR THE CLINICAL YEARS** ADVICE

## TAO LE, MD
*University of California, San Francisco, Class of 1996*
*Yale–New Haven Hospital, Resident in Internal Medicine*

## VIKAS BHUSHAN, MD
*University of California, San Francisco, Class of 1991*
*Diagnostic Radiologist*

## CHIRAG AMIN, MD
*University of Miami, Class of 1996*
*Orlando Regional Medical Center, Resident in Orthopaedic Surgery*

## ROSS BERKELEY, MD
*Student Editor*
*University of California, San Francisco, Class of 1997*
*University of Pittsburgh Medical Center*
*Resident in Emergency Medicine*

D1278424

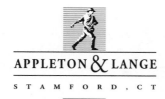

APPLETON & LANGE

STAMFORD, CT

Copyright © 1998 by Appleton & Lange
A Simon & Schuster Company

Information from the following title was adapted and incorporated with permission:
Segen JC, *Current Med Talk,* Appleton & Lange, 1995.

98 99 00 01 02 / 10 9 8 7 6 5 4 3 2

Prentice Hall International (UK) Limited, *London*
Prentice Hall of Australia Pty. Limited, *Sydney*
Prentice Hall Canada, Inc., *Toronto*
Prentice Hall Hispanoamericana, S.A., *Mexico*
Prentice Hall of India Private Limited, *New Delhi*
Prentice Hall of Japan, Inc., *Tokyo*
Simon & Schuster Asia Pte. Ltd., *Singapore*
Editora Prentice Hall do Brasil Ltda., *Rio de Janeiro*
Prentice Hall, *Upper Saddle River, New Jersey*

Acquisitions Editor: Marinita S. Timban
Production Service: Rainbow Graphics, Inc.
Cover design: Design Group Cook
Internal design: Ashley Pound Design

ISBN 0-8385-2595-4

90000

9 780838 525951

PRINTED IN THE UNITED STATES OF AMERICA

To all our contributors, who took time to share their experience, advice,
and humor for the benefit of students
&
To our families, friends, and loved ones, who endured and assisted in the
task of assembling this guide.

# Contributing Authors

Tim Abou-Sayed, MD
Resident in Surgery
Massachusetts General Hospital
*Surgery Chapter*

Taejoon Ahn, MD, MPH
Resident in Family Practice
University of California, San Francisco
*Psychiatry Chapter*

Shaun Anand, MD
Resident in Medicine
University of California, Los Angeles
*Medicine Chapter*

Catherine Lee, MD
Resident in Medicine
University of Pennsylvania
*Neurology Chapter*

Knef Lizaso
University of California, San Francisco
School of Medicine, Class of 1998
*Book Reviews*

Christine Pham, MD
Resident in Obstetrics & Gynecology
Johns Hopkins University
*Obstetrics & Gynecology Chapter*

Thao Pham, MD
Resident in Pediatrics
Yale-New Haven Hospital
*Pediatrics Chapter*

Diego Ruiz
University of California, San Francisco
School of Medicine, Class of 1999
*Book Reviews*

# Faculty Reviewers

Pauline Chen, MD
Chief Resident in Surgery
Yale-New Haven Hospital

G. Edward Fahy, MD
Chief Resident in Obstetrics & Gynecology
Yale-New Haven Hospital

James Longhurst, MD
Chief Resident in Psychiatry
Yale-New Haven Hospital

Daniel Lowenstein, MD
Assistant Professor of Neurology
University of California, San Francisco

Jarrod Post, MD
Chief Resident in Medicine
Yale-New Haven Hospital

Sadek Salloum, MD
Fellow in General Pediatrics
Yale-New Haven Hospital

# Contents

CONTENTS

# Preface

The change from the passive and controlled environment of the classroom to the fast-paced and active world of the wards can be stressful, confusing, and downright frightening at times. The purpose of *First Aid for the Wards* is to help ease the transition wards students must make as they begin their clerkship rotations. This book is a student-to-student guide that draws on the advice and experiences of medical students who were successful on the wards. It is our hope to familiarize you with life on the wards and to pass on some of the "secrets of success" that we picked up along the way in our training. The facts and wisdom contained within this book are an amalgam of information we, the authors, wished we had known at the beginning of our third year of medical school. *First Aid for the Wards* has a number of unique features that make it an indispensable guide for MD, DO and DPM students:

- Insider advice from students on how to succeed on your clinical rotations.
- Sample H&P notes, daily progress notes, procedure notes, postop notes, labor and delivery notes, and admission orders.
- Specific advice on how to give both concise and detailed oral patient presentations.
- Descriptions of typical daily responsibilities and interactions on each core rotation, including medicine, surgery, pediatrics, obstetrics and gynecology, neurology, and psychiatry.
- Key wards lingo with definitions courtesy of Dr. Joseph Segen and *Current Med Talk*.
- High-yield topics outlining the signs and symptoms, differential diagnosis, workup, and treatment of the important and commonly encountered diseases of each rotation.
- Student- and peer-reviewed evaluations of more than 140 commonly used handbooks, reference books, and texts, specifically addressing their usefulness to medical students on the wards.

*First Aid for the Wards* is meant to be a survival guide rather than a comprehensive source of information. It should supplement information and advice provided by other students, house staff, and faculty. It is designed not to replace reference texts as a source of information but rather to provide some essential background information for each core ward rotation. Although the material has been reviewed by medical faculty and students, errors and omissions are inevitable. We urge readers to suggest improvements and identify inaccuracies. We invite students and faculty to continue sharing their thoughts and ideas to help us improve *First Aid for the Wards* (see How to Contribute, page xvii).

New Haven
Los Angeles
Orlando
Pittsburgh

October 1997

Tao Le
Vikas Bhushan
Chirag Amin
Ross Berkeley

# Acknowledgments

This has been a collaborative project which would not have been possible without the thoughtful comments, insights, and advice of the numerous medical students and faculty whom we gratefully acknowledge for their support in the development of *First Aid for the Wards*.

Special thanks to Andi Fellows, our tireless editor, and Gianni Le Nguyen, our administrative assistant, for bringing the book together under constant pressure. Our eagle-eyed proofreading team included Dr. Jose Fierro, Laurie Hickey, Sundar Jayaraman, Warren Krackov, James Moak, Riva Rahl, Anne Rutledge, Dr. Kanwarjit Singh, Mark Tanaka, and Patricia Tsai. We also thank Dr. Joseph Segen for the use of several Med Talk terms from *Current Med Talk* in Chapter 1. For contributions to Chapter 1, we thank Dr. Lawrence Tierney, Jr. Thanks to Dr. Joanna Zell, Dr. Rita Suri, Dr. Sanjay Sahgal and Dr. Anthony Glaser for contributions to the Psychiatry chapter, to Dr. Angelica Go for contributions to the Pediatrics chapter, and to Dr. Steven Fleischman and Dr. Gaurang Daftary for reviewing the Obstetrics and Gynecology chapter. Also thanks to Cynthia Andrien for organizing Yale medical student reviews of the book. Thanks to the *Synapse*, UCSF, and Mona Lisa Valentin for the use of their computers.

Thanks to our publisher, Appleton & Lange, for offering a coupon for each new contribution used in future editions of this book, and for the valuable assistance of their staff. For enthusiasm, support, and commitment for this project, thanks to our editor, Marinita Timban. For editorial support, we thank Joan Kalkut. For speedy typesetting of all those last-minute changes, we thank Bennie, Jimmy, David, and the staff at Rainbow Graphics.

We would also like to thank the staff at Doody Publishing, the Milberry Union Bookstore, UCSF, and Discount Medical Books, San Francisco, for their time, patience, and help in obtaining book information and books for review.

For helping to review the books in this edition, we thank Paul Abrinko, Lisa Bardaro, Carrie Campbell, Jon Friedman, Erin Gourley, Praj Kadkade, and Mohan Viswanathan. And for fine-tuning and updating our book reviews, we thank David Bassler, Ayaz Bijivi, Charley C. DellaSantina, John Franco, Mark Goodarzi, Nicole Hartnett, Amy K. Howard, Wynne Hsieh, Mary Jung, Richard Kim, Robert E. Kuhn, James Lawrence, Lillian Lee, Nikki Levin, Tony Mosley, Ali Mesiwala, Ed Nguyen, Longhang Nguyen, Natalie Ong, Tom Ormiston, Jayana Patel, Uptal Patel, Michael Cahill Pickart, Bill Rhoads, Richard Roston, Simren Sangha, Patrick Suen, Chris Tang, Jeff Uller, David Vo, Paul Wallace, Steve Yao, Michael Yu, and Keren Ziv.

For field testing prepublication drafts of the book while on the wards, we thank Chris Aiken, Lee Akst, Alicia Arbaje, Ken Baum, Kirstin Boger, Wendi Brown, Deanna Chin, John Coombes, Alison Days, Elly Falzarano, Jessica Haberes, Daniel Hall, Laurie Hickey, Naomi Katz, Jennifer Kreshak, Yvonne Lui, Marlon R. Maragh, Aaron Milestone, Henry Nguyen, Gilbert R. Ortega, Abhijit A. Patel, Dan Rothbaum, Shahiam Salami, Jennifer Schutzman, Lisa Skinner, Tanya Smith, Vipal Soni, Deborah Steinbaum, Jakub Svoboda, Joy Weinberg, and Meher Yepremyan.

To all those we may have forgotten, please e-mail us for the second edition.

# How to Contribute

*First Aid for the Wards* is a work in progress—a collaborative project that was refined through the many contributions and changes received from students and faculty. The authors and Appleton & Lange intend to update *First Aid for the Wards* so that the book grows both in quality and in scope while continuing to serve as a timely guidebook to survival and success on the wards. We invite you to participate in this process by passing on your own insights.

Please send us:

- Tips for survival and success on the wards.
- New topics, diagrams, and tables that you feel should be included in the next edition.
- Mnemonics or algorithms you have used on the wards.
- Personal ratings and comments on books that you have used while on the hospital wards, including books that were not reviewed in this edition.
- Your medical school's handbook to the clerkships.
- Corrections and clarifications.

For each entry incorporated into the next edition, you will receive a $10 coupon (per entry) good toward the purchase of any Appleton & Lange medical book, as well as a personal acknowledgment in the next edition. Significant contributions will be compensated at the discretion of the publisher.

The preferred way to submit suggestions and contributions is via electronic mail, addressed to:

**Taotle@aol.com**

Vbhushan@aol.com
Chiragamin@aol.com

You can also use the contribution forms on the following pages. Feel free to photocopy these forms or attach additional pages as needed. Please send your contributions and corrections, neatly written or typed, to:

Attn: Contributions
First Aid for the Wards
Appleton & Lange
Four Stamford Plaza
P.O. Box 120041
Stamford, CT 06912-0041

Another option is to send in your entire annotated book. We will look through your additions and notes and will send you Appleton & Lange coupons based on the quantity and quality of additions that we incorporate into the next edition. Books will be returned upon request.

For corrections and updates, please visit the S2S Medical Website at:

**www.s2smed.com**

## NOTE TO CONTRIBUTORS

All entries are subject to editing and reviewing. Please verify all data and spellings carefully. In the event that similar or duplicate entries are received, only the first entry received will be used. Please follow the style, punctuation, and format of this edition if possible.

# Contribution Form I

For entries, facts, corrections, diagrams, etc.

Contributor Name:_____

School/Affiliation:_____

Address:_____

_____

Telephone:_____

E-mail:_____

Topic:

Signs & Symptoms:

Workup:

Treatment:

Notes, Diagrams, Tables, or Mnemonics:

Reference:

*You will receive personal acknowledgment and a $10 coupon toward selected Appleton & Lange books for each entry that is used in future editions.*

(fold here)

---

Return Address

_____

_____

_____

Postage
Required

Attn: Contributions
First Aid for the Wards
Appleton & Lange
Four Stamford Plaza
P.O. Box 120041
Stamford, CT 06912–0041

---

(fold here)

# Contribution Form II

For book reviews

Contributor Name:_____

School/Affiliation:_____

Address:_____

_____

Telephone:_____

E-mail:_____

We welcome additional comments on books rated in this edition, as well as reviews of texts not included in this edition. Please fill out each review entry as completely as possible. Please do not leave "Comments" blank. Rate all books using the letter grading (A⁺ to C⁻), taking into consideration the other books on that subject.

Title/Author: _____

Publisher/Series: _____   ISBN Number: _____

Rating: _____   Comments: _____

_____

_____

Title/Author: _____

Publisher/Series: _____   ISBN Number: _____

Rating: _____   Comments: _____

_____

_____

Title/Author: _____

Publisher/Series: _____   ISBN Number: _____

Rating: _____   Comments: _____

_____

_____

Title/Author: _____

Publisher/Series: _____   ISBN Number: _____

Rating: _____   Comments: _____

_____

_____

Title/Author: _____

Publisher/Series: _____   ISBN Number: _____

Rating: _____   Comments: _____

_____

_____

*You will receive personal acknowledgment and a $10 coupon toward selected Appleton & Lange books for each entry that is used in future editions.*

(fold here)

Return Address

_____

_____

_____

Postage
Required

Attn: Contributions
First Aid for the Wards
Appleton & Lange
Four Stamford Plaza
P.O. Box 120041
Stamford, CT 06912–0041

(fold here)

# User Survey

Contributor Name:_____
School/Affiliation:_____
Address:_____
_____
Telephone:_____
E-mail:_____

What student-to-student advice would you give to a student about to begin his or her clerkships?

Is there any advice in this book that you believe should be altered or amended? How can it be improved?

Have you experienced any "difficult situations" on the wards that were not covered in this edition or that you feel should be handled differently? Do you have any advice to others on how to deal with similar situations?

What would you change about the high-yield topics? Were the entries too superficial, too detailed, or just right?

How else would you improve *First Aid for the Wards*? Any other comments or suggestions? What did you like most about the book?

**You will receive personal acknowledgment and a $10 coupon toward selected Appleton & Lange books for each entry that is used in future editions.**

(fold here)

Return Address

_____

_____

_____

Attn: Contributions
First Aid for the Wards
Appleton & Lange
Four Stamford Plaza
P.O. Box 120041
Stamford, CT 06912–0041

(fold here)

# CHAPTER ONE
# Guide for Wards Success

## INTRODUCTION

For the past two years, you have been learning medicine in classrooms, labs, the library, and the floor of your bedroom. You may have spent some time on the hospital wards via an introductory clinical medicine class, observing, taking histories, and practicing physical exams. However, up to this point, your presence on the wards has largely been superfluous. All that is about to change. You are finally about to practice medicine. You will be an integral part of an organized team and will be given real responsibilities. And yes, you will have your own patients.

So relax.

The transition from the controlled environment of the classroom to the dynamic and often chaotic wards will be one of the most exhilarating periods in your training. The purpose of this book is to make your transition to the wards as smooth and stress-free as possible by familiarizing you with the inner workings of each service and the common pitfalls that many students encounter. Some common mistakes that students make when coming to the wards include:

- Not understanding the responsibilities and expectations for the rotation.
- Not seeking timely feedback.
- Utilizing inappropriate pocket references and clinical texts.
- Not knowing what to study on the wards.
- Inefficient organization and execution of daily work.
- Insufficient preparation for oral presentations for attending rounds.
- Not streamlining personal and family responsibilities.
- Scheduling key rotations too early or too late.

In this section, we will offer advice to help you avoid these pitfalls and be more productive in your clinical rotations. It is important, however, to first understand the wards experience itself.

A key to succeeding on the wards is understanding how your team works and how you fit in. Your goal should be to function as a productive team member,

**THE TEAM**

to care for your patients, and, of course, to learn. Winning friends and allies on the team can help ensure that you get the best teaching and support possible and that you **always** get the benefit of the doubt. For example, if you help the intern with the daily patient care, also known as SCUT WORK, he or she may prep you for the inevitable PIMP questions that the attending or resident may ask. On the other hand, making the intern or resident look bad in front of the attending will wreck the team's trust in you.

## CURRENT Med Talk

### CURRENT MED TALK

SCUT WORK: Menial, non-patient-care-related activities that are often passed to medical students (externs) or interns, although they are actually the responsibility of other health-care workers; the array of 'scut' details is vast and includes obtaining supplies, performing ward paperwork, going to the pharmacy, laboratory, and emergency room with specimens or paperwork, acting as an orderly, cleaning the nurses' station, going for pizza, and so on. Scut duties are often cited as a subtle form of 'medical student abuse.'

PIMPING: A practice in which persons in power ask esoteric questions of junior colleagues, usually with the sole purpose of publicly demeaning them, which most often occurs on ward rounds with a chief of service in a university hospital. The interrogating 'pimper' is theoretically interested in correct answers; the 'pimpee,' usually a medical student, is interested in self-esteem, although correct answers to the questions gain neither recognition nor relief from this form of harassment. Pimping serves to establish a 'pecking order' among the medical staff. DISADVANTAGE: It suppresses spontaneous or intellectual questions or pursuits, creates an antagonistic atmosphere, and perpetuates medical student abuse **(JAMA 1989; 262:2541-2; 263:1632c).**

A medical team typically consists of the following members:

### ATTENDING

As the head of the team, the attending is usually involved in the major treatment decisions affecting your patients, such as whether a patient needs chemotherapy versus radiotherapy for that tumor. The logistics (eg, scheduling, fine-tuning of treatment) are typically left to the resident and intern. On certain surgical services, the chief resident acts as the head of the team and reports to several "attending" surgeons. The attending is legally and morally responsible for the actions of each member of the team. Thus, the attending is ultimately responsible for educating and evaluating the resident, intern, and medical students on the team.

You will have far less contact with the attending than with the others on your team. Because the attending sees you mostly during attending rounds, buffed oral presentations are usually the key to winning points with the attending. The attending will also see your admit note and will often ask you questions at the patient's bedside. Therefore, knowing the patient inside out will keep you from falling on your face. You should also have a basic understanding of the patient's problem and the rationale behind the treatment plan.

## RESIDENT

The resident (PGY-2 and up) is a house officer who has gone through internship. As such, he or she works closely with the attending to devise and manage the treatment plan for your patient. The resident is also responsible for teaching you and the intern, via either didactics or informal pimping. Do not be afraid of pimp questions. No one expects you to be able to answer all of them. Junior medical students often report to interns, whereas subinterns usually report directly to the resident.

The resident monitors and sometimes supervises your daily activities. You can make a strong impression by making concise work-round presentations, demonstrating a strong fund of knowledge regarding your patient's illness and how it affects your treatment plan, maintaining an awareness of all events pertaining to your patient (eg, the latest CXR results), showing hustle and effort in scut work, and providing occasional review articles that address treatment issues affecting your patients. The best article is often a "review article" from a respected journal in the field. If the team has a conference scheduled, find out the topic ahead of time and copy articles for the team.

## INTERN

The intern (PGY-1) provides the "muscle" that gets the practical aspects of wards work done for the team and is responsible for executing the treatment plan under the direct supervision of the resident. Anything that does not get done on a patient falls in the lap of the poor intern. Because interns are usually the most overworked members of the team, they do little didactic teaching, but they can serve as excellent sources of information on how to get tasks done quickly and efficiently. While you are a physician-in-training, they are teachers-in-training. The junior clerk often reports directly to the intern.

Intern rules:
eat when you can,
sleep when you can,
leave when you can.

Inasmuch as he or she is a recent student, the intern is your most natural ally. You will, moreover, work very closely with the intern. Although the intern is usually not involved in your formal evaluations, he or she will let the resident know how you're doing. Keeping the intern up to date on patients will earn points. Lightening the scut burden on your intern will allow him or her to finish earlier and spend more time in the OR or reading about patients' problems. It should also give the intern more time to go through the patients with you. So volunteering for all the "thankless" duties not only earns the intern's gratitude but may also get you more one-on-one teaching in return. In contrast, neglecting the scut will force the intern to do everything himself to the detriment of your education.

Interns can be your best
friends; keep them
informed.

## SUBINTERN

The subintern is a fourth-year student who has the same responsibilities as the intern. Although the subintern has no responsibility for evaluating or teaching you and usually does not cover your patients, he or she can often be a valuable source of clinical pearls and practical information about the wards and applying for residency. Often, however, subinterns are overwhelmed by the amount of responsibility heaped upon them, so don't take it personally if they run past you in a frenzy down the hallway.

## NURSE

A good rapport with the nursing staff is one of the keys to a successful and enjoyable rotation. Ward nurses carry out the written physician orders and attend to the daily needs of the patient. Nurses are experienced in patient care and know a great deal about what is going on with patients. Accordingly, they can often give you the "scoop" on your patient when you pre-round in the morning.

Learn the names of the nurses caring for your patients and treat them as your equal. (Do not walk around barking orders rudely, or you will find out very quickly how critical it is to get along with the nurses, especially when you are trying to sleep on call.) Respect their opinions, but also double-check with your resident or intern. If something goes wrong, you will often take responsibility.

Never leave a mess for the nurse to clean up, and make sure you exchange relevant clinical information. If nurses like you, they may feed you extra information on your patient, clue you in on important treatment issues, and take the time to teach you important scut skills, such as placing Foley catheters or inserting IV lines. Be friendly yet assertive when asking for help.

**Nurses can make or break your rotation.**

**Never leave a mess.**

## CURRENT MED TALK

NURSE PRACTITIONER: A nurse certified to diagnose illness and physical conditions and perform therapeutic and corrective measures within a designated specialty area of practice. NPs may write orders for routine laboratory and clinical tests and prescribe routine drugs (ie, not controlled substances), devices, and immunizing agents as specified in his/her privileges in a particular health care environment or hospital; all such orders must be countersigned by an attending physician.

PHYSICIAN ASSISTANT: An individual who is qualified to perform a wide variety of medically related tasks under a physician's supervision, including taking a patient's history and performing physical examinations and autopsies. EDUCATION: Two postgraduate years beyond college or university, training as a physician assistant, surgeon assistant, or pathologist assistant. Physician assistants may then subspecialize for a one- to two-year period in various fields, including neonatology, pediatrics, emergency medicine, and occupational medicine.

## WARD CLERK

The ward clerk deals with many administrative issues affecting your patient. Specifically, he or she takes written orders off the charts, schedules procedures and lab tests, requests consults, and does discharge work on your patient. If the patient has gone somewhere for a diagnostic study, the ward clerk often knows where the patient is and when the patient will return (the only thing worse than not being able to find your patient's chart is not being able to find your patient).

## PHARMACIST

Sometimes staff pharmacists, residents, and/or students round with the team. Do not hesitate to hit them up for valuable information regarding toxicity, drug interactions, dosing in different disease states, and efficacy. Pharmacists are especially helpful on the medicine wards, where pharmaceuticals make up a large part of the internist's armamentarium.

## OTHER HOSPITAL STAFF

Other members of the hospital staff include PHYSICIAN ASSISTANTS, NURSE PRACTITIONERS, nutritional services, physical therapists, social workers, respiratory therapists, IV/blood draw (phlebotomy) teams, radiologic technicians, and laboratory technicians. All are important members of the hospital staff who are responsible for key aspects of your patient's care. Learning from their experience will thus make you a better ward clerk. For example, if you want to learn the finer points of IVs, you might want to tag along with the IV team on a day when you have extra time. Similarly, social workers are integral team members, often providing patient counseling, psychosocial assessment, and housing and transportation arrangements. Being on the wards is often the student's first exposure to the ubiquitous hospital "THREE-PIECE SUITS."

## CURRENT MED TALK

CURRENT *Med Talk*

'THREE-PIECE SUITS': A colloquial and nonspecific term for any businessperson, which in the health care industry includes 'medicrats' (MD/MPHs, ie, physicians with a master's degree in public health, hospital administrators), pharmaceutical representatives ('detail men'), and 'bean counters' (financial officers) who function in a medical center's bureaucracy.

SOAP: A mnemonic for the data that should be included in a problem-oriented medical record and in each entry in a patient's progress notes during hospitalization, including:

- SUBJECTIVE DATA, supplied by the patient or family
- OBJECTIVE DATA, ie, physical examination and laboratory data
- ASSESSMENT, a summary of significant (if any) new data
- PLAN of diagnostic or therapeutic action

## TYPICAL MEDICINE DAY

**A DAY ON THE WARDS**

The typical medicine day also applies to pediatrics, neurology, and psychiatry. Please refer to the chapters that follow for specific advice and information on each rotation.

**Prerounds:** 7:00–8:00 AM. As the primary caretaker of your patient, you note and evaluate during prerounds any event affecting your patient that occurred since you left the hospital the previous day (Table 1). Much of this information can be obtained by asking the overnight (cross-covering) house officer or the patient's nurse and by reviewing the chart. You can also discuss your plan prior to rounds with the intern who is following your patient. Note that interns are usually rushed in the morning, as they generally carry more patients.

**TABLE 1.**
**Preround checklist**

❏ Review the events since last night by checking the charts for new notes, talking to the cross-covering intern, and touching base with the nurse.

❏ Subjective status: ask the patient how he or she feels.

❏ Objective status: vital signs/brief physical exam focused on findings that are relevant to current problems.

❏ Check new labs, culture results, study results, and radiographs.

❏ Your plan for the patient for today (break it down by problem).

An intern will usually cosign everything you do—orders, notes, etc.

**Work rounds**: 8:00–9:30 AM. During work rounds, you round with the team minus the attending and give a very brief presentation (less than 30 seconds) on your patient to the resident in SOAP format. During work rounds, you also discuss your patient's problem and develop a plan with a to-do list for the day. Make sure to write down these chores immediately, as they may quickly be forgotten as you move on to the next patient. Most of the pimping you get is restricted to your patient's care—another reason to know your patient inside out.

**Work time, aka "Hour of Power"**: 9:30–11:00 AM. This is when you and the intern crank on the scut. Speed and efficiency during this critical period will determine what time you and the intern go home. Understand that studies and consults scheduled later in the day are often not accomplished until the next day. Typical tasks include:

- Placing orders in the chart
- Scheduling studies (eg, CT scans)
- Requesting consults
- Procedures (eg, paracentesis)
- Drawing blood for key labs
- Discharge paperwork
- Progress notes

**Attending rounds**: 11:00 AM – noon. During attending rounds, you meet with the entire medical team, including the attending physician, to discuss all newly admitted patients as well as to follow up on your current patients. On postcall days, you formally present your patient—a 4- to 6-minute ordeal—to the attending. As shallow as it may seem, acing the formal presentation is key to scoring points with the attending, since this may be the only chance you get to demonstrate your strengths face to face. Attendings depend on a smooth presentation to put a patient's story together and to formulate a diagnostic and therapeutic approach. A choppy or poorly organized presentation not only is painful to listen to but makes it difficult to concentrate on the patient's problems.

During attending rounds, you will receive didactic teaching related to patients' problems from the resident or attending. It can be very helpful to read up on your patients' problems before attending rounds. Do not hesitate to volunteer to organize a presentation on a disease or some aspect of its management; this is another chance to shine by demonstrating your sincere interest. Preparing handouts on your patient's disease (describing the clinical presentation, differential diagnosis, diagnostic findings and labs, complications, treatment, and prognosis) will make you a stellar student in the eyes of your team.

Radiology rounds are often part of attending rounds and occur with variable frequency. You may be asked to provide the radiologist with a 10- to 30-second bullet presentation prior to reviewing the films on each patient.

**Noon conference**: Noon – 1:00 PM. If your service offers a noon conference, don't miss it. First, there is often free food, courtesy of the service or a pharmaceutical representative. Second, noon conferences typically cover bread-and-butter topics that are geared toward house staff and medical students.

**Afternoon work**: 1:00 PM – ? In the afternoon, you plow through the rest of the to-do list and write your progress notes. During this time you will also check the results of any consults, studies, and labs that came back in the afternoon and adjust your treatment plan with the intern accordingly. On some days there will be additional conferences, some of which may be oriented toward medical students. If the service was light and you were a total stud(ette) during the Hour of Power, you may find yourself ready to go home by 4 PM.

**Signing out:** When the day is over and you have completed your daily chores, you have one critical responsibility left. "Signing out" involves a transfer of information to someone who will be responsible for your patients while you are home watching "Chicago Hope." Depending on your team, this may involve no more than an update of pending tests and your patient's condition to the resident or intern covering your patient. Alternatively, you may need to sign out to the cross-covering intern on call, who will be covering your patient overnight—in which case you will need to give a very brief description of your patient, current problems, medications and allergies, and any responsibilities you may be passing on to the cross-covering intern (eg, "Please check the patient's wound site at 10 PM"). This information is usually passed along on an index card. You should also document the patient's code status (full code vs. DNR), whether IV access is absolutely necessary (must it be restarted if it happens to fall out?), and whether you want blood cultures if the patient spikes a fever overnight.

A good sign-out is the mark of a good student.

## TYPICAL SURGERY DAY

The surgery day starts earlier and ends later than a typical medicine day. However, many of the same activities occur, but often at a quicker pace to make time for the OR. Differences are noted below.

**Prerounds:** 5:00–6:00 AM. Just like medicine prerounds—but in addition, you will be checking wounds and drains on postop patients. You may also be expected to write brief progress notes before work rounds.

**Work rounds:** 6:00–7:30 AM. If progress notes are not written during prerounds, they will be done here. Some services actually write notes during afternoon rounds or even twice a day. Otherwise, surgery work rounds are similar to medicine work rounds.

**Preoperative preparation:** 7:30–8:00 AM. During this period, you and a house officer work with the anesthesiologist to prepare the patient for the operation. This usually includes positioning the patient, placing a urinary catheter, and prepping the operative area.

**Surgery:** 8:00 AM–5:00 PM. This is where you have the most exposure to the attending. Depending on the needs and preferences of the team, your role may range from simple observation to retraction, suctioning, and tying and cutting sutures. The operating theater is often a place for rampant pimping, so bone up on your reading the night before the case. Alternatively, keep a pimp answer book in your locker for easy review.

Pimp questions often fly fast and furious in the OR.

**Floor work:** 8:00 AM–5:00 PM. If you are not in the OR during this period, you are getting the daily scut work done on your patients with a resident. This may include wound checks, pulling staples, pulling chest tubes, and getting consults. Often, you and another medical student will switch off between the OR and the surgical floors. Convey your relative desire to be in the OR and your case preferences to the chief.

**"Afternoon" rounds:** 5:00–7:30 PM. Sometimes more aptly called "evening" rounds, these rounds allow the team to review the day's events and plan the next day. Afternoon rounds usually start soon after the last surgery of the day has been completed. These presentations are generally more casual and abbreviated than the morning presentations.

**Postrounds work:** 7:30 PM–? Sometimes afternoon rounds generate a short list of tasks that the team must accomplish before going home.

This is just a sample schedule—times may vary depending on your institution, the number of patients on the service, and the number and length of operative cases. On clinic days, the morning schedule is usually similar, as rounds must be completed before the start of clinic. The evening schedule may be lighter depending on whether there is clinic scheduled in the afternoon and how many patients need to be worked up or admitted for surgery the next day.

## THE ADMISSION

As a third-year student, you will work with the team to admit one to three patients on a call night. This can be a scary experience for some, but it need not be if you follow a few simple rules. In general, the admissions process follows a loose sequence of events. Your resident receives the ER call. You both throttle to the ER to conduct a history and physical exam (H&P) on the patient, formulate an assessment and plan, write the appropriate admission orders, and then move the patient up to the floors (or the units). Generally, your resident decides which case(s) you will work up and admit, although you could try to request the *type* of case assigned to you (eg, cardiac, infectious).

### THE "CALL"

Patients are usually admitted through the emergency department. Others are admitted from clinic or transferred from an outside hospital or from other medical and surgical services. When the admission is called up from the ER, the resident is usually given a one-line description of the patient's complaint, like "33-year-old African-American female with abdominal pain" or "67-year-old Caucasian complaining of chest pain and dizziness." Immediately generate a differential diagnosis of possible etiologies (eg, skin, musculoskeletal, pulmonary, cardiac, GI) and use this to guide your initial approach to the patient's workup. Classic mnemonics like "MINT CANDY" will help you develop and organize a consistent differential diagnosis. You will then ask questions, look for physical signs, and review old records for information that will "tease out" a likely diagnosis.

### REVIEWING OBJECTIVE DATA

Patients will usually have had some workup tests done in the ER by the time you arrive, so read through the ER evaluation sheet to see what the ER doctors were thinking. Look up current laboratory values, chest x-rays, EKGs, etc., and compare them with previous findings. Do a quick chart review, paying close attention to the latest discharge summaries, past hospitalizations, and problem lists. Of course, you may have time for only some of the above if your patient is unstable or in critical condition.

---

**Quick framework for a differential diagnosis:**

**M**etabolic
**I**nfectious
**N**eoplastic
**T**rauma
**C**ollagen vascular disease
**A**llergies
**'N**'ything else
**D**rugs
**Y**outh (congenital)

## THE CHART REVIEW

Many of your patients have previously been admitted to the hospital. If so, the past medical records should be there when you arrive in the ER. If there is no old chart, ask the clerk if one exists and whether it has been ordered to the ER. A focused chart review before you see the patient can give you a good idea of your patient's previous health status and health issues. Concentrate on the discharge summaries from each admission, since they are typed, are concise, and provide a summary of the patient's hospitalization as well as a list of the patient's problems and discharge medications. Medical student admission notes are useful in that they often contain more detailed information on social history and physical exam. You should also look for studies such as an EKG, recent echocardiograms, radiology results, and past blood lab work. Knowing the patient's baseline will give you and your team a better understanding of how sick the patient currently is (eg, has the patient's chronic anemia worsened significantly? Are there new EKG changes?).

## INTERVIEWING THE PATIENT

At this point, you may have modified your differential diagnosis based on your review of the chart, labs, and diagnostic studies. Keep a mental note of these potential diagnoses as you begin the patient interview. Sometimes the H&P may be conducted as a team, with the medical student leading the history taking while your residents take notes. At other times you will evaluate the patient alone and then present the patient to the team before they conduct their own H&Ps. Remember, your H&P skills will be judged by your residents and almost always count toward your final clerkship evaluation. So be organized; try to prepare a mental outline of your questions before you see the patient.

If possible, avoid the "SHOTGUN APPROACH" to asking questions. The shotgun approach involves showering the patient with a barrage of nonfocused questions in the hopes of stumbling on a fact that will lead you closer to a diagnosis. Instead, ask about **pertinent** positives and negatives in the history. Admittedly, experience helps in developing a focused and directed H&P, and there is nothing wrong with being overly thorough. However, you will look sharper if you can conduct an interview that focuses on the pertinent issues at hand; you can ask your patient about nonurgent issues anytime after he or she has been admitted to the floor.

Remember to begin your interview with open-ended questions (eg, "What brought you to the hospital?"), thereby allowing the patient some control over the interview process. Then gradually move toward more structured questions (eg, "Was your pain dull or sharp?") if the interview loses focus or if the patient wanders off the subject. Above all, don't get discouraged if the interview does not go smoothly. The medical interview is an art form that can be mastered only through repeated practice.

## THE PHYSICAL EXAM

Conduct the physical exam as thoroughly as possible and in the same sequence every time. As a third-year student, you will need to develop solid physical exam skills. Each patient provides you with excellent practice, so time allowing, don't skimp on any part of the exam, including the rectal exam. You will soon enough

Focus on past discharge summaries and medical student admission notes.

Two reasons not to do a rectal exam:
(1) you don't have a finger, or
(2) the patient doesn't have a rectum.

be forced to do limited problem-oriented exams. Ask for supervision and feedback from a resident so you can fine-tune your examination skills.

## CURRENT MED TALK

'SHOTGUN APPROACH': A diagnostic method or technique in which every conceivable parameter is measured in order to detect all possible clinical or laboratory nosologies, however remote the possibility that a rare disease is present. An often-criticized result of practicing 'defensive medicine,' increasing the cost of health care without improving patient management.

SUTTON'S LAW: A guideline evoked to temper the enthusiasm of externs and other novices in clinical medicine who want to 'work up' an acute abdomen for porphyria, metastatic medulloblastoma or other esoterica, while ignoring a particular disease's most common causes. The 'law' is attributed to the noted bank robber, Willie Sutton, who, when asked why he robbed banks, reportedly replied, 'That's where the money is.' To apply Sutton's law, then, is to search for the most likely cause of a symptom, ie, to 'go where the money is.'

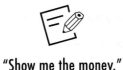

"Show me the money."

### PUTTING IT ALL TOGETHER

After conducting the H&P and reviewing all the medical records, labs, and studies, you will present the case to your resident(s) and formulate your assessment and plan. Give a short, 3- to 5-minute presentation similar in format to a full oral presentation, and present your most likely diagnoses. Include other, less likely considerations, as this shows depth and thoroughness in your evaluation of the case. Of course, if you can surreptitiously and quickly consult any pocketbooks about the diagnosis and management of your leading diagnoses, you will be better prepared for the impending onslaught of pimping questions. Sometimes you will be unsure of the diagnosis. But don't fret; your thought processes and reasoning ability are more important at this stage than hitting the exact diagnosis. Do, however, support your current diagnoses with both subjective and objective data; rank your differential diagnoses in order of likelihood (remember SUTTON'S LAW); and present a thorough plan for each diagnosis. This plan may include anything from more diagnostic studies to immediate and long-term therapy to obtaining further consultation from other services.

### ADMIT ORDERS

Admission orders are written soon after the patient's acute problems and management plans have been discussed with your team and at least a working diagnosis has been rendered. Orders are written in a standard format. "ADC VAANDIMSL" is one of a few versions of the mnemonic for admission orders. Here is an example of orders for a patient admitted for pneumonia:

ADMIT TO: Ward, service, your name/intern's name, beeper number.

DIAGNOSIS: If no clear diagnosis, give the two or three most likely suspects (eg, pulmonary embolism vs. CHF exacerbation) or the presenting complaint (eg, chest pain), or what diagnoses you are trying to exclude (eg, rule out MI).

CONDITION: Satisfactory, stable, fair, guarded, critical.

VITALS: Per routine, q4h, q1h, q shift.

ALLERGIES: Mention the specific reaction to the drug (eg, rash); NKDA if no allergies.

ACTIVITY: Ad lib, out of bed to bathroom (c̄ assist), out of bed to chair, strict bed rest, ambulation with crutches.

NURSING ORDERS: Strict I/Os, oxygen, daily weights, telemetry, glucose checks, Foley cath, NG tube.

DIET: Regular, 1800 cal ADA, low sodium, soft mechanical, NPO.

IV FLUIDS: Hep lock, KVO, type of solution (D5, NS, D5 1/2 NS, etc) and rate of infusion (eg, D5 1/2 NS + 20 mEq/L KCl at 125 cc/hr).

MEDICATIONS: Don't forget antibiotics and prn medications.

SPECIAL STUDIES: EKG, CXR, CT, etc.

LABS: AM labs: CBC, electrolytes, BUN, Cr, glucose, etc.

CALL HOUSE OFFICER: Temp > 38.4, pulse > 120 or < 50, SBP < 90 or > 180, resp rate < 8 or > 30 $O_2$ sat < 90%.

---

### COMMON PRN MEDICATION ORDERS

"Prn" is the abbreviation for *pro re nata*—Latin for "as the need arises."
Acetaminophen, 650 mg PO q4h prn temp > 101.5°F
Bisacodyl (Dulcolax) 10 mg PO/PR qd prn constipation
Diphenhydramine (Benadryl) 25 mg PO qhs prn insomnia
Maalox 10–20 cc PO q1–2h PO prn dyspepsia
Lorazepam 1–2 mg IM/IV q6h prn anxiety/agitation
Promethazine (Phenergan)25 mg PO/IM/IV q4h prn nausea

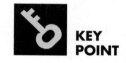

**KEY POINT**

**MEDICAL STUDENT ADMIT NOTE**

Depending on the policies of your medical service, you may be given varying amounts of time to get the admit note into the chart. Use that time wisely to learn more about your patients' problems. Regardless, you should have the admit note in the chart before work rounds the next morning. The HPI and the assessment and plan are the two most challenging portions to write. A well-written admit note is a testament to your thought processes and fund of knowledge.

**HPI.** Deciding which pieces of information belong in the HPI can be a difficult process at this stage of your career. Do not forget to characterize the chief complaint—quality, severity, location, duration, progression, things that make it worse or better, and what the patient was doing at the onset.

Also include the pertinent positives and negatives that support your diagnosis, and rule out the other main suspects. Present the information in chronological order. Information on the patient's past medical history, family history, health-related behaviors, or social history should be included in the HPI only if it is pertinent to the reason for admission.

**Assessment and plan.** Start off with a brief summary of the case. Give your presumed diagnosis at the end of the summary; then you can launch into a discussion of the case. Take the time to read up on your patient's diagnosis and management as well as his or her other important medical problems. Present your formulation of your patient's current health issues by a problem-list-based approach. Alternatively, you may use a systems-based approach if you have a more complicated patient (eg, in the ICU). Each problem has an assessment and plan. In the assessment of the primary problem, the reader wants to know (1) why you think this is the diagnosis, and (2) why the other possible diagnoses are less likely to be correct. Other incidental problems get a brief one-line assessment. In the plan, outline your initial treatment plans (eg, medications, procedures) and what additional workup needs to be done to further characterize the diagnosis or to clinch it if it is still unclear at this point.

A few other pointers on the admit note:

- As you write the admit note, you'll realize that there will be a few holes to fill in. Try to identify all the gaps at once so that you don't keep shuttling between the patient and your note.
- Be prepared to use the most common abbreviations. Avoid obscure abbreviations that may not be recognized or may be mistaken for something else. Don't coin your own.
- The admit note (like all your progress notes) becomes part of the legal record. Thus, opinionated comments that are not relevant to the patient's care are *faux pas*. "Chart wars" are unprofessional and create unwelcome medicolegal liability.
- Neat handwriting wins points. Messy handwriting can always be improved by slowing down. There is little point to writing an illegible note.

These tips should get you started. A more detailed discussion on admit notes can be found in any of a number of texts on medical history and physical examination.

CURRENT
*Med Talk*

## CURRENT MED TALK

CODE STATUS: The formally indicated (often through signed documents) status of a patient in a hospital with respect to his/her desire for resuscitative (ie, CPR) efforts, should the need arise; unless the patient specifically requests that he/she *NOT* be resuscitated, ie, DNR (do not resuscitate) status, CPR will be performed.

CODE: *(noun)* A widely used (albeit highly colloquial) term for a cardiopulmonary arrest which is invariably accompanied by a frenzied fracas and frenetic fray. *(verb)* To suffer a cardiac arrest in a hospital environment.

### A Sample Admit Note

**ID/CC:** 42-year-old Caucasian woman, former IV drug user, HIV+ $\bar{c}$ CD4 count of 250, complains of 3 days of painful neck rash and diffuse itching.

**HPI:** Patient has been HIV+ × 3 years, no opportunistic infections. She complains of sudden-onset painful neck rash 2 days prior to admit. Noted vesicle formation on L neck and deltoid $\bar{c}$ pruritus, as well as severe burning/stinging pain. Used warm compresses for symptomatic relief. She felt "drained" and stayed in bed × 2 days, denies any F/C/S, no N/V, no abdominal pain, no diarrhea. No arthralgias/myalgias, no cough, no SOB, no HA. She denies any vesicles on face, no ear pain, no eye pain or visual changes. She is unaware of any childhood history of chickenpox, denies any chemical or plant contacts or contact with others with similar symptoms.

**PMH:**

1. HIV+ × 3 years, CD4 of 250 3 months ago. Denies any OIs.

2. Pneumonia 3–4 × in past 3 years. Hospitalized but unaware of dates or specific diagnosis. Recalls having a chest CT in past and has never had to take prophylactic abx. Chart currently unavailable for review.

3. Cellulitis of extremities several times in the past. Patient unable to recall details or dates.

4. Hepatitis C Ab+.

**MEDS:** Ø

**ALL:** NKDA

**FH:** Noncontributory

**HABITS:** +tobacco: 1 ppd × 20 years

+EtOH 1 pint vodka per day, no h/o withdrawal

+h/o IV drug use, none × 6 years

**SH:** Patient is homeless. Moved from Chicago to San Francisco 4 years ago. She is unmarried and has 4 children, no family on the West Coast. She is intermittently followed by the HIV clinic at San Francisco General Hospital.

**ROS:** Negative, except as above.

**PE:** GEN: Somnolent, arousable to alertness, in mild distress due to pain & pruritus.

VS: T 37.1 BP 111/80 HR 112 RR 18, 99% $O_2$ sat on 2L NC.

SKIN/HAIR/NAILS: Vesicular rash $\bar{c}$ erythematous base, clustered, on L lateral and posterior neck and L deltoid, anteriorly to clavicle, stops at midline anterior and posterior.

HEENT: NC/AT, PERRL 4 → 3, EOMI, mild conjunctival injection bilat, TMs clear without vesicles, O/P is dry with poor dentition, no vesicles or open lesions, no thrush.

NECK: 1 posterior SCM node, supple neck.

BREAST: Deferred at this time per patient request.

---

ID = Identification

CC = Chief complaint

$\bar{c}$ = With

F/C/S = Fevers/chills/sweats

N/V = Nausea/vomiting

SOB = Shortness of breath

HA = Headache

OI = Opportunistic infections

ABX = Antibiotics

EtOH = Alcohol

NC = Nasal cannulae

NC/AT = Normocephalic/atraumatic

PERRL 4 → 3 = Pupils equal, round, responsive to light from 4 mm to 3 mm

EOMI = Extraocular movements intact

TM = Tympanic membrane

O/P = Oropharynx

SCM = Sternocleidomastoid

CTAB = Clear to auscultation bilaterally

M/R/G = Murmurs/rubs/gallops

NT = Nontender

NABS = Normal active bowel sounds

ND = Nondistended

HSM = Hepatosplenomegaly

C/C/E = Clubbing/cyanosis/edema

A&O × 4 = Alert & oriented

CN = Cranial nerves

MAE = Moves all extremities

DTR = Deep tendon reflexes

$$\text{WBC} \overset{\text{Hgb}}{\underset{\text{HCT}}{\Big|}} \text{Plts}$$

$$\overset{\text{Na} \mid \text{Cl} \mid \text{BUN}}{\text{K} \mid CO_2 \mid \text{Cr}} \Big\rangle \text{Glu}$$

O/W = Otherwise

*Remember*

*NABS   ND*

*DTR*

*NABS = Nml Active Bowel sounds*

*ND = Non distended*

*HSM = hepatosplenomegaly*

*O/W = Otherwise*

*RRR = Reg rate rythm*

*– M/R/G*

*murmurs/rubs/gallops.*

---

LUNGS: CTAB, no rales, no wheezes.

CV: Tachycardic, reg rhythm, normal S1/S2, no M/R/G. Good distal pulses.

ABD: Soft, NT, NABS, ND, no HSM.

GU: Deferred at this time per patient request.

EXT: No C/C/E. Cool and dry. Numerous old needle-track scars.

NEURO: A&O × 4. CN II–XII intact. MAE, DTRs 2+ & symmetric, sensation intact.

**LABS:**

$$8.2 \overset{\text{13.3}}{\underset{\text{40.0}}{\Big|}} 297 \qquad \overset{142 \mid 105 \mid 8}{4.0 \mid 29 \mid 0.8} \Big\rangle 92 \qquad$$ T. Bili 0.7; AST 38; ALT 20; Alk Phos 77

PT/INR/PTT: 12.4/1.2/32.2

Ca 8.3; Mg 2.3; Phos 3.9          Albumin 3.6; Amylase 82

**CXR:** Increased interstitial markings, o/w negative.

**A/P:** 42-year-old woman $\bar{c}$ HIV, presenting with likely herpes zoster in L C3/C4 dermatomal distribution.

1. **Herpes zoster:** The differential in this case is rather narrow given the history and presentation. A contact dermatitis is unlikely, although a possibility. Given the specific dermatome distribution, which stops at the midline, reactivation is far more likely than a primary varicella infection. The patient's HIV status places her at risk for zoster dissemination. Admit for involvement of 2 contiguous dermatomes and monitor for signs of dissemination.

    - Acyclovir 500 mg IV q 8 hours
    - Benadryl 25–50 mg PO q 6 hours prn pruritus
    - TyCo#3 1–2 tabs PO q 4 hours prn pain
    - Isolation protocol to protect other immunocompromised patients on floor

2. **HIV:** CD4 > 200, no h/o opportunistic infections.

    - Start AZT 500 mg PO TID and ddC 0.375 mg PO TID
    - Will arrange follow-up appointment with HIV clinic

3. **EtOH:** Monitor for signs of EtOH withdrawal.

    - Thiamine 100 mg IV
    - Folate 1 mg IV
    - MVI 1 amp IV
    - Ativan 1–2 mg IV q1–2h prn agitation

4. **Code status:** Patient is Full Code.

5. **Disposition:** Patient is homeless. Will consult social worker for discharge planning.

During your clerkships, no skill is more important to master than the delivery of a focused, fluent, and concise oral presentation. You will be called upon to present patients under varied circumstances and time constraints for the rest of your professional life, so getting a good handle on this skill early is critical to success on the wards. Indeed, it is the primary basis upon which you will be judged during attending rounds. When done effectively, the oral presentation approaches an art form that leaves your audience with a solid comprehension of your patient's health care issues. When it is done poorly, however, your audience is left confused and groping for further clarification. The ability to amass voluminous amounts of information is easily done, but to organize, synthesize, and tell a succinct story can be a challenging task. The story must make sense to you before you can tell it to anyone else. Don't expect to get away with just reporting snippets of data that you don't understand culled from old charts.

## THE FORMAL PRESENTATION

Classically, the formal oral presentation is given in 7 minutes or less. Although it follows the same format as a written report, it is not simply a regurgitation. A great presentation requires style as much as substance; your delivery must be succinct and smooth. No time should be wasted on superfluous information; one can read about such matters later in your admit note. Ideally, your presentation should be formulated so that your audience can anticipate your assessment and plan; that is, each piece of information should clue the listener into your thinking process and your most likely diagnosis.

More emphasis should be given to the patient's *current* state (CC, HPI, PE, labs, A/P) than to past events (PMH, FH, SH). Furthermore, body language, eye contact, posture, and the like all contribute to a polished presentation.

The following are the categories of information that you should be prepared to furnish during an oral presentation.

**Identification/chief complaint.** Ideally, this introductory portion of the oral presentation should be a one-line bullet presentation that includes identifying information and chief complaint (eg, "Mr. Veza is a 71-year-old diabetic Filipino male with longstanding hypertension who is admitted for a two-day history of dyspnea, bilateral pedal edema, and chest pain").

**HPI.** The HPI is the cornerstone of the medical presentation. The HPI you present will be very similar to the written HPI in that you are providing the pertinent positives and negatives that will move the audience toward your diagnosis. When done well, the HPI will have the feel of a story.

**PMH.** Do not repeat information already mentioned in the HPI. If any information is relevant to the patient's chief complaint, it should be included in the HPI. Omit any extraneous information from your oral presentation (eg, childhood chickenpox in a elderly man with an acute MI).

**Allergies/medications.** You need not present the dosage for each medication, but have it written down just in case you're asked.

**Practice, practice, practice your presentations!!**

**Social history.** Include at least a brief social history; it is always relevant. Remember, you are presenting another human being, not a disease.

**Health-related behaviors.** Again, this may be short or nonexistent if the information is included in the HPI. Usually includes tobacco, alcohol, and illicit drug use as well as a sexual history.

**Family history.** This section includes both positive and negative findings and should be very short, as any relevant information should have been mentioned in the HPI.

**A well-done presentation is like a riveting story.**

**Review of systems.** Often this section is omitted entirely; anything directly relevant should have been mentioned in the HPI.

**PE/labs/other tests.** Depending on your attending's preferences, you may present just the highlights or give a very thorough report of the physical findings. Ask your attending in advance what he or she prefers. Most will want just pertinent positives and negatives reported. Others may want a more formal approach detailing each physical finding and lab/other test values. In general, unless otherwise specified, present *all* the physical findings and lab/other test values; you will never be faulted for being too thorough. Always use simple declarative sentences when you present a physical finding, eg, "There were no murmurs, rubs, or gallops on cardiac exam" instead of "Cardiac exam was unremarkable."

**Assessment and plan.** Hopefully by this point, you have successfully "set the dinner table," and your audience sits hungry in anticipation; indeed, this section is the meat of the presentation. As in your admit note, you may give a short summary of the case, including only pertinent positives and negatives, as a preface to your assessment and plan; this is particularly useful in complicated cases with multifactorial diseases. Presumably you will have read as much as possible about each of your patient's preexisting illnesses and potential diagnoses. Know in advance how to differentiate each potential diagnosis and what each workup entails. Also know both the acute and long-term management of each diagnosis entertained, and incorporate this knowledge accordingly into your assessment and plan.

Again, you can present the A/P in the form of a problem or according to organ system; doing so makes it less likely that you will miss anything important. March through each problem on the list, give your assessment, and outline a plan succinctly. Finally, if you really want to impress your team, pose a question for discussion relating to, for example, the acute management of a problem. Of course, you should offer to give a short presentation on that topic based on a literature review!

## "BULLET" PRESENTATION

The 1-minute presentation is an extremely concise synopsis of the case presentation. You may give bullet presentations during work rounds and to consultants or other health care providers who are unfamiliar with your patient. Ideally, the history, physical exam, laboratory findings, and assessment and plan sections are each summarized into one sentence. You have time to include only the most pertinent positive and negative findings, usually anywhere from 15 to 20 facts about the case. Practice this skill with each patient you write up and present. Initially, you may try writing down the most important information from each of the write-up sections and then develop a cohesive 1-minute presentation. With practice, you will soon be able to filter the vast amount of information from memory.

## CURRENT MED TALK

PROGRESS NOTE: A brief summary of a hospitalized patient's current clinical status, which is usually written in sequential order in the patient's chart and reflects information provided by physical examination, laboratory tests, and imaging modalities; PNs serve to communicate perceived changes of the patient's condition among all members of the management team and serve as a public record of clinicians' rationale for performing certain procedures, and his/her expectations for outcome; PNs are thus critical 'documents' that may become legal substrate for determining liability.

## WRITING NOTES

A PROGRESS NOTE is a daily written record of all events pertaining to a patient. On medical-type services (including pediatrics, psychiatry, and neurology), progress notes are typically written in the afternoon. On surgical-type services (including OB/GYN), progress notes are written before work rounds in the morning. Make sure your intern or resident reviews and cosigns your notes. Most students write progress notes in the SOAP format described below.

**DAILY WARD ACTIVITIES**

- **Subjective.** This component includes the patient's own observations concerning changes in symptoms, any significant events in the last day, and any physical complaints.
- **Objective.** This includes vital signs, a focused, brief physical exam, and any laboratory and study results.
- **Assessment and plan.** This is your impression of the objective and subjective information and what the appropriate diagnostic and treatment regimen will be. Your plan should be concise and laid out so that someone else reading your note can easily understand the team's plan for your patient.

## WRITING ORDERS

Make it clear to your team that you want to write orders for your patients (they will be cosigned). This accomplishes multiple goals. First, you receive valuable practice in prescription writing and drug dosing. In addition, you will automatically stay current with your patient's treatment regimens. Things to keep in mind when writing prescriptions are as follows:

- Make sure your prescription has all of the following essential information:
  - Time and date
  - Generic drug name
  - Dose
  - Route of delivery (PO, IV, IM, SQ)

- Frequency
- Signature; include your printed name, title (eg, MS III), and beeper number
- Write legibly; do not use abbreviations.
- Have the prescription cosigned immediately by a house officer. Your signature alone is not sufficient.
- If it's an important order, also pass the order verbally to the nurse or the ward clerk.
- Just because a written order exists does not mean it was executed. Check nursing records frequently to be sure orders were properly carried out. Check the IV bag label to see if the correct IV meds are being given.

C/W = Compared with

RA = Room air

BR = Bathroom

I/O = Intake/output

RRR = Regular rate and rhythm

---

**Sample Progress Note**

Hospital Day #2: Medicine Service

**S:** No events overnight. Patient "feels OK," reports continued pruritis, although significantly improved c/w yesterday. Good sleep last night, good pain control. No other complaints. Has not noticed any progression of rash.

**O:** VS: T 36.6  BP 110/65  HR 90  RR 18  97% $O_2$ sat on RA

I/O: 950 cc/BR.

SKIN: No change in distribution or size of vesicles on L neck/shoulder, although some have crusted over. No new vesicles on body.

HEENT: PERRL, EOMI, no conjunctival injection, TMs clear, no vesicles, O/P moist and clear.

LUNGS: CTAB, no rales, no wheezes.

CV: RRR, nl S1/S2, no M/R/G.

ABD: Soft, NT, +BS.

LABS:

$$\begin{array}{c|c} & 12.8 \\ 7.9 & \\ & 37.2 \end{array} \Big< 260 \qquad \begin{array}{c|c|c} 134 & 103 & 8 \\ \hline 3.6 & 25 & 0.8 \end{array} \Big<$$

**A/P:** 42-year-old woman with herpes zoster, afebrile and comfortable, doing well.

1. **Herpes zoster:** No evidence of dissemination or spread to other dermatomes. Good pain control, tolerating IV acyclovir well.
   - Atarax prn pruritis.
   - Continue IV acyclovir, TyCo#3

2. **HIV**
   - Continue AZT and ddC.
   - Plan to speak with HIV clinic today to arrange follow-up care.

3. **EtOH:** No sign of alcohol withdrawal at this time. Continue to monitor.

4. **Dispo:** Social worker to speak with patient this afternoon re housing and $.

## COMMUNICATING WITH PATIENTS AND FAMILY MEMBERS

As the primary care provider for your patients, you should be the main communications link between the team and the patient and family. Becoming the information authority keeps you on top of your patients. Here are some tips to help you become the "Great Communicator":

- Your first duty is to respect the privacy and wishes of the patient. Never discuss patients in the elevator, the cafeteria, or other public places.
- Be as honest and direct as possible with family members. Update them appropriately regarding the progress of their loved ones. Think of how you would feel if a doctor were evading your questions about your hospitalized grandmother.
- Breaking major bad news may initially be done with a resident or an experienced intern at your side. They should guide you in helping the patient and the family weather the emotional repercussions of an illness. They can also help you deal with any possible backlash.
- Choose a quiet time to talk (ie, when nursing and ancillary staff is not around).
- Keep technical jargon to a minimum, and explain any medical terminology you use.
- Immediately inform the patient of any upcoming studies and events.
- Always finish with "Do you have any questions?"
- Never fudge an answer. If you are unsure, remind the family that you are in training and tell them that you will consult with a higher authority and get back to them promptly.

## PROCEDURES

Procedures are done for a variety of reasons. Some are diagnostic, while others are therapeutic and potentially lifesaving—but all are vital to the care of your patient (see Table 2). You can learn procedures by doing them under supervision or by carefully observing them while they are being performed. Reading about the procedure in a manual (see book reviews at the end of this chapter) beforehand maximizes your learning when you first see it and hear the explanation. At the same time, a procedure is not just technique; you should also have an understanding of its indications, contraindications,

| **TABLE 2.** Common procedures for a junior student | |
|---|---|
| **Basic** | **Advanced** |
| Venipuncture | Central line placement |
| Arterial blood gas | Lumbar puncture |
| Urinary (Foley) catheterization | Paracentesis |
| Blood culture | Thoracocentesis |
| IV placement | Obstetrical delivery |
| EKG | Chest tube insertion |
| NG tube placement | Arthrocentesis |
| Suturing | |
| Surgical knots | |
| Wound dressing change | |

potential complications, proper response to potential complications, and materials involved. A few tips about procedures:

- Before performing any significant procedure, you must obtain informed consent from the patient—meaning you must explain the procedure as well as its indications, its risks and benefits, any alternative options, and the risks/benefits of not having the procedure. Be sure to document the patient's consent or place a signed consent form in the chart. Some hospitals allow students to consent patients for simple procedures and operations while others do not.
- Have everything you need ready at the bedside (think through what you will require in advance).
- Gather enough materials for multiple tries (expect to miss the first IV or venipuncture).
- Position the patient and yourself for comfort (eg, raise the bed so you don't have to bend over; ensure adequate lighting).
- Always remember universal precautions.
- Prepare for a potential mess by having gauze and disposable dropcloths positioned as necessary.
- Clean up after yourself. Discard all of your sharps in the proper receptacle.
- Document the procedure and informed consent in the patient's records. A procedure note should be written for any invasive procedure performed on a patient, including lumbar puncture, thoracocentesis, paracentesis, and central line placement, etc. The note itself should be concise and should document the date and time, indications, consent, preparation of the patient, anesthesia used (if any), details of the procedure, yield, any studies sent, and any complications.

## CONSULTS

Often your team will have a diagnostic or treatment question regarding one of your patients that requires the expertise of a specialist. Requesting a consult involves filling out a consult request form as well as making a courtesy call to tell the consultant about the patient. Consultants dread receiving a consult request from a junior clerk who gives a rambling presentation and does not know why the request is being made. You can make the consultant's day much more pleasant (as well as impress him or her) by giving a concise, 1-minute bullet presentation that includes patient identification, pertinent present medical history, pertinent past medical history, medications, allergies, physical exam, key lab results, and study results. This brief presentation should then be followed by a clear question for the consultant.

Before calling the consultant, review the patient with your resident or intern to gain an understanding of why a consult is needed. If you don't understand why you need a consult you will often end up being bounced between an irritated consultant and an impatient resident. The more professional your interactions with the consultant are, the more likely it will be that the consultant will feed the recommendations and rationale to you rather than bypassing you for the intern or resident.

## CHECKING LABS AND STUDIES

During a typical ward day, labs and study results should be checked during prerounds, in the afternoon, and whenever stat labs or important studies are expected back. Anything pertinent should be reported to your intern or resident. If a patient is unstable, make sure you check more frequently to see if the labs are back. Whenever possible, look at the blood smear or chest x-ray yourself instead of reading the report.

## READING UP ON YOUR PATIENT'S PROBLEMS

Aside from one-on-one teaching and conferences, you are expected to learn through independent reading. It is critical to understand the rationale behind the treatment plan for your patients, so knowledge of the pathophysiology of their condition is necessary. The first priority is to read about your patients' problems. Next, read about other patients being carried by the team with active and interesting problems. Knowing about the other patients' problems keeps you involved in patient discussions during rounds. Depending on what you want to learn and when you can learn it, you will be using multiple sources of information.

**Pocketbooks and handbooks.** When you have 5 minutes before attending rounds, you can quickly read a pocket resource to get the "big picture" about a disease. A classic example is the *Washington Manual of Medical Therapeutics.*

**Compact reference books.** These books are generally meant to be read cover to cover during the course of a rotation. Whether that actually happens is anybody's guess. These texts cover diseases in moderate detail and are ideal for reading up on interesting patients.

**Textbooks.** These tomes comprehensively cover diseases in great detail. *Harrison's Textbook of Medicine* is an example. You should read about your own patients' problems in a clinical reference.

**Journal articles.** Sometimes even *Harrison's* can't tell you all you need to know about a patient's disease state. At this point, you should search MEDLINE to find a review or a study that answers your burning questions. Journal articles provide information on the latest treatment regimens and studies with information 2–4 years more recent than that in a reference book. For diseases in which our understanding is constantly evolving, such as HIV, a literature search may be mandatory. If you find a helpful paper, it is highly appropriate to photocopy that paper for your team. The truly enthusiastic student may also present the findings as well as a critique of the paper, perhaps in a one-page handout. A quick and helpful shortcut is to print several article titles along with abstracts for your resident or attending. Let them choose which ones to photocopy.

## BEING A "DISPENSER"

Sometimes the student serves as a mobile supply cart for the attending and house staff. This may sound demeaning, but it is actually a courtesy to the attendings and house staff. Attendings will often borrow your stethoscope and penlight. Simple things such as having extra gloves, 3 × 5 index cards, tongue blades, or pens will save time on rounds and make your team's life a little easier, so keep your pockets stocked. Make sure you get your pen back if borrowed (attendings are especially notorious for disappearing with them) or bring extras every day.

**TIPS FOR WARDS SURVIVAL**

## SCHEDULING ROTATIONS

In the spring of your second year, you will go through the process of scheduling your third-year clerkships. Many schools have rotations prescheduled on tracks. Your only task is to choose a track, usually by lottery. Fortunately, there are only a few guidelines you need to know when scheduling your third-year clerkships.

**Do not do your most likely specialty first.** During the first few weeks of your clerkships, you won't even know where the bathroom is, let alone competently function as a clerk. It is therefore important to allow yourself a chance to get the general feel of the hospital wards and understand your role, as well as to become comfortable presenting patients and writing notes. Your first rotation should be in a field that you are not likely to go into. For example, most students do not end up going into neurology; however, neurology (as opposed to psychiatry) has the look and feel of a medicine rotation. Make sure every member of your team knows that this is your first rotation; they will be more pleasant and forgiving.

**Do not do your most likely specialty last.** You will be scheduling your senior clerkships in the spring of your third year. If you're interested in pediatrics, you will want to have done your junior pediatrics before that crucial scheduling period so that you can decide if and when you will be taking any senior pediatrics rotations.

**Avoid back-to-back tough rotations.** This is a soft rule, especially if you've decided that you have no career interests in one of those specialties. However, you should be concerned about the possibility of burnout when "killer" rotations get scheduled together. Strategically place vacation time after especially difficult rotations to give yourself a chance to unwind.

**Schedule an easy rotation before your most likely specialty rotation.** Also a soft rule. This gives you time to relax and do some preemptive reading before you start that big rotation. Some students even recommend putting a little vacation time before a key rotation to do some heavy-duty reading.

## CHOOSING ROTATION SITES

Your rotations occur in a variety of hospital and clinical settings. Each type of setting has characteristics that will color your clinical experience. Consult senior students regarding the pros and cons of each site, including key attendings to seek out or avoid. The generalizations below don't always apply but should give you an idea of what to expect.

**County.** The county hospital is typically very busy yet understaffed. Chaos seems to be the baseline as interns and residents constantly battle high patient loads and constant fatigue. County hospitals usually serve the urban poor. In this "all hands on deck" state, you can expect to have more responsibility and more hands-on procedures but less guidance and didactic teaching. You can excel in this environment by being the perfect "SCUT MONKEY," taking care of all those little (but necessary) patient-care tasks. This helps get your team's census down before the next on-call onslaught. The discharge of county hospital patients tends to be more difficult and time-consuming owing to their social situations, so social workers will often become your best allies as you struggle to get your patients out of the hospital.

## CURRENT MED TALK

CURRENT
*Med Talk*

'SCUT MONKEY': A highly colloquial and demeaning term that usually refers to a medical student who is relegated to the bottom rung of a team involved in patient management in a university-affiliated health care facility, and performs so-called scut work.

**VA.** The VA system personifies the U.S. government in that things take twice as long to get done at twice the cost. Sometimes things don't get done at all without a little political back-scratching and schmoozing. Therefore, being savvy with regard to the political hierarchy definitely helps. The VA population is also unique, consisting mostly of older men with a lot of time on their hands. This makes for an entertaining and forgiving patient population, like the former Marine martial-arts instructor who lets you stick him five times for a blood draw and then teaches you block-and-kill moves after rounds. Female students should be prepared, if necessary, to be a bit more cautious with these patients. Because the population is somewhat demographically restricted, you will also see the same diseases over and over again, including:

At the VA, know how to
work the system.

- Congestive heart failure
- Myocardial infarction
- COPD
- Lung cancer
- Diabetes
- Arrhythmias
- GI bleeding
- Peripheral vascular disease

Definitely read up on these diseases before you go to the VA. Often patients remain in house owing to placement issues (where will the patient go after discharge) rather than medical issues. You may end up with a large yet inactive census if you neglect discharge planning.

**Academic/university center.** Ivory-tower medicine has its own unique approach to treating patients. Medical and surgical services are top-heavy with consultants and fellows. As a result, residents and interns are often deprived of procedures, leaving even less for you to do. In addition, university hospitals are often tertiary and quaternary referral centers; thus, they get the patients that stump the community physicians. This is where you will see "ZEBRA" cases. So be prepared to spend time with MEDLINE.

The high staff-to-patient ratio also means that a lot of time is spent rounding and discussing the latest treatment for your patient's disease. You can stay ahead of the game by pulling current review papers in the literature for yourself and for the team. The quality of didactics is typically best in the academic center but can sometimes stray into the realm of cutting-edge research and basic science. Finally, a lot of the bigwigs at your school can be found in the academic center. Many students schedule key core and senior rotations there to rub elbows with the academic gods. Scoring an enthusiastic letter of recommendation from them can help make your residency application more impressive.

CURRENT
*Med Talk*

## CURRENT MED TALK

'ZEBRA': A somewhat hackneyed aphorism often quoted to wide-eyed medical students during their clinical rotations is, *'when you hear hoofbeats, don't think of zebras'*; this variation of 'Sutton's law' is designed to teach students a logical approach toward achieving a diagnosis, since common things occur commonly and when one hears hoofbeats, one usually thinks of horses. (Note: In the Republic of South Africa, zebras are more abundant and the word 'canary' is substituted.)

IVORY-TOWER SYNDROME: A highly colloquial ad hoc term for the blatant disregard that academic physicians have for economic realities when teaching medical students the practice of medicine; in the academic construct, information that is deemed extraneous to learning the foundations of medicine is regarded as unnecessary or unworthy of a medical student's time **(Am Med News 24 April 1995, p 15).**

However, it should be noted that this form of medicine is currently under siege. Rising managed-care competition plus dwindling Medicare and Medicaid reimbursements are forcing prestigious academic centers to forge new alliances and scramble for managed-care contracts. Because academic centers have a concurrent and vital teaching mission, they are inherently more costly (IVORY-TOWER SYNDROME) and less efficient than HMOs. Many centers will adopt managed-care strategies to survive, but not all centers will be successful at balancing the bottom line and your education.

**Community hospital.** Community hospitals are the antithesis of the academic center in that the focus here is on the patient's treatment and the bottom line. Patients thus tend to come in with bread-and-butter diagnoses, and the populations tend to be more skewed toward the middle class. Many of the physicians are, in addition, private community types—so if residents are present, they are sometimes relegated to "water-boy" status, carrying out orders rather than formulating treatment plans. In many cases, you will be working with a different private physician for each patient. Again, schmoozing is key to participating in a meaningful learning experience as well as to getting things done on your patients. Teaching is more relaxed and deals with the practical treatment approach. Nobody really cares if the long QT syndrome is linked to the Harvey ras (H-*ras*-1) oncogene on the short arm of chromosome 11 as long as you know what to do when a patient with a more common problem walks (or rolls) through the door.

**Outpatient clinic.** Reforms in medical education will lead to more time spent seeing patients in the outpatient clinic. Residents can blow through half a dozen patients in an afternoon. You'll be lucky if you manage to see three patients in the same amount of time. Keys to being a well-regarded outpatient clerk include obtaining a focused H&P guided by past clinic notes and studies and making a succinct presentation with pertinent positives and negatives that allow your resident or attending to clearly assess the problem. It is also crucial to learn the important things to ask and document as well as the nonessential information that is better left out, since time and efficiency are of the essence. Outpatient medicine is very different from inpatient care in that the patients are not "prisoners," so you cannot order all the tests at once and expect to get them back the same day. In this setting, you will also learn the frustration of patient noncompliance and missed appointments (think about that the next time you decide to blow off your dental appointment).

## EFFICIENT TIME AND PATIENT MANAGEMENT

Getting out at a reasonable hour ultimately depends on your ability to work closely with your team and to organize and efficiently execute your duties, although complicated patients will certainly make your days longer. Here are some tips that will help you take better care of your patients without depriving you of sunlight (unless you're on surgery):

**Commit all tasks to a to-do list.** Write each task down immediately. You will be bombarded with multiple responsibilities, so it is inevitable that you will forget something. Add even the "smallest" tasks to your to-do list. When it comes to your patient's care, there is no such thing as a small task. Check off your chores as they are accomplished, and roll over any unfinished ones to the next day's to-do list.

**Prioritize your tasks.** You will have time to get things done in the morning and the afternoon. In medicine, if key tasks don't get done during the Hour of Power, you won't have a chance to work on them until the early afternoon. Think about what needs to get done first to make sure your patient does not stay any longer than necessary. For example, requests for consults and studies must be done in the morning or they often have no chance of getting done that day (see Table 3). If you are planning to discharge a patient, take care of the paperwork and placement issues early.

**Organize tasks by location when possible.** Always think about what tasks can be done while you are in a particular location. If you are in the radiology

| TABLE 3. Example of prioritized tasks | |
| --- | --- |
| **Do Now** | **Do Next** |
| Request consults | Progress notes |
| Schedule studies | Check routine labs |
| Do discharge paperwork | Follow-up consults |
| Check stat or crucial labs | Follow-up studies |

department to look at Patient A's CXR, for example, you might as well take care of any radiology-related tasks, such as seeing Patient B's head CT and Patient C's abdominal films. If Patient B is on a different floor from your other patients, take care of tasks related to him while you're there, such as requesting that cardiology consult and scheduling him for a CXR.

**Learn to maximize the HIS.** A good hospital information system (HIS) can be your friend. Some systems can handle custom patient lists, print labs, and problem lists and can even perform literature searches.

**Keep scut essentials on board.** Supply carts are always in the third place you look. If you find a mother lode of supplies, load up on the suture removal kits, blood-draw supplies, and other essentials you need to get through your scut so that you won't have to look for a supply cart every time you go to a different floor to get something done on a patient.

**Carry a beeper.** Ideally, the medical school or hospital should provide you with a permanent beeper for the third and fourth year. If they do not, many students advise getting your own anyway. The easier you are to reach, the more you will stay involved with patient care. Also, there is nothing worse than hanging around waiting for an admission without a pager, when you could be in the library or call room.

## ORGANIZATIONAL AIDS ("PERIPHERAL BRAINS")

Another key to being an efficient and effective ward clerk is to have and use the right organizational aids. The pros and cons of the most popular organization aids, ranging from the lowly clipboard to high-tech personal digital assistants, are discussed below. Regardless of the type of aid you choose, you should remember to come prepared on day one; don't wait until halfway through your first rotation to start your system. If a given system doesn't work for you, you can always change it, but you need to be organized from the very start.

**Clipboard.** Many students start out with the clipboard as the preferred mode of organization. The clipboard gives you lots of surface area to organize patient information and tasks. It also gives you the ability to hold additional items such as progress notes, journal articles, and lab requests. However, a clipboard gets lost easily. There will be many times during the day when you'll put your clipboard down to do a physical exam or pull sutures. The clipboard can also get overstuffed with miscellaneous papers. Most fashion-conscious students eventually lose the clipboard when they come to feel comfortable with note cards.

**Note cards.** Most house staff and senior students use note cards to organize their patients, scut lists, and clinical cheat sheets. Note cards are compact and slide easily into your pocket. Because of space considerations, note cards force you to organize your thoughts about the patient and decide what to record and what to leave out. In addition, they are much less obtrusive when you are presenting. However, note cards may force you to use abbreviations and tiny print to the point where they are barely legible. Here are some more pointers regarding note cards:

- Blank note cards can often be found at the nurses' station.
- A ring binder or a ring clip prevents you from scattering loose cards and allows you to keep more cards together. You will need to punch holes in the cards. An alternative is to maintain a small pocket spiral-bound notebook.
- Use a high-quality, fine-point pen (eg, Pilot fine ballpoint) to minimize "microglyphics." Do not use felt-tip pens, as they may run if the card gets wet.
- Consider using a different color card for the patient's admission history and physical.
- Create an "if found" card with your name and pager number. Losing your cards is like having an unscheduled lobectomy. You have not known true fear until you have misplaced your patient cards.
- Create a card with key phone numbers on it (team pagers, lab, x-ray, nursing stations of each ward, etc.). This is key. It will save you time and will often help members of your team.

True fear is misplacing your patient cards before a presentation.

**Personal Digital Assistants (PDAs).** Also known as electronic organizers, these handheld computers have recently gained popularity among well-equipped house staff and medical students. PDAs not only handle telephone numbers, addresses, schedules, and to-do lists but can also record as a document file the clinical pearls you pick up during conferences and on the wards. Unlike note cards and pocket-binder-based collections of clinical cheat sheets, PDA cheat sheets can easily be edited and modified with supplemental information either from a text or from a subsequent conference. In addition, some PDAs, like the Apple MessagePad (Newton), can run specialized software for managing in-house patients and hospital activities. Most PDAs also have infrared ports that allow you to easily exchange information with similar PDAs. Newer-generation PDAs use MS Windows CE and offer modems and easy synchronization with a desktop PC. Unfortunately, PDAs are expensive, and some are bulky. Also keep in mind that technology such as this is often outdated by the time you purchase it. Moreover, you may find that you do not have the obsessive-compulsive disposition required to maintain a PDA. Unlike note cards and clipboards, PDAs can require a significant investment in both time and money. Also, since PDAs are a small but valuable piece of equipment, they are always at risk of being misplaced and even stolen—so you'll need to be very careful about having it in sight at all times. There are several PDAs offered in a variety of configurations, including:

PDAs are convenient for maintaining current clinical cheat sheets.

- Apple MessagePad
- Casio BOSS
- Casio Cassiopeia
- Hewlett-Packard Palm Top

- Psion 5
- Sharp Zaurus
- US Robotics Palm Pilot
- Philips Velo

Talk with several PDA users before you make the commitment.

**Practice what you preach: stay healthy.**

## STRATEGIES FOR MENTAL AND PHYSICAL HEALTH

Clinical clerkships are a very taxing time, but you have to make a conscious effort to balance work and rest, as ignoring your body's needs will eventually compromise your clinical performance. Besides, how can you possibly tell your patients how to stay healthy if you do not care for yourself? (Actually, that is fairly easy, as most medical professionals do not practice what they preach.) Remember that your own health must come first, as you are no help to the team if you are ill. Most of the following advice is considered so basic that it is actually ignored.

**Streamline and/or delegate household chores when possible.** Consider using an automatic bill payment service. Chip in for a bimonthly cleaning service. Eat out or use paper plates when possible (don't forget to recycle). Schedule household chores while on an easier rotation in exchange for your roommate's doing them during the more time-consuming rotations. Make sure your roommate understands how difficult your schedule will be on the wards.

**Stay grounded in friends and family.** They've been there for you during the preclinical years. You'll need their support and companionship more than ever during the clerkships. Given the hours you may be keeping, it can become difficult to stay in touch at times, especially since many of your friends may be classmates who are equally overwhelmed. But make sure you make a solid attempt to return phone messages and remember birthdays, anniversaries, etc.

**Eat well.** It is a well-known fact that hospital food and most lunches at noon conferences are considered risk factors for cardiovascular disease. You can still be picky without sacrificing speed. In addition, eat when you can. Being well fed is the key to a high energy level. Load up with complex carbohydrates instead of fat and sugar snacks.

**Exercise.** "No kidding," you say, but this can be especially tough when you're exhausted from a long day on the wards. It's even worse if you view exercise as another chore. You must find an activity that you enjoy, whether it be walking or basketball. Exercising with a friend keeps you more committed and makes it more social. Consider joining a 24-hour gym so you can work out at the odd hours that you are free. Another option is to have a treadmill or a bike at home so you can work out while watching TV or reading.

## SURVIVING CALL NIGHTS

A travel alarm is essential on call nights. Do not rely on the hospital operator to wake you up. Also make an "on-call" bag with a toothbrush, a hairbrush, a razor, and a change of clothes if working in a clinic the next day. Sleep whenever possible; eat whenever possible. Order in food every now and then so you don't get completely sick of the cafeteria food (this is, of course, inevitable). Hang out in the residents' lounge to watch TV, and bring a review/mini-reference book to learn about your patients' problems.

## GETTING OFF TO A GOOD START

To further maximize your wards experience, here are some preparatory measures you can take the weeks and months before your first rotation starts.

**Months before starting on the wards.** A few months prior to your rotation, you should consider the following:

- Order an extra white coat or two from the AMA catalog. They have great, big pockets both inside and out.
- Gather your medical supplies. Find a stethoscope that is light, yet one you can actually hear with. Test them out in the bookstore on your own heart, lungs, and belly; you're sure to get some strange looks, but doing so will help you decide whether you really need the Littmann Cardiology II.

Remember, too, that equipment is less pricy when ordered in bulk through medical schools—and you might even get a stethoscope for free if you can wrangle one from a pharmaceutical company. If your medical school does not have a deal with a pharmaceutical company and if it is compatible with your ethics and your financial status, you can try calling around to the marketing divisions of pharmaceutical companies yourself; you might just get lucky. You should also buy a cheap stethoscope to have as an "extra" in case your good one walks off one day and you have no time to go to the bookstore to replace it.

**Weeks before.** As soon as you know your schedule, find out from the department secretary who the chief residents and attendings will be during that rotation. Then find out from fourth-years and fellow classmates which residents and attendings are excellent teachers, which ones have a tendency to give unfair evaluations, which ones have a chip on their shoulder, etc. Having done so, ask the secretary to put you on a team with a satisfactory combination of the above; chances are that other students will be doing the same thing. So do the legwork as early as possible, and be prepared with alternate choices. During this time, you should also do a practice H&P.

**One week before.** You will feel less lost on the first day if you follow these general rotation-specific guidelines:

- If you're starting neuro, practice the neuro exam.
- If you're starting psych, practice or review the psych interview.
- If you're starting medicine, review normal values and the H&P.
- If you're starting surgery, review knots, sutures, and what goes in a preop, brief-op, postop, and progress note.

**The night before.** On the night before your rotation starts, you should do the following:

- Get your white coat (leave it home if you're doing psych) and/or your fanny pack together. Chances are that there is no safe place to leave anything in the hostial on your first day, so don't bring too much. Remember to bring your ID, your name tag, some money, extra pens, your stethoscope, *Pharmacopoeia* (for all rotations because it is tiny and will quickly translate all those brand names into generic names), your beeper (memorize the number so you can give it out), and a set of car or apartment keys.

- Set your alarm half an hour early, especially if you're not sure how to get either to the hospital or to your floor.
- Make sure you know where to go and when to get there. If in doubt, ask classmates who are on your team, or page a resident on the team.
- Recheck your alarm, especially the volume and the AM/PM settings.

**The first day.** On the first day of your wards experience:

- Eat a big breakfast.
- Arrive early.
- Make sure every member of your team knows this is your first rotation. That way, they are likely to be more tolerant toward you and to pay more attention to teaching you hospital basics, such as how to read a nursing chart, get labs or cultures off the computer, or page someone.
- Don't leave until the chief resident says to leave.
- If in doubt, ask when and where rounds will be the next day. Especially for surgery and medicine, bring an on-call bag with a toothbrush and toothpaste, underwear, socks, any medication you are on, and earplugs. Leave this gear in your car in case you are on call that first night.

## EVALUATIONS

Your third-year evaluations are critical, as they make up the majority of your dean's letter. Residency directors looking to recruit the best medical students look at third- and fourth-year evaluations first. Unfortunately, preclinical performance does not always predict clinical success. During the first two years, your fund of knowledge is everything; during the clinical years it is only one of many criteria by which you will be judged. As a result, doing well during the first two years provides little guarantee that you'll be successful on the wards.

### WRITTEN EVALUATIONS

Written evaluations are usually subjective assessments written by the attending or the senior resident. They should include a compilation of comments and observations from evaluation forms filled out by all residents and attendings who worked with you during the rotation. Written evaluations are easily influenced by personal factors and can be dangerous, since they are often quoted verbatim in the dean's letter. A single interaction (both positive and negative) can easily be seen by the attending as representative of your performance during the entire rotation.

### MAXIMIZING YOUR EVALUATIONS

It is critical to stay on top of your evaluations by getting feedback from your attendings and residents early, before potentially negative material ends up in your written evaluations. At the beginning of the rotation, ask both the attending and the resident what their expectations are. Two weeks into the rotation, meet with your attending and with your resident one-on-one to see if you are meeting their expectations and if there are any areas in which you can improve (eg, notes, rounds, procedures, communication). Sit down with your attending and resident at the end to review your performance. Your persistence will not only provide invaluable feedback but also demonstrate initiative that will not go unnoticed.

Within weeks, the clerkship office should have written evaluations on file. Visit the office to review them; hopefully the results will be pleasant. However, if you believe the evaluation is an inaccurate representation of your performance, now is the time to bring it to the attention of the clerkship director or the dean of students. It may be too late to change them when dean's letters are written during the summer of your fourth year.

Do not allow evaluations to affect your self-perception. Evaluations can vary widely. However, do not ignore trends or patterns in your evaluations, as they more or less reflect the consensus perception of your performance.

**Third-year evaluations are crucial to a successful residency application.**

## HONORS/GRADES

Most schools have a grading system of one sort or another, such as "Honors/Pass/Fail" or the traditional letter grading system, to gauge your clinical performance. Make sure you have a clear understanding of the criteria for achieving honors and "A's," as clerkship directors often fail to volunteer this information (sometimes intentionally). Note that objective standards (eg, mini-boards exams) and subjective standards (eg, Did the student fit in well with the team?) are often used together. Looking at an evaluation form can also tell you what specific skills and performance criteria you'll be judged on. Keep in mind that getting honors is not necessarily everything. Although it is certainly helpful for residency (icing on the cake), it is more important to consistently perform well on rotations, which will be reflected in your dean's letter.

## LETTERS OF RECOMMENDATION

If your attending wrote you a glowing evaluation or has given you very positive feedback, you may ask for a letter of recommendation while details of your valor are still fresh. Letters of recommendation are used when you apply for residency positions. If you ask for a letter early in the third year, have the attending update the letter when your career path becomes clearer.

The junior clerk is faced with a host of situations for the first time that require social and political savvy. Unfortunately, the junior clerk is typically at the bottom of the totem pole and has little political leverage. Failure to handle these situations can lead to anything from simple embarrassment to patient endangerment.

Do not hesitate to seek help if things become overwhelming. The wards can be a very stressful environment. Remember that getting help is not a sign of failure; rather, it is a testament to your ability to understand your limits. Most institutions will have discrete counseling available at little or no cost. Remember that your fellow classmates are in the same situation as you and may be having similar concerns. So this is a time to reach out to others and talk about your feelings, concerns, and fears.

**DIFFICULT SITUATIONS**

**Confidential counseling is available.**

**CURRENT**
*Med Talk*

UNIVERSAL PRECAUTIONS: A method of infection control in which all human blood, certain body fluids (to wit, amniotic fluid, CSF, pericardial, peritoneal, pleural, and synovial fluids, saliva in dental procedures, semen, vaginal secretions, and any fluid grossly contaminated with blood) as well as unfixed organs or tissues of human origin, HIV-containing cell or tissue cultures, and HBV-containing culture media or other solutions are treated as if known to be infected with HIV, HBV, and/or other blood-borne pathogens **(Federal Register Dec 6, 1991, p 64107, col 2);** in the absence of knowledge of the nature of the fluid, it should be treated as if potentially infectious. UPs consist of the constellation of safeguards for handling materials, tissues, and fluids that may contain human pathogens; exposure to blood and body fluids is minimized by using isolation materials and removable and disposable barriers (latex and vinyl gloves, protective eyewear, masks and gowns, and 'disposable sharps' containers). Body fluids that require 'universal precautions' include blood (serum and plasma) and all body fluids containing visible blood as well as maternal milk, semen, vaginal secretions, and cerebrospinal, synovial, peritoneal, pleural, pericardial, and amniotic fluids.

## NEEDLESTICKS

Being stuck by a needle or other sharp is probably the most feared incident that can happen to any health care worker. As a medical student, you are at a higher risk for being stuck because of your inexperience at handling sharps as well as your limited knowledge as to where things are in the hospital. Here are some useful tips:

**Never recap, bend, or break a sharp.**

- Always practice UNIVERSAL PRECAUTIONS. You won't always know and certainly can't guess a patient's HIV or HBV/HCV status. So wear gloves whenever handling any blood products or starting IV lines. Protect your eyes with a face shield or glasses to guard against splashes (eg, vomiting patient, arterial spray in surgery, or a trauma case in the ER). Wear a gown to protect other exposed areas (as well as your clothing) from contamination.
- Don't rush. Slow down and think about what you are doing. Be especially careful in the ER and in surgery, where needles and other sharps are being passed around you.
- Plan ahead. Have all of the necessary materials for the procedure you are about to perform at the bedside. Anticipate needing more than one needle for blood draws in case you miss (ditto for IVs). Find the sharps container ahead of time so you do not have to walk around the room with a needle in your hand.
- Dispose of contaminated sharps immediately (like a loaded gun) into the nearest sharps container. You are responsible for your own sharps. Never simply leave a needle on a table or a bed, as you may forget it is there or someone else may be stuck by it (you could easily forget about the needle if you suddenly leave the room for a Code Blue). If you absolutely have to put a contaminated sharp down, announce it ("sharp on the table") so that others are aware. If others are in the room when you are carrying a sharp to the disposal con-

tainer, let them know you are carrying a sharp and protect them as well as yourself.

- Never recap, bend, or break any needles/sharps.
- Don't force a needle into a sharp container that is full.
- Get vaccinated against HBV!

Despite your best efforts, the unthinkable may still occur. If you are ever stuck by a contaminated sharp, try to remember the following:

- Don't panic. Take a deep breath. You cannot change what has already occurred, but your actions now are still very important.
- Make sure the patient is safe, and discard the sharp properly.
- Wash the involved area with soap and water or Betadine.
- Call the Needlestick Hotline as soon as possible and inform one of your team members. Report exactly what has happened and follow the appropriate protocol. The hotline will give you information and facilitate blood testing, counseling, and possible HIV prophylactic treatment.

Do not hesitate to speak with team members, fellow students, friends and family, or counselors about what has happened. A needlestick can be extremely traumatizing (in many ways, it can be like a brush with death). If you feel you need to leave early to go home, tell your resident.

Always report a needlestick.

## CURRENT MED TALK

MEDICAL STUDENT ABUSE: A widely extant practice in which medical students are psychologically 'abused' by superiors (interns, residents, fellows, and attending physicians) in the form of badgering, belittling, and being forced to perform menial, degrading tasks; see pimping, scut work. Note: The opinion has been privately voiced by some health care workers that abuse is part of the medical student experience, which helps 'harden' them for the realities of practicing medicine (JAMA 1996; 275:414-6).

## ABUSIVE OR INAPPROPRIATE HOUSE OFFICERS

House staff typically work long hours and lead hectic lifestyles. However, that does not give them an excuse to vent their frustrations on you (MEDICAL STUDENT ABUSE). If the situation does not resolve, you should bring it to the attention of the clerkship director, ombudsperson, or student dean. Of course this is a very awkward situation, since you are being evaluated by the house officer. Avoid bringing this to the attention of the attending, as this can further disrupt the dynamics of the team.

On the other hand, you may receive unwanted attention, such as the resident who asks you out for a drink. You may avoid an awkward situation by suggesting that perhaps the entire team should go out for drinks. If the resident is insistent, you may have to be more direct. If this leads to a negative working relationship, you may have to bring it to the attention of the clerkship director or the student dean to resolve the situation as well as to protect yourself from any unfair evaluations.

## INAPPROPRIATE PROCEDURES

Be aggressive in volunteering for any procedures appropriate to your skill level (residents love highly motivated students). However, do not be pushed into performing any procedure with which you are not comfortable. This is dangerous for both you and the patient and is not an optimal learning situation. Good house officers will recognize your maturity in saying, "I'm not comfortable with this procedure. Can you walk me through it, or can I watch this one and perform the next one?"

**Learn to trust and depend on your classmates.**

## OVERLY COMPETITIVE CLASSMATES (AKA "GUNNERS")

The desire to achieve recognition and high marks can cloud the better judgment of your classmates (and sometimes your own). When there is more than one student to a team, a sense of do-or-die competition may arise, leading to excessive "brown-nosing" or back-stabbing behavior. This way of thinking must be curbed at the very start of any rotation. Your classmates are some of your most valuable resources, so make it clear that cooperation and support are key to learning and doing well on the rotation. Also, residents and attendings have all been junior students, so they can spot "brown-nosing" and back-stabbing behavior easily. Take the initiative; keep your classmates informed of scheduled events, share procedures, teach each other, and share information. Address back-stabbing behavior immediately and firmly. As they say in psychiatry, set clear limits. If the pattern persists, bring it to the attention of your intern or resident. Always maintain the moral high ground; you'll sleep better at night.

**The first few patient deaths are often very disturbing to the student.**

## PATIENT DEATH

Despite the best efforts of you and your team, some of your patients will die under your care. The first patient death can be particularly disturbing, especially if you developed any personal attachments. You should consider discussing the patient's death with your team or other students if they are receptive. Good social and family support also helps. Seek confidential counseling if necessary. As you continue your clinical training, you will learn to deal more effectively with patient death. However, do not distance yourself so much from the patient as to lose the human perspective.

**Document the harassment. Then see your student dean.**

## SEXUAL HARASSMENT

The power structure of a medical team can lead to abuses of attending and house staff privileges. Female students are especially vulnerable to snide remarks and outright inappropriate behavior. Confront the offender immediately only if you feel that you can handle it. In any case, document the event(s) clearly and unambiguously. Record the exact circumstances and the nature of the incident(s), and identify any witnesses. Then, make an appointment to see your student dean as soon as possible. Review the school's written policies. Your dean should be able to confidentially evaluate the information and determine the best course of action. Your school may have a sexual harassment prevention office or a dean or ombudsperson in charge of a sexual harassment protocol. Sexual harassment is a highly charged issue; you want to have as many backers as possible before you confront an offender. If you decide that the degree of harassment is mild, you may elect to tolerate the situation or wait until the rotation is finished for the sake of preserving your evaluation and team dynamics. This is a personal decision. However, continue to document all offending incidents in case you do change your mind and decide to act. At the end of the rotation, consider using evaluation forms to state your case so that you can help prevent this behavior in the future.

## DIFFICULT OR VIOLENT PATIENTS

Not all patients are pleasant and enjoyable to work with. Sometimes patients can be manipulative, hostile, verbally abusive, and even violent. Often such negative behavior is a physical manifestation of the patient's anger and frustration. Do not take anything personally. You need not like every patient you care for, but every patient deserves your best efforts and respect. Use common sense when dealing with difficult patients. Never hesitate to call on more experienced house staff to intervene when situations escalate. Never, ever retaliate against a patient. When dealing with agitated or potentially violent patients, keep the following in mind:

Personal safety is a priority with potentially violent patients.

- Remember that your own safety must come first.
- Never let the patient get between you and the door.
- Keep the door open.
- Visit the patient only with a nurse or house officer.
- Assess restraint status.
- Rule out reversible causes of increased agitation and lability.

## DIFFICULT FAMILY MEMBERS

Having a sick loved one in the hospital places considerable stress on family members and friends. Sometimes the anger, frustration, and sadness are redirected toward you. Again, do not take anything personally. When dealing with family members, find out who the chief decision maker is, especially if the patient is incapacitated or not competent to make decisions. Do not let family members push you into speculating about a treatment course. If you are unsure about anything, check with your team before giving the family a definitive answer. Again, know when to seek help from your team or a social worker in order to defuse highly charged or emotional situations.

## "NARCOLEPSY"

During your preclinical years, no one would notice if you fell asleep after lunch in a roomful of people. On the wards, however, everyone knows when you doze off, as you tend to be in much smaller gatherings. Although occasionally falling asleep is understandable given your state of frequent exhaustion, constant snoozing will leave a bad impression and will deprive you of valuable learning in attending rounds and conferences. The best remedy is to get more sleep. Other students become believers in coffee; however, be aware that caffeine withdrawal is a real clinical syndrome! You can also remain standing during rounds and conferences (although for some, even standing will not prevent a quick snooze). Although this may raise a few eyebrows, remember it's your learning (and to some extent your evaluation) which is at

Do whatever it takes to stay awake!

stake. Finally, if all else fails, sit behind or to the side of the attending. He or she will then be less likely to notice that you're sleeping unless you snore.

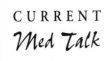

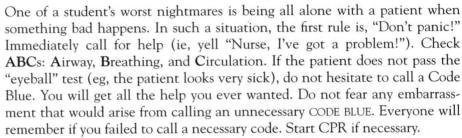

## CURRENT MED TALK

'CODE BLUE': A message announced over a hospital's public address system indicating that a cardiac arrest requiring medical attention is in progress; in a similar context, to be 'coded' is to undergo cardiopulmonary resuscitation.

## PATIENT EMERGENCIES

One of a student's worst nightmares is being all alone with a patient when something bad happens. In such a situation, the first rule is, "Don't panic!" Immediately call for help (ie, yell "Nurse, I've got a problem!"). Check **ABC**s: **A**irway, **B**reathing, and **C**irculation. If the patient does not pass the "eyeball" test (eg, the patient looks very sick), do not hesitate to call a Code Blue. You will get all the help you ever wanted. Do not fear any embarrassment that would arise from calling an unnecessary CODE BLUE. Everyone will remember if you failed to call a necessary code. Start CPR if necessary.

By the time you check the ABCs, there should be hordes of physicians and other health care professionals who will take over. The patient's code status will be ascertained, and the resulting resuscitation will be driven by established ACLS protocols. In a full code situation, the medical student often does the chest compressions, places an IV, or helps defibrillate (A-B-C/D-E-F sequence).

In a patient emergency:
1. Don't panic.
2. Get help.
3. Check ABCs.
4. CPR if necessary.

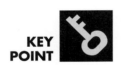

KEY POINT

| A-B-C/D-E-F SEQUENCE | |
|---|---|
| AIRWAY | Ensure airway patency (clear bronchotracheal tree) |
| BREATHING | Ensure breathing by intermittent positive pressure ventilation |
| CIRCULATION | Compress chest at 60/minute |
| DRUGS/Fluids | Place intravenous line |
| EKG | Monitor cardiac rhythms |
| FIBRILLATION | Defibrillate |

## PERSONAL ILLNESS

As students slip into the role of health care provider, they often come to believe that they are not allowed to get sick. In fact, it is a wonder that students do not get sick more often given the long work hours and relentless stress they face. When you get sick, your first priority has to be your own health. You cannot provide good patient care while sick, and you may transmit your illness to your patients. Do not dwell on your clinical responsibilities while you are ill; your team will likely get the job done just fine without your help. When sick, immediately page your resident or intern and let them know when you hope to return. If you are out for more than one day, try to keep track of events with your patients by speaking to your team once a day.

This will help you slide back into the ward routine with minimal confusion. Use the down time to catch up on reading.

## TIME OFF FOR PERSONAL OBLIGATIONS

When you need time off to attend to personal obligations such as a wedding, make arrangements with your resident as far in advance as possible, preferably at the beginning of the rotation. Arrange your call nights around the event if possible. If not, make up the call day elsewhere in the rotation. Try to limit major time off to once a rotation. Of course, there will be situations when you suddenly need time off, such as a family illness or a death. Again, give your team as much advance notice as possible, even if it is just one day. Everyone will understand. As with personal illness, try to keep track of your patients' events if possible. Otherwise, come in the evening before or very early in the morning of your next work day to review patient notes.

Although you may think that starting on the wards is akin to getting tossed to the wolves, you are not going in empty-handed. You need to be aware of several advantages that you can maximize to work in your favor.

## ENTHUSIASM

House staff may have a deeper fund of knowledge and more experience, but you can easily match or even surpass them when it comes to hustle, effort, getting there early, and staying late. Team members are often impressed by enthusiastic students, as are patients.

## TIME

The house staff's time is very precious. You, on the other hand, have plenty of time available. While the house officers have to do brief histories and physicals, you have the opportunity and privilege to really learn about your patients. This often allows you to ferret out bits of information on history and physical that can contribute to—or sometimes drastically change—patient management. If your patients are frustrated at having to repeat their entire histories again, let them know that you will be able to give them more of your time than anyone else on the team.

## BASIC SCIENCE KNOWLEDGE

Not too long ago, you completed one of the most arduous tasks of medical school: passing the USMLE Step 1. Believe it or not, some of the minutiae that you memorized are still buried somewhere in your unconscious and will surface when you least expect it. The interns and residents are years away from their basic science classes, so don't be surprised when you show them a thing or two on rounds in front of the attending (of course, don't make a habit of making your resident look dumb, or you may be less than happy with your evaluation). Discreetly feeding the tired intern or resident factoids for attending rounds helps them look good. This can build your reputation as a "team player."

Nobody can blame you for getting sick.

# YOUR ADVANTAGES

## "LOW" EXPECTATIONS

You are *not* expected to know the answer to every question, nor are you expected to know the set of orders written for a rule-out-MI protocol with your first patient. You will find to your surprise that residents are often impressed by your level of knowledge, even when you consider a question to be a relatively simple one. You *are* expected to care about your patients and to make a sincere effort to be a contributing member of the team. As long as you show your resident that you are trying to be productive, regardless of how inefficient you are, your resident will be satisfied.

# TOP-RATED BOOKS

Although each of the chapters that follow includes a listing of top-rated books specific to that rotation or specialty, the following list outlines books that are of potential use to you on all your rotations.

## GENERAL

### Guide to Antimicrobial Therapy
Sanford
J. P. Sanford, 1997, 131 pages, ISBN 093377530X, $8.95

The gold-standard pocket antimicrobial reference guide, updated yearly. Includes dosage, coverage, sensitivities, length of therapy, and drugs of choice for common infections. Presented in table format. Often available free from drug reps.

### Tarascon Pocket Pharmacopoeia
Tarascon, 1997, 56 pages, ISBN 1882742060, $6.95

The gold-standard pocket antimicrobial reference guide, updated yearly. Includes drug class, dosage, tables, and conversion factors. Compact and inexpensive. An absolute must-have for the wards.

### Current Clinical Strategies: Diagnostic History and Physical Exam in Medicine
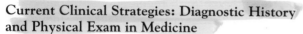
Chan
Current Clinical Strategies, 1996, ISBN 096203062, $8.75

**A**

Concise outline pocketbook. Contains guidelines to help you avoid missing pertinent positives and negatives on H&Ps that you will be asked about on rounds. Useful for writing admit notes. Limited coverage of diseases. An excellent investment for the price.

### Pocket Guide to Diagnostic Tests
Nicoll
Appleton & Lange, 1997, 457 pages, ISBN 0838581005, $19.95

Provides a concise reference for common diagnostic tests in quick-flip table format. Includes physiologic bases for and interpretation of lab results as well as nomograms, excellent algorithms on common diseases, and a useful section on EKG interpretation.

### Clinician's Pocket Reference
Gomella
Appleton & Lange, 1997, 593 pages, ISBN 0838514766, $27.95

Good overall orientation for the wards. Excellent use of tables, graphs, and diagrams to explain concepts. Includes useful protocol algorithms for medical emergencies, interpretation of abnormal lab values, and a chapter on commonly used drugs. Includes sections on basic EKG reading and critical care medicine. Differential diagnoses are provided; however, pathophysiology is not emphasized, and there is little information regarding patient workup. Overly basic and best suited for the newcomers on the wards.

**A-** **Current Pocket Reference**
Shepherd
Specialty Cards, 1997, 92 pages, ISBN 0964219336, $8.75

A compact pocket database featuring a comprehensive pharmacopoeia as well as medical notes spanning most medical fields. The medical notes are useful in many cases, but as a pharmacopoeia this database falls short of *Tarascon* with respect to oncology, metabolism, excretion, and safety in pregnancy.

**A-** **Diagnostic Examination**
DeGowin
McGraw-Hill, 1994, 1033 pages, ISBN 0070163383, $37.00

A classic handbook divided into physical exam, lab tests, and common disease patterns. Gives clear explanations of the pathophysiology of nearly any physical finding imaginable. Too big to carry around with you. Explains the pathophysiology behind laboratory values.

**A-** **Intern Pocket Survival Guide**
Masterson
IMP, 1992, 70 pages, ISBN 0963406302, $7.59

Practical, inexpensive pocket guidebook to day-to-day chores, writing H&Ps, admissions, discharge, workup and interventions. Includes only the most essential facts and numbers. Written for the intern, but useful for subinterns and medical students as well.

**A-** **Interpretation of Diagnostic Tests**
Wallach
Little, Brown, 1996, 1093 pages, ISBN 0316920487, $39.95

Excellent encyclopedic coverage of diagnostic tests organized by diseases, systems, and abnormal lab values. Includes sections on specific lab exams, drugs, and lab values.

**B+** **Facts & Formulas**
Rollings
McNaughton & Gunn, 1985, 82 pages, ISBN 0181120690, $6.50

Compact compilation of key facts, formulas, graphs, and tables of basic topics encountered in medicine. Most of the information can be found in larger pocket references, but this tiny pocketbook provides quick, easy access. Very popular.

**B+** **Handbook of Commonly Prescribed Drugs**
DiGregorio
Medical Surveillance Inc., 1995, 270 pages, ISBN 0942447158, $15.50

An alternative to *Tarascon*. Lengthier, but includes indications for use and additional drug-related information.

### On Call: Principles and Protocols
Marshall
Saunders, 1993, 393 pages, ISBN 0721639828, $28.95

**B+**

A practical guidebook to tackling common on-call problems. Designed for interns, but may be valuable for subinterns and junior clerks. Compact coverage of the myriad potential on-call problems, but inevitably incomplete. Divided into phone-call management, elevator thoughts, threats to life, and bedside care.

### Handbook of Clinical Drug Data
Anderson
Appleton & Lange, 1997, 976 pages, ISBN 0838535615, $44.91

**B**

Extensively referenced, current, and comprehensive drug guide including mechanisms of action, detailed clinical information, and abundant tables. Useful, but too bulky to be used as a pocket drug manual.

### An Introduction to Clinical Medicine: A Student-to-Student Manual
Macklis
Little, Brown, 1994, 308 pages, ISBN 0316542431, $29.95

**B**

A practical handbook featuring many tables and illustrations as well as an appendix listing common drugs by generic and trade name. Lacks in-depth discussion of therapy.

### Maxwell's Quick Medical Reference
Maxwell
Maxwell, 1996, 15 cards, ISBN 0964519100, $7.95

**B**

Compact, spiral-bound fact cards primarily detailing ACLS algorithms, various in-house notes, normal lab values, H&P, and the neurologic exam. Information appears to target different levels, keeping this database from being universally useful to anyone.

### Medi-Data
Rodriguez
Rodram Corporation, 1995, 58 pages, ISBN 9686277087, $8.95

**B**

Small, concise pocketbook with extensive listings of normal lab values and diagnostic tests.

### Pocket Guide to Commonly Prescribed Drugs
Levine
Appleton & Lange, 1996, 422 pages, ISBN 0838580998, $16.95

**B**

Unlike most other drug references, this pocketbook contains pearls, side effects, and cost ranges. However, the drug list is not as extensive as that of *Tarascon*.

### Rapid Interpretation of EKG: A Programmed Course
Dubin
Cover Press, 1996, 342 pages, ISBN 0912912022, $29.99

Presented as a "workbook," this reference facilitates rapid acquisition of EKG fundamentals. Emphasizes active learning with fill-in-the-blanks and visual aids accompanying each page. An excellent, quick reference summary of each section provided at the end. Can be easily read in a weekend. Although the content has not changed significantly in several years and it may be overly simplistic (only a starting point), most agree that it is still the best basic stepping stone for the junior student.

### Marriott's Practical Electrocardiography
Wagner
Williams & Wilkins, 1994, 434 pages, ISBN 0683086049, $35.00

A thorough EKG reference, including normal and abnormal EKG findings. May be too detailed for a third-year clerkship level. Includes illustrations, literature references, EKG tracings, and a glossary. Excellent for cardiology subinterns.

### Clinical Electrocardiography: A Simplified Approach
Goldberger
Mosby, 1994, 341 pages, ISBN 081513620X, $49.95

A very basic approach to EKG interpretations with many EKG examples, 12 leads, and rhythm strips. Includes practice problems at the end of each chapter and a final section with self-assessment problems and case presentations. Useful as a home reference book, and provides enough depth for good understanding of basic principles and correlation of cardiac pathophysiology with EKG findings. A bit too expensive.

### The Only EKG Book You'll Ever Need
Thaler
Lippincott, 1994, 293 pages, ISBN 0397514085, $34.95

Stresses basic electrophysiology and simple EKG interpretation organized by problems. Includes useful end-chapter summaries and a comprehensive summary of important principles. Also includes 8 case presentations, tables, graphs, and a few 12-lead EKGs. Concise and highly readable.

### Understanding Electrocardiography
Conover
Mosby, 1996, 528 pages, ISBN 0815119275, $34.95

A reference providing an in-depth overview of EKG interpretation. Includes 12-lead EKGs, rhythm strips, tables, and charts. The dense and lengthy writing style limits its usefulness on the wards. Includes references for further study.

### ECG Made Easy
Hampton
Churchill Livingstone, 1992, 106 pages, ISBN 0443045070, $16.95

**B+**

A simple and practical quick-reference pocketbook that emphasizes basic EKG interpretation. Includes tables and a few rhythm strips, but lacks practice problems or case discussions. Not as comprehensive or detailed as other books, but easily read in a few hours.

### ECG Workout: Exercises in Arrhythmia Interpretation
Huff
Lippincott, 1997, 336 pages, ISBN 0397553714, $24.95

**B**

A practical workbook with more than 500 EKGs. Emphasizes arrhythmias, but lacks discussion of MI, ischemia, or hypertrophy. Includes good tables, illustrations, and self-assessment problems. Best used in conjunction with a primary EKG reference.

### How to Quickly and Accurately Master ECG Interpretation
Davis
Lippincott & Raven, 1992, 402 pages, ISBN 039751106X, $34.95

**B**

A reference lacking a basic discussion in EKG electrophysiology and the pathophysiology of EKG findings. Provides excellent practice for EKG interpretation, with numerous EKG tracings included. Useful as a secondary source but not as a primary text.

### Recognition and Interpretation of ECG Rhythms
Ochs
Appleton & Lange, 1997, 425 pages, ISBN 0838543235, $29.95

**B**

Spiral-bound introductory manual featuring tons of sample strips but sparse explanatory text. Contains limited coverage of topics other than dysrhythmias.

### Lessons in EKG Interpretation
Summerall
Churchill Livingstone, 1991, 214 pages, ISBN 0443087784, $34.95

**C+**

Does not devote enough time to basic pathophysiology of EKG findings. Moderate to poor readability; tends to be too wordy. Poor presentation style.

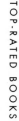

# Notes

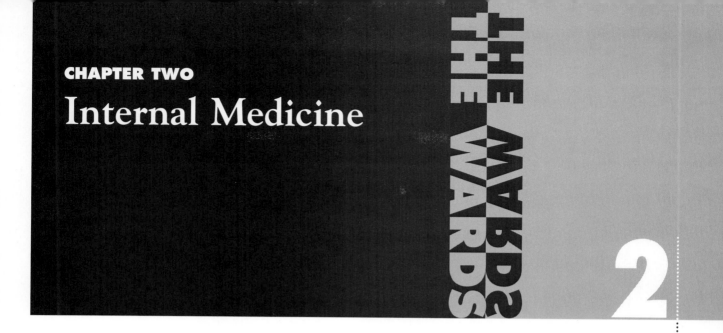

## CHAPTER TWO

# Internal Medicine

THE WARDS

2

# WARD TIPS

## WHAT IS THE ROTATION LIKE?

The internal medicine clerkship ranges from 8 to 12 weeks in duration and will serve to broaden your scope in the areas of cardiology, pulmonary medicine, gastroenterology, endocrinology, hematology, and infectious disease in both an outpatient and an inpatient setting. Given the sheer scope of the field, internal medicine will serve as a strong foundation for all of your other rotations when done early and, when done later, will shore up your fund of knowledge. The internal medicine rotation is thus an invaluable experience, regardless of when it is done and what specialty you eventually choose. So enjoy the rotation.

## WHO ARE THE PLAYERS?

**Attendings.** Consisting of clinical and academic faculty, the attendings are in charge of the ward team and are ultimately responsible for patient care. Attendings are also the source of most of the didactic learning that takes place during attending rounds. Your interaction with attendings consists mostly of making formal patient presentations in attending rounds and participating in didactic teaching. Thus, it is crucial to read up on your patients' problems before attending rounds, especially if you are presenting the patient.

**Residents.** Since residents are at least a year ahead of interns, they supervise the ward team and help formulate patients' treatment plans. Residents also serve as a major teaching resource, dispensing clinical pearls on work rounds and bringing in pertinent review articles. Your interaction with the resident will vary depending on his or her style; some remain aloof and serve only to answer questions while others are more interactive, giving informal lectures and taking you to patients' bedsides to teach physical findings. Residents also love to pimp as a means of teaching and assessing your knowledge base. They may even take the time to give you organized lectures on EKG reading or to lend you recent journal articles that are pertinent to patients on the team.

**Interns.** Interns are the cogs that make the hospital machinery move by performing most of the primary patient care. As they will co-follow your patient,

Internal medicine dilemmas are faced by practitioners in all specialties.

you will probably have the most interaction with your intern. All questions and management issues regarding your patient should initially be directed toward the intern. You should also remember that interns were recently medical students themselves, so they can be an invaluable resource for practical information as well as survival tips. You can use them for feedback on your progress notes and presentation style. If they have time, consult with them before rounds to discuss your plan for your patients so that you can have a more coherent plan in your mind when presenting on rounds.

## HOW IS THE DAY SET UP?

The typical day on a medicine rotation starts at about 7 AM and usually runs until 4–5 PM.

| | |
|---|---|
| 7:00–8:00 AM | Prerounds |
| 8:00–9:00 AM | Work rounds |
| 9:00–10:30 AM | Work time |
| 10:30–12:00 noon | Attending rounds |
| Noon–1:00 PM | Noon conference |
| 1:00 PM – ? | Work time, student conferences |

## WHAT DO I DO DURING PREROUNDS?

Please refer to "Prerounds" in "Typical Medicine Day" on p. 5 of Chapter 1.

## HOW DO I DO WELL IN THIS ROTATION?

Learning the material well does not always correlate with doing well on the clerkship. Often your grade will depend on subjective forces beyond your control, such as whether your personality matches that of your residents. But the following tips will help stack the deck in your favor.

**Know your patient.** You should know the very latest clinical information on your patient, be it the most recent laboratory values, the planned studies of the day, or simply how the patient is feeling. Relay this information to the intern so that management plans can adapt. Keep on top of consults and tests you have ordered. Speak with the consulting service about their recommendations: consultants can give you valuable information and may even have time to give you a short tutorial on your patient's disease process. Another important part of knowing your patient is a daily check of the nurses' log of medications given. This will allow you to ensure that the antibiotics ordered were given (not always the case) as well as to gauge whether the patient is receiving symptomatic relief. For example, is the pain well controlled, or is the patient asking for a lot of pain medication? You should also be aware of a patient's social situation so you can keep the family up to date regarding his or her progress. Finally, be aware of special circumstances to be considered on discharge (eg, getting a hotel room for a homeless patient).

**Develop differential diagnoses.** The search for the etiology of a patient's problem begins with knowing the differential diagnosis. Therefore, a critical goal of

**You cannot diagnose what is not in your differential diagnosis.**

this rotation is to learn the basic differential diagnoses of common patient signs and symptoms. The differential can often be broken into three groups: common etiologies, uncommon etiologies, and etiologies you don't want to miss (because they're either highly treatable or life-threatening). Mastering the differentials of common problems will serve you well in any specialty.

**Care about your patients.** Perhaps the single most important thing you can do on *any* rotation is to be genuinely concerned about your patients. Nothing is more highly respected by faculty and your team. Don't simply leave at 5:00 PM if your patient is crashing. Remember why you decided to go to medical school in the first place.

**Medicine is more than a 9-to-5 job.**

**Getting along with your team.** It is critical to remember that you are part of a team. Even though you may be low on the totem pole, you still have an integral role to play and are a genuine asset to your team. Medical students who make life easier for the interns and residents through diligent and efficient work will also be rewarded in their evaluations. It is thus important to be personable and affable to ensure that the members of your team work as a cohesive unit. By contrast, a sure-fire way to effectively shoot yourself in the foot is to openly conflict with others on your team. If you feel uncomfortable with another team member or sense any kind of personality problem developing, it is crucial to nip it in the bud as early as possible. If you are unable to smooth things over, do whatever it takes to avoid conflicts so that the team can continue to work together without problems. A serious rift in the team is an uncommon situation, but when it does occur, it can be devastating to patient care, team morale, and your evaluation.

**Be early.** Never underestimate the importance of punctuality. Attendings and residents probably won't take notice when you show up on time, but they *will* remember if you walk in late.

**Work independently.** Try to work as independently as your talent permits. The easier you make your intern's life, the more he or she will appreciate you. If you can call the consults, order the lab tests, and determine if the patient is comfortable, you will go a long way. Expect to be very dependent initially; this is perfectly normal. But as you become more experienced, you will feel the desire and have the confidence to work more independently.

**Read, read, read.** Keep both a pocket manual and a home reference book handy. As a third-year student, you have a responsibility to read about your patients and all their issues. This will save you when the inevitable pimping starts. Reading will also help you ask intelligent questions about the diagnosis and treatment of your patient and will ultimately move you toward making management decisions. Performing MEDLINE searches for current literature pertaining to your patient's problem is also important. You will have to gauge how many searches you can do in accordance with your time constraints.

**Ask for feedback.** Midway through the course, have the attending and resident set aside time so that they can give you feedback; "you're doing fine" is not an acceptable answer. Be persistent, and ask about your weaknesses. This will help you identify areas needing improvement and will also notify them that you are a responsible student.

If you are sincerely interested in pursuing a career in internal medicine, you need to take additional steps. First, let the members of your team know of your interests. They may make a special effort to teach and help you. However, don't lie; insincerity is easily sensed and is definitely looked down upon. Second, the status of your attending becomes crucial; it is ideal to have at least one block of your clerkship with a senior attending (ie, a big shot). In residency applications, the person writing your letter of recommendation is often almost as important as what is said about you in the letter. Performing well will virtually assure you of a good letter of recommendation from a senior faculty member. Talk to your resident and the course scheduler to see if you can work with a senior faculty member in at least one block of your clerkship.

### Presentations

**Work rounds.** Presentations during work rounds consist of an oral version of your SOAP note. Here the team will focus on brevity and efficiency, with emphasis on the assessment and plan. A well-thought-out assessment and plan takes extra time during prerounding, so start early. Do not be discouraged if your assessment and plan is completely wrong—you are there to learn, and the team will appreciate the fact that you are trying. It is better to come up with a well-thought-out plan that is incorrect than to simply say "I don't know" when you are asked about your next move in patient management.

**Attending rounds.** This is your time in the spotlight, when you really need to shine. Your attending will probably want a more lengthy formal oral presentation than on work rounds. Although they will primarily want to learn about the patient, attendings will also be observing your presentation style and how well you understand the patient's problems. One key means of demonstrating your knowledge is to include all pertinent positives and negatives relating to your patient's condition. This is not easy at first, especially since it requires an understanding of the presentation of the other possibilities in the differential. It is okay, however, if you leave out something from the history, since the attending will simply ask for additional information if it is important. Don't panic if your attending asks you several additional questions about your patient; instead, make a mental note of the specific tidbits that your attending likes to hear so that you can include them in your next presentation. You should also make sure you understand why the attending considers certain pertinent positives or negatives to be relevant to your patient.

Remember that your attending's comments weigh heavily in your final grade. Formal oral patient presentations comprise a large part of how the attending perceives you, so you will want to shine in this arena. Ask the attending how he or she would like you to present the patient. Practice your presentation before attending rounds, even running it by your resident for feedback.

## KEY NOTES

Please refer to the prototypical medicine admit note and progress note in Chapter 1 on pp. 11–14, 17–18.

## KEY PROCEDURES

Explanations for the basic procedures that follow can be found in any pocket ward manual, such as Gomella's *Clinician's Guide to Patient Care*.

- Phlebotomy
- IV line placement
- Arterial blood gas
- Foley placement

If you're lucky, your resident may allow you to perform the following advanced procedures on your patient:

- Thoracocentesis
- Paracentesis
- Lumbar puncture

## WHAT DO I CARRY IN MY POCKETS?

**Checklist**

- ❑ Stethoscope
- ❑ Eye chart
- ❑ Tuning fork (the big one)
- ❑ Penlight
- ❑ Reflex hammer
- ❑ Tongue blades

Remember
Reflex hammer
penlight

# TOP-RATED BOOKS

## HANDBOOK/POCKETBOOK

**A**

**Practical Guide to the Care of the Medical Patient**
Ferri
Mosby, 1995, 893 pages, ISBN 0815133901, $32.95

Well-organized and easy-to-read pocketbook for management and treatment of common diseases. Includes sections on etiology, differential diagnosis, approach to diagnosis, laboratory values and interpretation, treatment, and commonly used drugs. Some sections are better covered in more specialized pocketbooks.

**A**

**Saint-Frances Guide to Inpatient Medicine**
Saint
Williams & Wilkins, 1997, 533 pages, ISBN 0683075470, $19.95

Excellent, cheap, and concise pocketbook with an emphasis on developing an organized approach to many common diseases. Good use of tables and charts. Includes a unique section devoted to medical mnemonics. Cannot be used as primary source because it lacks extensive discussion of pathophysiology, diagnostic evaluation, management, or treatment. Best used as prerotation reading, as it gives a nice overview of differential diagnosis and simplifies the approach to complex medical issues.

**A-**

**Current Clinical Strategies: Medicine**
Chan
Current Clinical Strategies, 1996, 89 pages, ISBN 1881528324, $12.75

Compilation of admission orders for commonly encountered diseases, including detailed pharmacologic treatment options. Useful and inexpensive pocketbook for third-year students doing their medicine rotation.

**A-**

**Manual of Medical Therapeutics (The Washington Manual)**
Ewald
Little, Brown, 1995, 641 pages, ISBN 0316924334, $34.95

Unique handbook outlining the pathophysiology and diagnosis of common diseases. Contains excellent, detailed descriptions of various therapeutic options. Aimed toward medical residents, but very useful for medical students as well. Tight fit in most lab coat pockets.

**B+**

**Internal Medicine: Diagnosis and Therapy**
Stein
Appleton & Lange, 1993, 654 pages, ISBN 0838511120, $28.95

A 5.5″ × 8.5″ pocketbook written in an expanded outline format. Includes pathophysiology, diagnosis, and treatment but contains limited discussion of differential diagnosis. Designed for residents; however, useful for students. Compare to *The Washington Manual*.

### Internal Medicine on Call
Haist

Appleton & Lange, 1997, 593 pages, ISBN 0838540562, $24.95

Quick reference guidebook to the approach of most commonly encountered medical "on-call" problems. Includes sections on wards procedures and drugs. More appropriate for subinterns. Compare with Marshall's *On Call*.

### Harrison's Principles of Internal Medicine Handbook
Isselbacher

McGraw-Hill, 1995, 940 pages, ISBN 0070709106, $32.00

"Baby" pocket version of parent book focusing on commonly encountered diseases. Useful for quick reading on established diagnoses. Not particularly practical for day-to-day wards problems.

### Internal Medicine Companion
Ferri

Mosby, 1994, 349 pages, ISBN 0801678250, $29.95

Small, quick-flip collection of lists, tables, and great flowcharts of the diagnostic evaluation of numerous conditions. Covers the etiology of common diseases, differential diagnosis, diagnostic approaches, therapeutics, medication comparison tables, and lab evaluations. Friendly format with useful content, but contains many gaps. An interesting book, but not adequate as a sole reference on the wards.

### The Portable Internist
Zollo

Hanley & Belfus, Inc., 1995, 704 pages, ISBN 1560530669, $41.95

Broad but superficial coverage of various disease processes. Good for quick reading, but not as a primary reference source. Given its dimensions (6" × 9"), not quite as portable as the name implies.

## REVIEW/MINI-REFERENCE

### Current Medical Diagnosis & Treatment
Tierney

Appleton & Lange, 1997, 1587 pages, ISBN 0838514898, $45.00

Clinically oriented reference that is concise yet detailed and very readable. Well organized with excellent descriptions of pathophysiology and specific treatment of diseases. Revised annually and complete with useful tables and up-to-date references. Strong coverage of ambulatory care relative to more conventional texts.

### Clinical Medicine
Greene

Mosby, 1996, 965 pages, ISBN 0815140266, $45.95

A sizable softcover text which gives a broad overview of medicine and primary care. It has an excellent, readable format that emphasizes clinical decision making. It also contains abundant figures, tables, and color illustrations as well as an index of algorithms outlining the evaluation of common problems.

**Pathophysiology of Disease: An Introduction to Clinical Medicine**
McPhee
Appleton & Lange, 1997, 604 pages, ISBN 0838576788, $32.95

A concise interdisciplinary reference text of the pathophysiology of common diseases, organized by system. Excellent explanations of disease processes. Not designed for the wards, but useful as an adjunct to a more traditional textbook.

**Principles and Practice of Medicine**
Stobo
Appleton & Lange, 1996, 921 pages, ISBN 0838579639, $41.95

Organized by organ system, this text gives a useful "how-to approach" discussion for each disease process and a summary of key points at the end of each chapter. Level of detail is moderate and manageable, placing this text in between a primary reference and a pocketbook.

**Cecil Essentials of Medicine**
Andreoli
Saunders, 1993, 921 pages, ISBN 0721632726, $39.95

Great condensed version of parent book. Excellent for understanding pathophysiology, but not as useful for treatment reference or for differential diagnosis. Contains many great tables and charts. Not portable.

**Medical Secrets**
Zollo
Mosby, 1997, 516 pages, ISBN 156053172X, $38.95

Interesting but dense compilation of useful and not-so-useful facts presented in a question-and-answer format. Designed for surviving wards pimping sessions, although one is inevitably never asked the majority of these questions. Excellent tables that may be useful for quick reviews or "spiffing up" presentations. Well indexed and referenced. A must for the "Jeopardy" fan, but otherwise not a prudent buy.

**Medicine**
Fishman
J. B. Lippincott, 1996, 654 pages, ISBN 0397514646, $32.95

Organized by system. Very readable and approachable. Sometimes simplistic and lacking in detail. Good use of tables, but with few illustrations. Not a replacement for a medicine reference book.

**NMS Medicine**
Myers
Williams & Wilkins, 1994, 600 pages, ISBN 0683062336, $27.00

Not quite a reference book, but organized by system with easy-to-read chapters in outline form. Includes questions at the end of each chapter to solidify concepts just learned, and a comprehensive exam at the very end. Geared more toward the USMLE Step 2. Scarce diagrams, tables, and illustrations.

INTERNAL MEDICINE

**Internal Medicine, Oklahoma Notes Series**
Jarolim
Springer-Verlag, 1993, 240 pages, ISBN 0387979603, $16.95

**B-**

Quick but dry reading. Outline format, but with poor presentation of material. Questions are too simplistic and answers are sometimes lacking in depth and detail. Geared more toward USMLE Step 2.

**Internal Medicine Pearls**
Marsh
Mosby, 1993, 271 pages, ISBN 1560530243, $49.95

**B-**

Compilation of clinical case presentations of commonly encountered diseases. Requires considerable reading time for limited amount of information. Good leisure reading, but not a useful reference book for the wards.

**Internal Medicine: Rypin's Intensive Review**
Frohlich
Lippincott, 1996, 282 pages, ISBN 0397515480, $19.95

**B-**

Paragraph-style review of common diseases with exam questions. Simplistic and not appropriate for the wards.

**Phantom Notes Medicine**
Glickman
Phantom Notes, 1992, 900 pages, ISBN 1880934000, $29.95

**C**

This review book is written in a dry, boring outline format. Mediocre coverage of workup and treatment of diseases; lacks graphics; requires too much reading time.

## TEXTBOOK/REFERENCE

**Cecil Textbook of Medicine**
Wyngaarden
Saunders, 1996, 2300 pages, ISBN 0721635733, $110.00

**A**

One of the classic textbooks of medicine. Comparable to and easier reading than *Harrison's,* but not quite as comprehensive or detailed. Great index organization. Available as single- or double-volume text.

**Harrison's Principles of Internal Medicine**
Fauci
McGraw-Hill, 1997, 2496 pages, ISBN 0070202915, $99.00

**A**

An excellent "classic" comprehensive medical reference text. Excellent use of tables, graphs, illustrations, and radiographs. Not for quick reference but rather for in-depth home reading on specific topics. It is incredibly detailed and can be overwhelming to the junior student. Requires serious concentration and reading time.

**The Merck Manual of Diagnosis & Therapy**
Merck
Merck, 1992, 2844 pages, ISBN 0911910166, $26.00

Clear discussions of a wide variety of diseases, but with limited use of tables, charts, and illustrations. May be used as a reference book, but is not nearly as extensive as *Harrison's*. Useful as an adjunctive, quick home-reference textbook. A great buy.

**Internal Medicine**
Stein
Mosby, 1994, 2861 pages, ISBN 0801669111, $99.95

Comprehensive reference book. Not of the same level of detail as *Harrison's*, but more approachable and friendly. Good explanations of pathophysiology, with good sections on diagnostic evaluation.

**Essentials of Internal Medicine**
Kelley
Lippincott, 1994, 826 pages, ISBN 0397512724, $39.95

Boring, dry review of medicine topics presented in outline form. Too much text and not enough graphs, tables, or illustrations. Limited discussion of workup and treatment of diseases.

# HIGH-YIELD TOPICS

## ROTATION OBJECTIVES

Because internal medicine covers so many domains, you should set achievable goals in your bid to attain a solid fund of knowledge. The following is a list of common diseases that you may want to review during the rotation. Remember, you will face these diseases regardless of the specialty you choose, so learn away. (Disease entities that are discussed in this chapter are listed in italics.)

**Cardiology**
- *Angina pectoris*
- *Unstable angina* (rule out myocardial infarction)
- *Prinzmetal's (variant) angina*
- *Acute myocardial infarction*
- *Congestive heart failure*
- Arrhythmias (eg, *atrial fibrillation*)
- Cardiac arrest
- Cardiomyopathies
- Hypertension
- Valvular heart disease
- Endocarditis, pericarditis, and myocarditis

**Pulmonology**
- *Pneumonia*
- *Pleural effusion*
- *Pulmonary embolism*
- *Pneumothorax*
- *Asthma*
- *Chronic obstructive pulmonary disease*
- *Bronchogenic carcinoma*
- Interstitial lung disease
- Acute respiratory failure
- Pulmonary nodules and masses

**Gastroenterology**
- *Gastrointestinal bleeding*
- *Peptic ulcer disease*
- *Inflammatory bowel disease (eg, Crohn's disease, ulcerative colitis)*
- *Pancreatitis*
- Abdominal pain
- Acute hepatitis
- Portal hypertension
- Gastrointestinal cancer
- Disorders of swallowing (eg, achalasia, esophageal cancer)
- Diarrhea
- Malabsorption

**Infectious disease**
- *Tuberculosis*
- *HIV and AIDS*
- *Fever of unknown origin (FUO)*
- CNS infections (eg, meningitis, encephalitis)
- Respiratory tract infections (eg, pneumonia, URI)
- Intra-abdominal infections (eg, spontaneous bacterial peritonitis)
- Urinary tract infections
- Sexually transmitted diseases (eg, syphilis, gonorrhea, herpes)
- Animal-borne diseases (eg, Lyme disease, rabies, malaria)

**Nephrology**
- *Acute renal failure*
- *Glomerulonephritis*
- Chronic renal failure
- Electrolyte disorders
- Acid-base disturbances
- Kidney stones

**Endocrinology**
- *Diabetes mellitus (types I and II)*
- Pituitary disorders (eg, Cushing's disease, acromegaly)
- Thyroid disorders (eg, Graves' disease, Hashimoto's thyroiditis)
- Gonadal disorders (eg, testicular feminization)
- Hyperlipidemias (eg, familial hypercholesterolemia)

**Rheumatology**
- *Systemic lupus erythematosus*
- Rheumatoid arthritis

### Rheumatology (cont'd)

- Osteoarthritis
- Vasculitis (eg, polyarteritis nodosa, temporal arteritis)
- Ankylosing spondylitis
- Gout and pseudogout
- Polymyositis
- Fibromyalgia

### Hematology

- Anemia
- Bleeding disorders (eg, hemophilia)
- Hypercoagulable states

### Oncology

- Paraneoplastic syndromes
- Breast cancer
- Lymphomas
- Leukemias
- Prostate cancer

### General medicine

- Health maintenance issues
- Cancer screening
- Medical ethics issues
- Outpatient management

---

## ANGINA PECTORIS

Angina is the hallmark of myocardial ischemia and infarction and is usually due to atherosclerotic disease. Recognition of this symptom is key to the early management of myocardial disease.

### Signs and Symptoms

Classic symptoms include exertional substernal chest pressure radiating to the lower jaw/left shoulder/left arm that may be associated with nausea, vomiting, dyspnea, and diaphoresis. It is relieved promptly by rest or nitroglycerin and lasts less than 30 minutes. Chest exam may reveal an S4 heart sound due to a stiff left ventricle and, rarely, mitral regurgitation murmur secondary to papillary muscle ischemia.

### Differential

In the emergency room, you must always consider potential causes of chest pain that can kill your patient. Otherwise, a number of conditions mimic angina, including costochondritis (Tietze's syndrome), gastroesophageal reflux disorder, peptic ulcer, and intercostal neuritis (eg, from herpes zoster and diabetes mellitus).

### Workup

In the emergency room, the EKG may show ST-segment depression or T-wave flattening. Get three creatine phosphokinase levels with MB fractions every 8 hours to rule out an MI. Look for electrocardiographic or scintigraphic evidence of ischemia during pain or stress testing once an MI has been ruled out (see Figure 1).

### Treatment

- **Initial treatment.** The initial treatment of angina assumes possible infarction. Therefore, the patient should receive aspirin, oxygen, beta blockers, telemetry monitoring, and possibly anticoagulation with heparin. Consider thrombolytic therapy or emergency percuta-

---

**Deadly causes of chest pain— "TAPUM"**

**T**ension pneumothorax

**A**ortic dissection

**P**ulmonary embolism

**U**nstable angina

**M**yocardial infarction

---

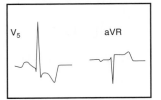

**FIGURE 1.** ST depression typical of ischemia. Note that the "ST elevation" in aVR is really depression, as it goes in the opposite direction of the QRS. Nicoll et al., *Pocket Guide to Diagnostic Tests*, Second Edition, Stamford, CT: Appleton & Lange, 1997, page 294.

neous transluminal coronary angioplasty (PTCA) if an evolving MI is apparent. The heparin and telemetry may be stopped when CK with MB fractions come back negative.

- **Risk factor modification.** The patient must quit smoking. Treat underlying hypertension, diabetes, hypercholesterolemia.
- **Medical.** Sublingual nitroglycerin, long-acting nitrates, beta blockers, and calcium-channel blockers decrease myocardial $O_2$ demand by reducing the amount of work performed by the heart.
- **Surgical.** Coronary revascularization, like coronary artery bypass grafting (CABG) and PTCA, increases oxygen delivery to the myocardium by increasing blood flow.

*$O_2$ B. blocker.*
*TELEMETRY*
*Aspirine (anticoagulant.*

---

## KEY CARDIAC DIAGNOSTIC EXAMS

### Exercise Electrocardiography

The patient is EKG monitored while exercising. Exercise often takes the form of a treadmill according to the Bruce protocol: an increase in treadmill speed and elevation every 3 minutes. You attempt to detect signs of myocardial ischemia precipitated by exercise by looking for angina, ST-segment changes on EKG, exercise intolerance, or decreased systolic blood pressure. A positive test should be further evaluated with cardiac catheterization.

### Myocardial Perfusion Scintigraphy

In order to assess myocardial perfusion, radionuclides (eg, thallium, Tc-MIBI) are injected into the blood and are preferentially taken up by the myocardium. The amount of radionuclide uptake is directly related to the amount of blood flow. Areas of diminished uptake indicate relative hypoperfusion. When combined with exercise or dipyridamole (Persantine)-induced vasodilation, coronary vessels vasodilate, giving the most blood flow to those vessels without lesions. Areas of radionuclide defect indicate hypoperfusion. These defects may fill in over time as coronary vessels return to their initial state and the relative blood flow equalizes. Defects that then fill in indicate reversible ischemia, whereas fixed defects signify areas of dead tissue (ie, post-myocardial infarction). Areas of reversible ischemia may be rescued with PTCA or CABG surgery.

### Echocardiography

A real-time ultrasound of the heart, the echocardiogram (aka "the echo") reveals ischemic or infarcted portions of the heart by the inability of that portion of the heart to move as compared to intact segments (ie, a segmental wall motion abnormality). Echo gives the additional benefit of assessing left ventricular function and estimating the ejection fraction, an important predictor of prognosis. Normal ejection fraction is around 55%.

*Handwritten margin notes:*

*READ. Intern. MED. chp*

*READ on syncope.*

*Angina = Arthrosclerosis*

*Goals:*
*d HrP finding*

**DIAGNOSTIC TESTS**

*indication for stress "stress test" - chest pain.*

*you are looking for Myocardial ischemia ST seg changes.*

*→ (+) cardiac cath*

*as you do the stress test also do myocardial perfusion test.*

*So your looking at the heart.*

*? what causing "chest pain"*

*is it ischemia not enough $O_2$*
*- perfusion study*
*- during exercise*

*Angina → Pectoris - stable = when you exert yourself.*
*→ unstable -*

Obje. of student: know about your pt. admit note labs.
go see pt, write note on pt. orders
Round

Difinitive procedure
for Coronary artery
disease

## Coronary Angiography

An invasive procedure that visualizes the coronary vasculature by injecting dye into the vessels, coronary arteriography is the definitive diagnostic procedure for CAD. Stenotic lesions in the vessels will be visualized and quantified with respect to the amount of obstruction (most lesions causing symptoms are greater than 70% stenotic) as well as their location. While this procedure gives anatomical information, it does not indicate whether any given stenosis is clinically significant; that is, a 50% stenotic lesion may be the cause of the patient's symptoms as opposed to the 70% lesion in another vessel. This procedure also gives an estimate of the ejection fraction. Catheterization is typically used to (1) confirm the presence and map the extent of CAD, and (2) define the method of revascularization (PTCA vs. CABG) if appropriate.

## UNSTABLE ANGINA

Angina is considered "unstable" if it does one of three things:

1. It is new.
2. It is accelerating—occurs with less exertion, lasts longer, or is less responsive to medications.
3. It occurs at rest.

Unstable angina is worrisome because it often signifies a stenotic lesion which has suddenly enlarged via plaque rupture, hemorrhage, or thrombosis. Such an unstable lesion may acutely progress to complete occlusion.

### Treatment

Therapy consists of admission to the hospital for aggressive management. Antianginal medications (nitrates, beta blockers, calcium-channel blockers) decrease myocardial $O_2$ demand, while aspirin and IV heparin inhibit further plaque formation (shoot for PTT = 60–90 seconds). After the patient is stable, his or her coronary vasculature should be evaluated by the diagnostic methods discussed above. If the patient cannot be made ischemia-free and still has angina despite the above measures, he or she should be considered for urgent coronary arteriography and revascularization.

## PRINZMETAL'S (VARIANT) ANGINA

Prinzmetal's angina mimics angina pectoris but is caused by vasospasm of coronary vessels (eg, clean coronary vasculature). It often affects young women and classically occurs at rest in the early morning.

### Workup

The EKG shows ST-segment elevation (not depression). The diagnosis is confirmed by coronary angiography that is free of stenotic lesions and that displays coronary vasospasm when the patient is given ergonovine.

## Treatment

Therapy consists of vasodilators (nitrates, calcium-channel blockers).

## ACUTE MYOCARDIAL INFARCTION

Myocardial infarction (MI) is usually caused by an occlusive thrombus in a coronary artery resulting in myocardial ischemia and ultimately tissue death. The area of infarct depends on the vessel occluded as well as on where the occlusion occurred along the vessel's path. The size and location of the area of infarct will determine the patient's acute clinical picture, complications, and long-term prognosis. Patients usually have a history of CAD as well as cardiac risk factors. Twenty percent present with sudden death due to a lethal arrhythmia (often ventricular fibrillation).

## Signs and Symptoms

Pain is similar to anginal pain but is much more severe, lasts for more than 30 minutes, and does not resolve with nitroglycerin. Signs that may be present include diaphoresis, "clutching chest" sign, pulmonary rales, heart failure, gallop rhythms, and mitral regurgitation secondary to papillary muscle dysfunction.

---

### CORONARY ARTERY DISTRIBUTION

- **Left anterior descending:** Supplies anterior LV, interventricular septum (see Figure 2).
- **Left circumflex:** Supplies anterolateral and posterolateral LV.
- **Right coronary:** Supplies interventricular septum, RV, posteroinferior LV, SA, and AV nodes.

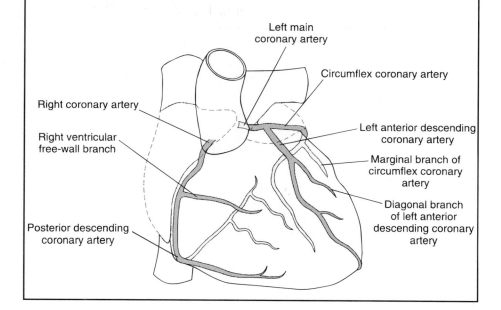

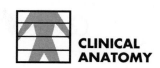

**CLINICAL ANATOMY**

*(handwritten margin notes:)*

indication for ⊕ urinary tract infection
- ⊕ nitrites.
- ⊕ ~~lympho~~ leuko. esterase
- ⊕ bacteria in urine
- ⊕ WBC.

Tx: Bactrim
Trimethoprin
sulfamethox.

Signs of MI
- diaphoresis (sweating)
- clutching chest
- pulmonary rales

**FIGURE 2.**  Coronary arteries and their principal branches. Stobo et al., *Principles and Practice of Medicine,* Twenty-third Edition, Stamford, CT: Appleton & Lange, 1996, page 17.

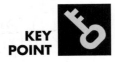

**KEY POINT**

---

### Q-WAVE VS. NON-Q-WAVE MI

A Q wave on EKG in the presence of infarction indicates that the infarction extended through the full thickness of the myocardial wall (transmural).

A non-Q-wave MI (NQWMI) involves the subendocardium, not the full thickness. NQWMIs are dangerous in the sense that the patient is still at risk for a full-thickness infarct in that area.

---

### Workup

**EKG.** EKG changes in acute myocardial infarction generally follow a specific sequence (see Figure 3):

Peaked T waves → T-wave inversion → ST-segment elevation → Q waves

EKG changes in the anterior leads (V1–V4) usually indicate an **anterior** MI, whereas changes in II, III, and aVF are consistent with an **inferior** MI.

**Cardiac enzymes.** The death of myocardium releases cardiac enzymes into the blood which can be measured (see Figure 4).

- Creatine kinase (CK) is the first of the cardiac enzymes to rise. Measure serum CKs every 8 hours for 24–48 hours to detect an elevation. It is ideal to detect an infarct in the last 2 days. This measure is of low specificity, since CK has many origins (myocardium, skeletal muscle, brain).
- CK-MB is an isozyme of CK which is very specific and sensitive to myocardium. It appears 4–6 hours post-MI, peaks at 12–24 hours,

*[Handwritten margin notes: "Qwave mi goes thru the entire wall. Non Qwave does not go thru the entire wall." "Non Qwave" "Qwave" "Ischemia enzymes releases." "Q wave." "Creatine kinase first 8hrs → 24-48hrs. 4-6 hrs → 12-24hrs."]*

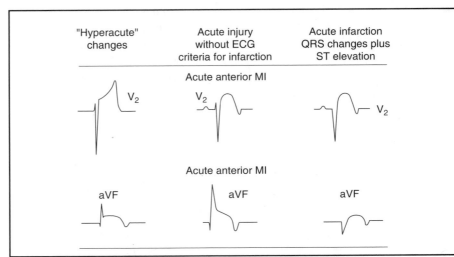

| "Hyperacute" changes | Acute injury without ECG criteria for infarction | Acute infarction QRS changes plus ST elevation |
|---|---|---|
| Acute anterior MI | | |
| V$_2$ | V$_2$ | V$_2$ |
| Acute anterior MI | | |
| aVF | aVF | aVF |

**FIGURE 3.** Classic evolution of the EKG in MI. Normal waveform is seen in lead V$_2$. Follow the EKG change from left to right. Note the elevated ST segments and peaked T waves that evolve into rounded "tombstones" with new Q waves and T-wave inversions. Nicoll et al., *Pocket Guide to Diagnostic Tests*, Second Edition, Stamford, CT: Appleton & Lange, 1997, pages 291, 296.

INTERNAL MEDICINE

**60**

and disappears over 48–72 hours. It is ideal to detect an infarct in the last 2 days.

- LDH-1 is a cardiac muscle-specific isoenzyme of the ubiquitous enzyme. It is elevated at 1–2 days, peaks at 3–6 days, and declines until day 8–14. An LDH-1/LDH-2 ratio greater than 1.0 suggests an MI. It is ideal to detect an infarct on day 3–6.
- Troponin-I and troponin-T are emerging tests that can detect infarction as early as 2–4 hours after the event.

## Treatment

Your job is to increase $O_2$ supply and to decrease $O_2$ demand of threatened myocardium. Often the patient will present early enough that the myocardium is still viable if the vessel is somehow opened; hence the rationale for thrombolytics and emergent PTCA. The best predictor of survival is LV ejection fraction.

- **Increase $O_2$ supply:** Supplemental $O_2$, emergent angioplasty vs. thrombolytics.
- **Decrease $O_2$ demand:** Bed rest, pain meds, stool softeners, beta blockers, nitrates, ACE inhibitors, and anxiolytics.
- **Thromboprophylaxis:** Prevent stenotic lesion from enlarging with aspirin and heparin.
- **Thrombolytics:** Also known as "clot busters," thrombolytics dissolve thrombotic plaque. Thrombolytics (eg, tPA and streptokinase) achieve the greatest benefit early (achieving 50% mortality reduction 1–3 hours after chest pain) but are still effective up to 10 hours after chest pain onset (10% mortality reduction). The choice of tPA vs. streptokinase remains controversial despite the GUSTO trial. Thrombolytics are indicated in patients under 80 years old, presenting within 6–12 hours of chest pain and EKG evidence of infarct (ST elevation > 1 mm in two contiguous leads). Intracerebral hemorrhage can complicate up to 1% of all cases using thrombolytics.
- **Emergent angioplasty:** Cardiologists in many academic centers now physically open up the clotted vessel with balloon angioplasty during an acute MI. The results have been shown to be as good as or better than thrombolytics. However, angioplasty is a much more costly procedure and requires a skilled interventional cardiologist as well as a catheterization lab that can be fired up quickly.

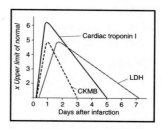

**FIGURE 4.** Myocardial enzymes. Time course of serum enzyme concentrations after a typical myocardial infarction. CK-MB = isoenzyme of CK. LDH = lactate dehydrogenase. Harvey AM et al [editors], *The Principles and Practice of Medicine*, Twenty-second Edition, Stamford, CT: Appleton & Lange, 1988.

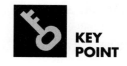

**KEY POINT**

## GO FOR THE GUSTO

GUSTO was a recent randomized trial comparing four thrombolytic strategies for acute myocardial infarction (*N Engl J Med* 1993:329, 673). This study with 41,000 patients demonstrated a modest increase in survival with accelerated tPA followed by IV heparin compared to streptokinase regimens. You'll hear a lot about this trial, so be familiar with the results.

## Complications

- **Infarct extension:** This occurs especially in those with non-Q-wave infarcts and in those treated with thrombolytics. Suspect infarct extension if you see postinfarction angina.
- **Arrhythmias (eg, V-tach, V-fib):** Most common cause of sudden death following an MI.
- **Myocardial dysfunction:** Acute CHF that may result in cardiogenic shock.

Less common complications include papillary muscle rupture, ventricular rupture, LV aneurysm, mural thrombus, and fibrinous to hemorrhagic pericarditis.

## CONGESTIVE HEART FAILURE

Congestive heart failure is an end-stage condition that leads to insufficient cardiac output (CO) as well as to congestion of the pulmonary vasculature. Insufficient CO leads to increased preload as a compensatory mechanism to increase systolic contraction (Frank-Starling relationship). Think of a rubber band—the more you stretch it, the greater the force with which it will recoil. Increased sympathetic firing, which increases preload, also increases CO by elevating the HR. However, these compensatory mechanisms are only temporarily effective and ultimately lead to hypertrophy, ventricular dilation, and increased myocardial work. In CAD, this is problematic, as the increased work (with a limited $O_2$ supply) can lead to further ischemia and, possibly, infarction.

## Etiology

Poor left ventricular systolic function (LVEF less than 40%) is usually due to inappropriate contractility, preload, afterload, or heart rate. Ischemic heart disease is the most common cause of poor systolic function.

- **Decreased contractility:** Myocardial infarction, myocardial ischemia, infiltrative processes, and alcoholic and viral myocarditis cause loss of functional myocardium.
- **Excessive preload:** Mitral or aortic valvular regurgitation.
- **Excessive afterload:** Aortic stenosis, severe HTN.
- **Inappropriate heart rate:** Tachyarrhythmias (not enough filling time), bradyarrhythmias (too slow).

Poor left ventricular diastolic function results from decreased relaxation, decreased elastic recoil, or increased stiffness of the ventricle. This leads to high filling pressures and to a small end-diastolic volume. Other causes include chronic HTN, IHSS, and cardiomyopathies.

## Signs and Symptoms

In LV failure, insufficient output and increased filling pressure cause congestion of pulmonary vasculature. Early symptoms include dyspnea on exertion and exercise intolerance. Later the patient presents with orthopnea, dyspnea

---

### CHF exacerbation

Previously stable CHF patients (on meds) who present with worsening CHF. Causes include **FAILURE.**

**F**orgot medication

**A**rrhythmia/**A**nemia

**I**schemia/**I**nfarct/ **I**nfection

**L**ifestyle (too much Na+ intake) = most common cause

**U**pregulation (increased CO) = pregnancy, hyperthyroidism

**R**enal failure → fluid overload

**E**mbolus (pulmonary)

---

ischemic heart disease most common cause of poor systolic function.

systolic dysfunction Pumping problem muscle not getting $O_2$ = dead

The most common cause of RV failure is LV failure.

ischemia → systolic problem

at rest, paroxysmal nocturnal dyspnea, chronic cough, nocturia, pulmonary congestion (rales, pleural effusion, wheezing), and an S3 gallop.

In RV failure, increased filling pressure causes congestion of systemic veins manifested by increased abdominal girth, lower-extremity pitting edema, elevated JVP, and congestive hepatomegaly.

## Workup

CBC, BUN, creatinine, and TSH can rule out severe anemia, renal failure, and thyrotoxicosis, respectively, as underlying causes. CXR may show cardiomegaly and pulmonary vascular congestion (plump vessels, interstitial or alveolar edema, Kerley-B lines). Echocardiography provides information on the size and function of both ventricles and valves and can be useful in pinpointing an underlying cause (eg, ischemia [segmental wall motion abnormalities], valvular disease). If ischemic heart disease is suspected, the patient should be ruled out for an MI, and cardiac catheterization may indicate whether cardiac bypass graft (CABG) surgery is an option.

## Treatment

Any reversible underlying cause should be addressed first. Then, the treatment goal should be to decrease the workload of the heart and increase cardiac function by:

- **Increasing contractility:** Digoxin, IV dobutamine.
- **Decreasing preload:** Nitrates, diuretics, sitting upright, morphine, salt restriction.
- **Decreasing afterload:** Hydralazine, ACE inhibitors, IV nitroprusside, oxygen.

Patients with CHF related to ischemia should strongly consider cardiac bypass surgery if appropriate, since CABG patients tend to do better than those on medical management alone.

## ATRIAL FIBRILLATION

In atrial fibrillation, chaotic atrial activity (multiple atrial pacemakers) leads to an atrial rate of 400–600 beats per minute (bpm) and to an irregularly irregular ventricular response rate of 80–160 bpm. This is the most common form of chronic arrhythmia.

## Etiologies

- Pulmonary embolism
- HTN
- CAD
- Valvular disease (rheumatic heart disease, mitral valve prolapse)
- Dilated cardiomyopathy
- Pericarditis
- Cardiothoracic surgery postoperatively
- Hyperthyroidism
- Alcohol withdrawal ("holiday heart")
- Pulmonary disease (COPD)

---

heart disease MI angina, etc can lead to CHF

Echo can tell you if valvular dz ischemia by wall motion

**CHF treatment**
**L**asix (diuretic)
**M**orphine
**N**itrates
**O**xygen
**P**ressors (dobutamine, nitroprusside)

*Atrial fib*
*· Can lead to stroke*

*LABS*
*order echocardio gram*
*to see how the valves are working*

### Signs and Symptoms

The patient may experience palpitations, dizziness, dyspnea, angina, and/or syncope. When you palpate the radial pulse, you should detect the classic irregularly irregular rhythm, usually with a rate greater than 100. Irregular heartbeats of varying loudness can be heard on cardiac auscultation.

### Differential

A number of cardiac rhythms can yield an irregular heartbeat. These include frequent paroxysmal atrial contractions, paroxysmal ventricular contractions, multifocal atrial tachycardia, and atrial flutter with variable AV conduction. These can be distinguished through careful analysis of the EKG.

### Workup  *→ shows the irreg. irreg. rythm*

The EKG will be your primary diagnostic tool. You should see a narrow complex rhythm (QRS complex less than 120 msec) with no consistent interval between the QRS complexes. There is a conspicuous absence of P waves in leads II, III, aVF, and V1–2; instead, you should see fibrillatory waves (irregular wavelets going at a rate of 300–500 in those leads) or simply a wavy baseline without distinct P waves (see Figure 5). Otherwise, the workup should be directed toward any suspected underlying etiologies.

Although most common causes of atrial fibrillation are apparent with a good H&P, you may want to send off a TSH and order an echocardiogram to assess the valves, ventricular function, and left atrium.

### Treatment

*control rate*
*∓ Cardzem*
*or diltiazem*
*which is a Ca*
*channel blocker*

**Control ventricular rate.** Rapid ventricular rate can lead to inadequate LV filling and to insufficient cardiac output. Emergent rate control with a calcium-channel blocker (diltiazem IV) or a beta blocker (metoprolol IV) is in-

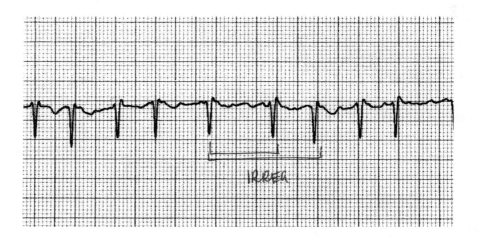

*IRREG*

**FIGURE 5.** Atrial fibrillation in V1. Note absence of P waves and irregularly irregular rhythm. Stobo et al., *Principles and Practice of Medicine*, Twenty-third Edition, Stamford, CT: Appleton & Lange, 1996, page 78.

INTERNAL MEDICINE

dicated if there is myocardial ischemia, CHF, or rapid tachycardia. Hypotension is an emergency that may require immediate DC cardioversion. Otherwise, use nonemergent rate control with digoxin (in an outpatient setting) if the patient is tolerating the arrhythmia.

**Cardiovert rhythm.** Cardioversion to sinus rhythm is the ultimate treatment goal in atrial fibrillation. Electrocardioversion (initially start with 100 J DC) is the most successful form of cardioversion. Quinidine is usually the drug of choice in chemical cardioversion. Prerequisites for success include recent onset (< 12 months) and lack of severe left atrial dilation (chamber measures < 45 mm by echocardiography). Because cardioversion can cause embolization of atrial intramural thrombi, the patient is usually anticoagulated with warfarin for 3–4 weeks before and after or receives an echocardiogram to exclude an atrial thrombus.

**Prevent embolization.** Left atrial dilation leads to blood stasis, which can form intramural thrombi that may embolize to the brain. Patients with chronic atrial fibrillation have an annual stroke risk of 4%. Cardioversion to normal sinus rhythm is the most desirable form of thromboprophylaxis. However, if cardioversion is unsuccessful or is not an option, prophylaxis with warfarin (or aspirin in younger patients) is appropriate.

## PNEUMONIA

Pneumonia is an infection of the bronchoalveolar unit that leads to inflammation and to inflammatory exudate. This is one of the "bread-and-butter" diagnoses in medicine and its causes include bacteria, viruses, atypical bacteria (eg, mycobacteria, mycoplasma), parasites, and fungi.

### Signs and Symptoms

In pneumonia the patient reports cough productive of purulent yellow or green sputum together with dyspnea, fever/chills, night sweats, and/or pleuritic chest pain. Physical exam is typically significant for areas of decreased breath sounds, dullness to percussion, increased tactile fremitus, and wheezing (Table 1).

### Workup

The standard workup for pneumonia includes CBC, electrolytes, blood cultures, ABG, sputum Gram stain and culture, and chest x-ray.

**TABLE 1.** Pulmonary diagnostic tips

|  | Pneumonia | Pleural Effusion | Pneumothorax |
|---|---|---|---|
| Breath sounds | Decreased | Decreased | Decreased |
| Abnormal sounds | Inspiratory rales | Egophony (E→A changes) | None |
| Percussion | Dull | Dull | Hyperresonant |
| Tactile fremitus | Increased | Decreased | Decreased |

*Handwritten margin notes:*

BP = slant to ↓ may cardiovert to sinus rythm

Pt is anticoagulated c̄ warfarin for 3-4 wks.

Atrial fib > 300

CARDIOVERSION c̄
- Quinidine
- Digioxin
- CARDIZEM (diltazem) (cca channel :)
- B blocker

RALES crepitus
Rhonchi : caused by air passing thru
Wheezes. inflamed bronc

↓ CBC = WBC H+H platlets

↓ Electrolytes : chem 7

Pneumonia
CBC
lytes
CXRay
↓ ABG
sputum stain C+S

- **CBC:** Typically seen are leukocytosis and left shift (immature form of WBCs present) with bands.
- **Sputum Gram stain and culture:** Identifies the pathogenic organism as well as an organism's sensitivities/resistances to antibiotics. A good sputum sample has many PMNs and few epithelial cells. Otherwise, suspect contamination by oral flora.
- **Blood culture:** If the patient appears very ill, suspect bacteremia from pneumonia.
- **ABG:** Poor oxygen saturation and acid–base disturbance characterize an ill patient.
- **CXR:** Look for lobar consolidation with patchy infiltrates (see Figure 6).

Tx for Pneumonia
antibiotic

**Alcoholic? Think anaerobes. COPD? Think *H. flu.***

### Treatment

Your initial choice of antibiotics will be directed against what you judge to be the most likely pathogens affecting your host given his or her risk factors and environmental exposures. If you want to look really smart, you can quote the American Thoracic Society (ATS) guidelines for community-acquired pneumonia. We added a fifth category for hospital acquired (nosocomial) pneumonia in Table 2. Your patient should fall into one of the five categories listed in that table. Once Gram stains, cultures, and sensitivities return, you can adjust your antibiotic coverage.

Consider hospitalization in patients older than 65 or in those with comorbidities, immunosuppression, altered mental status, aspiration, malnutrition, alcohol abuse, tachypnea, hypotension, sepsis, hypoxemia, and/or multilobar involvement.

Any patient sick enough to be admitted probably deserves IV antibiotics. However, if a patient is afebrile for greater than 24 hours, you may

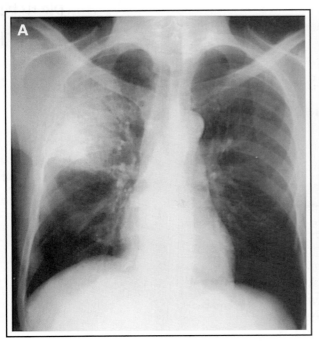
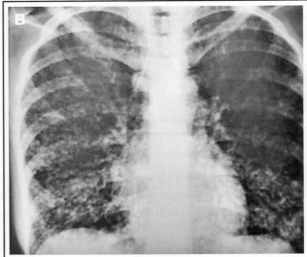

**FIGURE 6.** Typical CXRs in pneumonia. (A) Acute lobar pneumonia in RUL. (B) Interstitial (atypical) pneumonia. Stobo et al., *Principles and Practice of Medicine*, Twenty-third Edition, Stamford, CT: Appleton & Lange, 1996, page 127.

**TABLE 2.** Initial antibiotic treatment of pneumonia

| Patient Type | Suspected Pathogens | Initial Coverage |
|---|---|---|
| Outpatient community-acquired pneumonia, less than 60 years of age, otherwise healthy | *Streptococcus pneumoniae, Mycoplasma pneumoniae, Chlamydia pneumoniae, H. flu,* viral | Erythromycin, tetracycline. Consider clarithromycin or azithromycin in smokers to treat *H. flu,* viral. |
| As above except greater than 60 or with comorbidity (COPD, heart failure, renal failure, diabetes, liver disease, EtOH abuse) | *S. pneumoniae, H. flu,* aerobic gram-negative rods (GNRs—*E. coli, Enterobacter, Klebsiella), S. aureus* | Second-generation cephalosporin (cefuroxime), TMP/SMX, amoxicillin. Add erythromycin if atypicals *(Legionella, Mycoplasma, Chlamydia)* are suspected. |
| Community-acquired pneumonia requiring hospitalization | *S. pneumoniae, H. flu,* anaerobes, aerobic GNRs, *Legionella, Chlamydia* | Third-generation cephalosporin (ceftriaxone, cefoperazone). Add erythromycin if atypicals are suspected. |
| Severe community-acquired pneumonia requiring hospitalization (generally needs ICU care) | *S. pneumoniae, H. flu,* anaerobes, aerobic GNRs, *Mycoplasma, Legionella* | Erythromycin and third-generation cephalosporin (ceftriaxone, cefoperazone). |
| Nosocomial pneumonia—patient hospitalized > 48 hours | GNRs including *Pseudomonas, S. aureus, Legionella* | Third-generation cephalosporin and aminoglycoside (gentamicin). |

want to consider switching to an oral antibiotic. If the patient remains afebrile on the oral antibiotic, he or she may be able to finish the course of antibiotics (7–14 days total) as an outpatient.

While the patient is in the hospital, think about incentive spirometry, chest physical therapy, hydration, and ambulation to loosen consolidation and improve aeration.

## PLEURAL EFFUSION

Pleural effusion is defined as an abnormal accumulation of fluid in the pleural space. It is normally classified as transudative or exudative.

### Signs and Symptoms

The patient may complain of dyspnea and pleuritic chest pain but often has no symptoms. On physical exam, there may be decreased breath sounds, dullness to percussion, and decreased tactile fremitus.

### Differential

The causes of effusion can generally be categorized according to the type of pleural effusion they cause.

**Transudative effusion.** Intact capillaries lead to protein-poor pleural fluid. Common causes of pleural fluid transudates include CHF, nephrotic syndrome, cirrhosis, and protein-losing enteropathy.

**Exudative effusion.** Inflammation leads to leaky capillaries which result in protein-rich pleural fluid. Common causes of exudative pleural effusion include tuberculosis, bacterial infection (parapneumonic effusion and empyema), viral infection, neoplasm, pulmonary emboli with infarct, collagen vascular disease, pancreatitis, chylothorax, and traumatic tap.

## Workup

CXR may show blunting of the costophrenic angles. A decubitus CXR can tell you whether the fluid is free-flowing or loculated. The definitive diagnostic test is thoracocentesis (tap the pleural space for fluid). Send for CBC, differential, protein, LDH, pH, glucose, Gram stain, and possibly cytology.

|  | Transudate | Exudate |
|---|---|---|
| Pleural/serum protein | < 0.5 | > 0.5 |
| Pleural/serum LDH | < 0.6 | > 0.6 |

## Treatment

Treatment targets the underlying disorder and varies with the effusion itself.

**Transudative.** Treat the underlying condition; do a therapeutic lung tap when massive effusion leads to dyspnea.

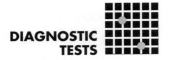

**DIAGNOSTIC TESTS**

---

**PLEURAL FLUID TIP-OFFS**

**Bloody:** Neoplasm, TB, traumatic tap, pulmonary embolus, hemothorax.

**Low glucose:** Neoplasm, TB, empyema, rheumatoid arthritis (extremely low glucose).

**Lymphocytic:** Viral infection, TB, malignancy.

**Milky (triglyceride-rich):** Chylothorax.

---

**Malignant.** In malignant effusion, the pleural surface and fluid are invaded by malignant cells from an unresectable tumor. Consider pleurodesis in symptomatic patients who are unresponsive to chemotherapy and radiation therapy. Therapeutic thoracocentesis, pleuroperitoneal shunting, and surgical pleurectomy are alternatives.

**Parapneumonic.** This is pleural effusion in the presence of pneumonia. If you suspect infected or "complicated" parapneumonic effusion, you should consider immediate drainage via a chest tube. Signs of a "complicated" effusion include puslike appearance, a positive Gram stain, low pH (< 7.1), low glucose (< 50 mg/dL), and high LDH (> 1000 IU/L).

**Hemothorax.** Place a chest tube to control bleeding by the apposition of pleural surfaces, determine the amount of blood loss, and determine the risks of infection and fibrothorax.

All parapneumonic effusions need a diagnostic tap.

## PULMONARY EMBOLISM

A pulmonary embolus is a body originating elsewhere that lodges in the pulmonary arterial vasculature, often leading to life-threatening complications such as pulmonary infarction, right heart failure, and impaired oxygenation of blood. The embolus often originates from a deep venous thrombosis above the calf.

## Signs and Symptoms

Patients often report dyspnea, chest pain, cough, anxiety, and, rarely, hemoptysis or syncope. Signs include tachycardia, tachypnea, low-grade fever, accentuated $S_2P$, evidence of DVT and, rarely, RV heave, right-sided S3, or rales.

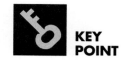

---

### VIRCHOW'S TRIAD

Risk factors for thrombus development include:

- **Blood stasis:** Immobility, CHF, surgery.
- **Venous endothelial injury:** Surgery of the pelvis/lower extremity, trauma.
- **Hypercoagulable state:** Pregnancy/postpartum, oral contraceptive use, coagulation disorder (protein C/protein S deficiency, Factor V mutation), malignancy, severe burns.

---

## Workup

Although PE is a difficult diagnosis to make because of the nonspecific signs and symptoms with which it is associated, you should have a high clinical suspicion for PE because it is life-threatening. Table 3 outlines the diagnostic tests for PE.

The PIOPED study is the classic paper that studied the use of V-Q scans and clinical suspicion in the diagnosis of PE. Data from that study have been used to develop diagnostic algorithms (Figure 8). Trust your clinical judgment. Even a patient with a low-probability V-Q scan still has a 40% chance of PE if the clinical suspicion is high.

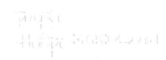

Sudden onset of dyspnea in the setting of a clear chest x-ray is suspicious for PE.

| TABLE 3. Diagnostic tests for PE | |
|---|---|
| **Test** | **Findings/Comments** |
| CXR | Usually normal. Rarely see Hampton's sign (wedge-shaped infarct) or Westermark's sign (decreased vascular markings in embolized lung zone). |
| EKG | Usually sinus tachycardia and/or nonspecific ST-T wave changes (pathognomic: SI, QIII, TIII). |
| ABG | Respiratory alkalosis (↑ pH, ↓ $pCO_2$), $pO_2$ less than 80 mm (90% sensitive). |
| V-Q scan | Segmental area(s) of mismatch in the lung (ie, well ventilated but not perfused) suggest PE (Figure 7). Results reported as normal or low/intermediate/high probability of PE: <br> • Normal result rules out PE. <br> • High probability: 85–90% incidence of PE. <br> • Low probability: does not rule out PE (14–31% incidence). |
| Pulmonary angiogram | Gold standard. However, invasive and inherently risky. |
| Doppler ultrasound | Visualize if deep venous thrombosis present in lower extremity. |

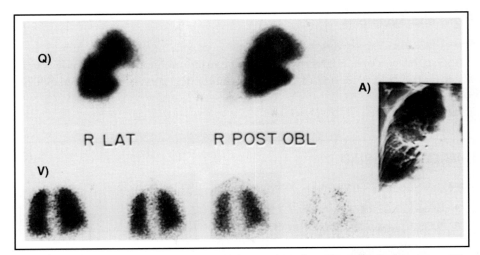

**FIGURE 7.** V-Q scan shows unmatched defects in the right midlung. The perfusion scan (Q) of the right lung (seen from the right lateral view and the right posterior oblique view) shows defects in right anterior midlung, while the ventilation scan (V) is normal. Pulmonary angiogram (A) of the right lower lobe shows an embolus to the right midlung field. Stobo et al., *Principles and Practice of Medicine,* Twenty-third Edition, Stamford, CT: Appleton & Lange, 1996, page 174.

## Treatment

The initial treatment of a PE consists of anticoagulation with heparin (for a PTT of 60–90) to prevent extension of the clot in the lung and at the source. You should start warfarin as well (INR goal of 2–3) for long-term anticoagulation. You can discharge the patient on warfarin after he or she has been stable on therapeutic levels of warfarin and heparin together for 1–2 days.

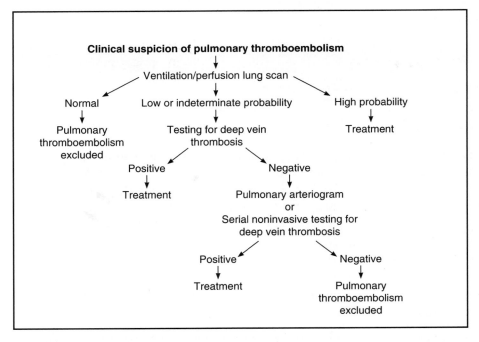

**FIGURE 8.** Diagnostic approach to pulmonary embolism. Tierney et al., *1997 Current Medical Diagnosis & Treatment,* Stamford, CT: Appleton & Lange, 1997, page 292.

Consider thrombolysis (with tPA) if the patient has a large embolus on angiogram and is hypotensive or very hypoxemic. Consider the placement of an IVC filter (aka a Greenfield filter) in large and repeated PEs to prevent future PEs originating from the legs or if anticoagulation is contraindicated. Surgical embolectomy is sometimes attempted in a crashing patient, but the procedure is usually not successful.

## PNEUMOTHORAX

Pneumothorax can have primary, secondary, or iatrogenic causes:

- **Primary:** Subpleural apical blebs (usually in thin, tall young males).
- **Secondary:** COPD, asthma, tuberculosis, trauma, *Pneumocystis* pneumonia.
- **Iatrogenic:** Thoracocentesis, subclavian central line placement, positive-pressure mechanical ventilation, bronchoscopy.

Tension pneumothorax is a deadly variant in which the defect in the chest acts like a one-way valve, drawing air into the chest during inspiration but trapping it during expiration.

### Signs and Symptoms

The patient reports pleuritic chest pain and dyspnea. Examination can reveal areas with diminished breath sounds, hyperresonance to percussion, and decreased tactile fremitus. You should suspect tension pneumothorax if you also see respiratory distress, falling $O_2$ saturation, hypotension, and tracheal deviation.

Turn the CXR on its side to help you focus on the lung parenchyma edge.

### Workup

CXR reveals a strip of blackness between the pleura and the edge of the lung parenchyma (seen best with end-expiratory film in upright position). Don't wait for the CXR if you suspect tension pneumothorax.

### Treatment

Small pneumothoraces are allowed to resolve spontaneously. Large, severely symptomatic ones are treated with a chest tube and/or pleurodesis (the injection of an irritant into the pleural cavity to scar the pleura together). A tension pneumothorax requires the immediate action of needle thoracostomy if the patient is unstable. A large-bore needle (14-gauge Angiocath) is inserted into the second or third intercostal space at the midclavicular line. A hissing sound signals the decompression of the pneumothorax. A chest tube can then be placed.

## ASTHMA

Asthma is characterized by bronchospasm, inflammation, and mucus plugging. Triggers include allergens (dust, animal hair, odors), upper respiratory infections, cold air, exertion, and stress.

**Signs of bad asthma:**
- Frequent ER visits
- History of intubation
- Corticosteroid use

*"All that wheezes is not asthma."*

Asthma
tv c̄ O₂ and albuterol

## Signs and Symptoms

The patient will complain of cough, dyspnea, wheezing, and/or chest tightness. On exam, look for tachypnea, tachycardia, and decreased $O_2$ saturation. Signs include decreased breath sounds, wheezing, hyperresonance, and accessory muscle use (intercostals, sternocleidomastoid). Lack of wheezing can result from very mild asthma or from extremely severe asthma to the point at which the patient cannot move air.

## Differential

Some of the many conditions that can mimic asthma include congestive heart failure ("cardiac asthma"), COPD, gastroesophageal reflux, PE, foreign bodies, tumors, sleep apnea, and anaphylaxis.

## Workup

- With a peak flowmeter, you can see low peak expiratory flow rates. The patient should be admitted if the peak flow is less than 60 L/min or does not improve to greater than 50% of the predicted value after 1 hour of treatment.
- An ABG commonly shows respiratory alkalosis and mild hypoxemia. A rising $PaCO_2$ can be a sign of tiring and impending respiratory failure, which may require intubation.
- Although the CXR does not usually help in the initial management of asthma, it can detect conditions associated with asthma (eg, pneumonia, atelectasis) or conditions that mimic asthma (eg, cardiac asthma with pulmonary edema and cardiomegaly).

## Treatment

The initial management of asthma includes oxygen and albuterol nebulizers (see Table 4). Patients who do not respond adequately to inhalers are given

| TABLE 4. Therapeutic management of asthma | | |
|---|---|---|
| **Treatment** | **Mechanism of Action** | **Typical Drugs** |
| Oxygen | | |
| Beta agonists | Bronchodilator | Albuterol (Proventil) |
| Steroids | Reduction of airway inflammation; potentiation of the effects of beta agonists | Methylprednisolone (Solu-medrol) IV Prednisone PO Beclomethasone inhaled |
| Xanthines | Bronchodilation, possibly anti-inflammatory effect, improved ventilatory drive and diaphragm contractility | Theophylline (Theo-Dur), aminophylline |
| Antibiotics | If underlying bronchitis suspected | TMP/SMX, cefuroxime |
| Hydration | Loosens any consolidation; presumed dehydration from illness | |

IV steroids (eg, methylprednisolone). If the patient does not require intubation, then he or she will be admitted to a regular ward bed and given oxygen, round-the-clock albuterol nebulizers, IV steroids, hydration, and pulmonary toilet.

*Admit Note*
*Admit orders*

*look up*
*theophylline*
*aminophylline*

## CHRONIC OBSTRUCTIVE PULMONARY DISEASE (COPD)

Years of cigarette smoking lead to damaged and obstructed airways. The damaged airways lead to prolonged expiration or obstructed outflow. Unlike asthma, this obstruction is minimally reversible with bronchodilators. Chronic bronchitis is a *clinical* diagnosis of excessive bronchial secretion defined by productive cough for over 3 months over a 2-year period. Emphysema is a *pathologic* diagnosis of terminal airway obstruction. The term *chronic obstructive pulmonary disease* (COPD) covers both chronic bronchitis and emphysema.

*Chronic bronchitis:*
*> 3 mo over a 2 yr*
*" Chronic cough "*
*productive*
*(flem)*

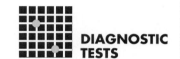

**DIAGNOSTIC TESTS**

### PULMONARY FUNCTION TEST (PFTS)

PFTs consist of spirometry, diffusion capacity for carbon monoxide (DLCO), and ABG. They are used primarily to detect the presence and to quantify the severity of obstructive and restrictive pulmonary disease (see Table 5).

- **Obstructive dysfunction:** Decreased expiratory airflow/increased air trapping in lung secondary to obstructed airways. Seen in asthma, chronic bronchitis, emphysema, and bronchiectasis.
- **Restrictive dysfunction:** Decreased lung volume. Seen in extrapulmonary (chest wall disorders, neuromuscular disease, pleural disease) and pulmonary diseases (pulmonary infiltrates and diffuse interstitial lung disease).

| **TABLE 5.** PFTs in obstructive and restrictive lung disease | | |
| --- | --- | --- |
| Measurement | Obstructive | Restrictive |
| Spirometry | | |
| $FEV_1$ | ↓ | N or ↓ |
| $FEF_{25-75}$ | ↓ | N or ↓ |
| $FEV_1/FVC$ | ↓ | N or ↓ |
| Lung volumes | | |
| FVC | N or ↓ | ↓ |
| VC | N or ↓ | ↓ |
| TLC | N or ↓ | ↓ |
| RV | ↑ | N, ↓ or ↑ |

Adapted with permission from Tierney et al., *1997 Current Medical Diagnosis & Treatment*, Stamford, CT: Appleton & Lange, 1997, page 239.

## Signs and Symptoms

Signs and symptoms of COPD include productive cough, progressive dyspnea, decreased breath sounds, rhonchi, and pursed lips with expiration. Exacerbations are characterized by acute worsening of dyspnea and are usually triggered by bronchitis (*H. flu, S. pneumoniae, Moraxella*), pneumonia, PE, and LV failure.

## Workup

CXR classically shows clear lung fields (or diminished vasculature) with flat diaphragms, hyperinflated lungs, increased AP diameter, and a thin mediastinum (see Figure 9). Peak flows are also decreased. An ABG during an acute exacerbation should show hypoxemia with an acute respiratory acidosis (increased $pCO_2$). You should get blood and sputum cultures if there is a fever or increased sputum production.

## Treatment

The management of COPD is very similar to that of asthma. Patients are treated with oxygen (carefully, see below), nebulized beta agonists like albuterol, IV steroids, anticholinergic agents like ipratropium bromide, hydration, and antibiotics (eg, TMP/SMX, cefuroxime) if bronchitis is suspected. When the patient is stabilized, consider pulmonary function testing to assess the severity of the COPD. At discharge, also consider the following: smoking cessation, flu and pneumococcal vaccines, home oxygen therapy if the patient's rest $pO_2$ is less than 55 mm or $O_2$ saturation less than 88%, and alpha$_1$-antitrypsin therapy in patients with alpha$_1$-antitrypsin deficiency.

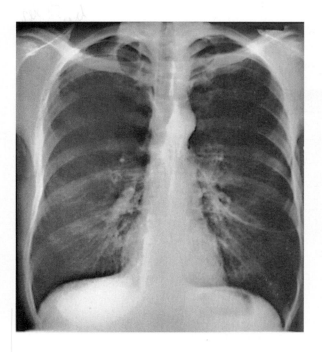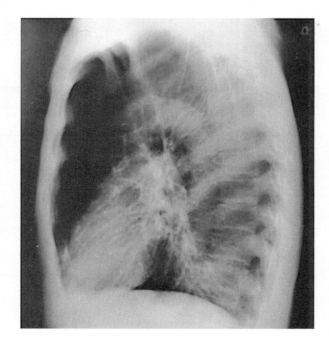

**FIGURE 9.** CXR with COPD. Note the hyperinflated and hyperlucent lungs, flat diaphragm, increased AP diameter, and narrow mediastinum. Stobo et al., *Principles and Practice of Medicine*, Twenty-third Edition, Stamford, CT: Appleton & Lange, 1996, page 135.

## Complications

- **Chronic respiratory failure:** Chronic hypoxemia with a compensated respiratory acidosis (high $pCO_2$). Beware of "$CO_2$ retainers" who occasionally do **worse** with supplemental $O_2$ because they lose their hypoxemic drive to hyperventilate and acutely increase their $pCO_2$.
- **Destruction of pulmonary vasculature:** Leads to pulmonary hypertension, resulting in right heart failure (cor pulmonale).

## BRONCHOGENIC CARCINOMA

Lung cancer is the most common cause of cancer death in the U.S. Most cases present between the ages of 50 and 70. To no one's surprise (except the

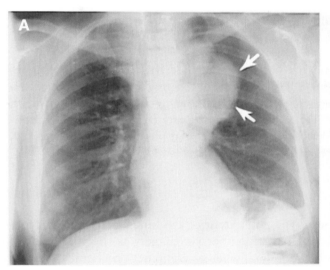

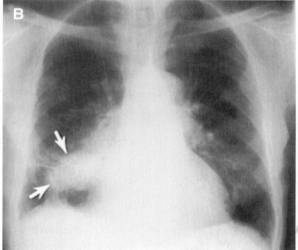

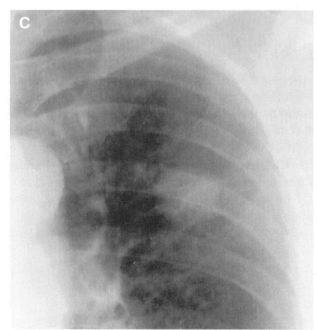

**FIGURE 10.** CXRs in lung cancer. (A) Small-cell cancer in the left hilum. Note the left hemidiaphragm paralysis secondary to phrenic nerve involvement. (B) Squamous cell cancer in the right lower lobe. (C) Adenocarcinoma in the left upper lobe. Stobo et al., *Principles and Practice of Medicine*, Twenty-third Edition, Stamford, CT: Appleton & Lange, 1996, page 180.

tobacco companies), smoking is the most important cause of lung cancer in both men and women in the U.S.

### Signs and Symptoms

Patients often present with cough, dyspnea, hemoptysis, anorexia, and/or weight loss. Only 10–25% of patients are asymptomatic at the time of diagnosis. Physical examination is often unremarkable. You may hear decreased breath sounds and increased fremitus with postobstructive pneumonitis and pleural effusion. Keep an eye out for the more striking clinical complications, such as superior vena cava syndrome, Horner's syndrome, Pancoast tumor, and paraneoplastic syndromes.

### Workup

Initial blood work should include a CBC with differential, electrolytes, LFTs, and serum calcium. CXR may show hilar and peripheral masses, atelectasis, infiltrates, or pleural effusion (see Figure 10). A CT scan (or MRI) of the chest can better characterize involvement of the parenchyma, pleura, and mediastinum.

A histologic diagnosis is important because the treatment approaches for small cell and non–small cell lung carcinoma are different. Sputum cytology is easy to do and highly specific for malignancy but is not very sensitive. If the sputum is negative, a biopsy sample can be obtained from bronchoscopy, lymph node biopsy, thoracocentesis (if pleural fluids are present), mediastinoscopy, sites of metastases, or thoracotomy.

### Treatment

Treatment depends on the type and extent of the lung cancer and includes surgery, chemotherapy, and radiation therapy. Surgery is the treatment of choice in non–small cell carcinoma, whereas combination chemotherapy is preferred in small cell carcinoma.

## GASTROINTESTINAL BLEEDING

Patients with GI bleeding often have a history of PUD, prior GI bleeds, NSAID use, EtOH use, liver disease, varices, severe vomiting/retching, anticoagulant use, bleeding disorder, or steroid use. GI bleeding is usually classified as upper or lower GI (UGI and LGI) bleeding; classification is dependent on whether the suspected source is proximal or distal to the ligament of Treitz. Common causes of UGI bleeds include PUD, esophageal varices, Mallory-Weiss tears from retching, erosive gastritis, vascular ectasias/AVMs, and gastric cancer. In LGI bleeds think about hemorrhoids, diverticulosis, vascular ectasias, inflammatory bowel disease, ischemic colitis, and malignancy.

### Signs and Symptoms

Hematemesis and melena support a UGI source, whereas hematochezia is usually (but not always) secondary to an LGI source. If bleeding is severe,

- **Hematemesis:** vomiting bright red blood or coffee-ground emesis
- **Hematochezia:** bright red blood per rectum (BRBPR)
- **Melena:** black, tarry stool

the patient may also complain of dizziness and weakness and may exhibit signs of hypovolemia and shock. On physical exam, look for pallor, tachycardia, orthostatic hypotension or frank hypotension, heme-positive stool, melena, and/or hematochezia.

## Workup

The initial workup consists of merely evaluating volume status and vital signs as described above. Orthostatic vital sign changes indicate significant volume loss and usually requires ICU monitoring. A systolic blood pressure less than 90 mmHg signifies shock. The rest of the workup occurs while treating the patient.

## Treatment

The management of GI bleeding is as easy as "**ABCDE.**"

**"ABCs" for stabilize and resuscitate if necessary**. In someone with a significant bleed, IV access is essential. Start normal saline (NS) through two large-bore IVs. Send for stat CBC and coagulation studies and cross-match for 4 units of blood. The degree of transfusion and hydration should be based on vital signs, HCT, and signs of continued bleeding. Drop a nasogastric tube in all cases of UGI and severe LGI bleeding. A bloody lavage that does not clear with 2–3 L of cold NS may necessitate emergent upper endoscopy. If only bilious fluid is aspirated, you probably have an LGI source only. Most cases of GI bleeding resolve spontaneously. A patient requiring more than 5 units of blood should have a surgical consult.

**"D" for define source**. The source should be designated as upper or lower. All UGI bleeds, when stabilized, get an upper endoscopy. If the bleeding is continuous, the patient may need angiography and embolization to locate and control the bleeder. LGI bleeds need anoscopy and sigmoidoscopy for small bleeds in young, healthy patients; otherwise, the patient receives colonoscopy. Continued significant LGI bleeding can be evaluated by angiography or nuclear bleeding scans.

**"E" for eliminate source**. Any aspirin or NSAID use should be discontinued and the patient should be started on an IV H$_2$ blocker. UGI bleeds are usually treated with endoscopy. Varices can be sclerosed and rubber-banded. Ulcers, angiomas, and Mallory-Weiss tears can be cauterized, sclerosed, or injected with epinephrine. Vasopressin and octreotide can be used in severe variceal bleeding. In more complicated and/or severe cases, embolization by angiography or emergent surgery are options. LGI bleeds may be treated with colonoscopic cauterization, intraarterial vasopressin or embolization by angiography, or surgery.

## PEPTIC ULCER DISEASE

Peptic ulcer disease is a break that occurs in the gastric or duodenal mucosa when damaging mechanisms (eg, acid) to the gastric mucosa outweigh protective mechanisms (eg, mucus and bicarbonate) (see Figure 11). Duodenal ulcers are five times more common than gastric ulcers. The three major causes of peptic ulcer disease are NSAID use, chronic *H. pylori* infection, and acid hypersecretory states such as Zollinger-Ellinger syndrome.

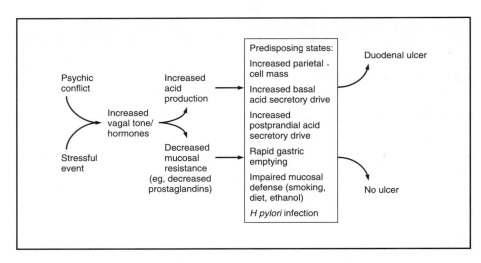

**FIGURE 11.** Pathophysiology of peptic ulcer disease. McPhee et al., *Pathophysiology of Disease*, Stamford, CT: Appleton & Lange, 1995, page 234.

## Signs and Symptoms

Patients with PUD usually present with a periodic chronic, burning epigastric pain. The pain is often temporarily alleviated with eating and antacids (especially with duodenal ulcers) but usually recurs about 3 hours later. Pain from gastric ulcers can worsen with food. Less common symptoms of peptic ulcer disease include nausea/vomiting, early satiety, and a positive guaiac test for fecal occult blood loss.

## Differential

Other GI disorders such as GERD, chronic cholecystitis, and biliary tract disease can all cause dyspepsia. Severe epigastric pain is consistent with PUD complicated by perforation or penetration but can also be caused by acute pancreatitis, acute cholecystitis, choledocholithiasis, esophageal rupture, ureteral colic, ruptured aortic aneurysm, angina, or acute MI.

## Workup

Lab work may reveal microcytic anemia consistent with iron deficiency anemia. The definitive diagnosis of peptic ulcer disease is made with endoscopy and concurrent biopsy of the lesion to determine the presence of malignancy or *H. pylori* infection. *H. pylori* can also be detected by serologic testing and breath tests. A barium upper GI series can also be used to diagnose peptic ulcer disease. A gastrin level can rule out Zollinger-Ellison syndrome.

## Treatment

Treatment of the ulcer focuses on keeping the stomach pH greater than 3.5 with the use of antacids, H$_2$ blockers, and omeprazole. In addition, concurrent antibiotic treatment for *H. pylori* infection has proven to be extremely beneficial in preventing recurrence of peptic ulcers (see Table 6). Gastric ulcers are associated with an increased risk of gastric carcinoma and thus should be biopsied.

PUD **perforates** into the peritoneal space and **penetrates** into adjacent organs.

*ulcer is due to acid build up in the stomach*

| TABLE 6. Treatment of *H. pylori* infection | |
|---|---|
| **Treatment Regimen** | **Comments** |
| Metronidazole (or amoxicillin), tetracycline, bismuth for 2 weeks | First-line "triple therapy." |
| Clarithromycin, tetracycline, bismuth for 2 weeks | Useful in patients with prior exposure to metronidazole. |
| Clarithromycin, omeprazole for 2 weeks | More expensive and slightly less effective than "triple therapy," but may yield higher compliance and fewer side effects. |

## Complications

Complications of peptic ulcer disease include hemorrhage (erosion into the gastroduodenal artery), gastric outlet obstruction, perforation, and penetration.

## INFLAMMATORY BOWEL DISEASE

Chronic inflammatory bowel disease (IBD) includes ulcerative colitis and Crohn's disease. Table 7 compares the two entities side by side. It is usually difficult to differentiate between ulcerative colitis and Crohn's disease on initial presentation.

## ACUTE PANCREATITIS

Acute pancreatitis commonly results from alcohol abuse or passed gallstones. Other causes include hypercalcemia, hyperlipidemia, and drugs (such as sulfonamides and thiazides).

## Signs and Symptoms

Acute pancreatitis is characterized by sudden onset of deep epigastric pain, often radiating to the back, with nausea, vomiting, sweating, and weakness. The patient may be febrile, tachycardic, and/or hypotensive. The skin is often cool, pale, clammy, and/or jaundiced. There is severe epigastric pain and tenderness, typically without guarding and rebound (as in appendicitis).

## Differential

Perforated duodenal ulcer, acute cholecystitis, acute intestinal obstruction, leaking aortic aneurysm, renal colic, and ischemic colitis should be kept in mind.

## Workup

You may see an elevated white count, BUN, glucose, LDH, bilirubin, AST, alkaline phosphatase, amylase, and/or lipase. Serum calcium may be low, and the hematocrit may drop later on. The laboratory criteria have been incorporated into the infamous Ranson's criteria, which are used to assess prognosis. The mortality rate correlates with the number of Ranson's criteria (three or more is

**Ranson's criteria** *the likelihood of death — Ranson's criteria*

**At presentation—BAG the LAW**

**B**ase deficit > 4 mEq/L

**A**ge > 55 years

**G**lucose > 200 mg/dL

**L**DH > 350 IU/L

**A**ST > 250 IU/L

**W**BC > 16,000/mm³

**After 48 hours—BACH in F major**

**B**UN rise > 5 mg/dL

**A**rterial pO₂ < 60 mmHg

**C**alcium < 8 mg/dL

**H**CT drop > 10 points

**F**luid sequestration > 6 L

**Sentinel loop:**
A segment of air-filled small intestine most commonly seen in the left upper quadrant.

**TABLE 7.** Classic comparison of ulcerative colitis and Crohn's disease

| | Ulcerative Colitis | Crohn's Disease |
|---|---|---|
| Site of involvement | The rectum is always involved. May extend proximally in a continuous fashion to involve some or all of the colon. Inflammation and ulceration are limited to the mucosa and submucosa. | May involve any portion of the GI tract, usually the ileocecal region in a discontinuous pattern. The rectum is often spared. Inflammation is transmural. |
| Symptoms and signs | Bloody diarrhea, lower abdominal cramps, and urgency. Exam may reveal orthostatic hypotension, tachycardia, abdominal tenderness, frank blood on rectal exam, and extraintestinal manifestations (see below). | Abdominal pain, abdominal mass, low-grade fever, weight loss, watery diarrhea. Exam may reveal fever, abdominal tenderness or mass, fistulas, and extraintestinal manifestations (see below). |
| Extraintestinal manifestations | Aphthous stomatitis, episcleritis/uveitis, ankylosing spondylitis, sclerosing cholangitis, thromboembolic events, erythema nodosum, and pyoderma gangrenosum. | In addition, you may see nephrolithiasis and fistulas to the skin, biliary tract, or urinary tract or between bowel loops. |
| Differential | Crohn's disease, infectious colitis (ie, bacterial, amebic, *C. difficile*), ischemic colitis, proctitis secondary to radiation therapy or STDs. | Ulcerative colitis, ischemic colitis, irritable bowel syndrome, appendicitis, intestinal lymphoma, diverticulitis. |
| Workup | Severe disease characterized by anemia, elevated ESR, and low albumin. Send stool cultures, ova and parasites, and stool assay for *C. difficile*. Sigmoidoscopy shows diffuse and continuous rectal involvement, friability, edema, pseudopolyps. Plain abdominal x-rays rule out toxic megacolon. | Crohn's has the same laboratory workup as colitis. Colonoscopy may show aphthoid, linear, or stellate ulcers, strictures, "cobblestoning" and "skip" lesions. Noncaseating granulomas are seen on biopsy. A barium UGI series with small bowel follow-through typically shows ulcerations, strictures, and fistulas. |
| Treatment | Sulfasalazine, 5-aminosalicylate (mesalamine), corticosteroids, immunosuppression. With fulminant disease and toxic megacolon, consider NG suction, broad-spectrum antibiotics, steroids, rehydration. Total colectomy is curative. | Sulfasalazine, corticosteroids, metronidazole, TPN with bowel rest, immunosuppression. Ileectomy, but Crohn's disease may recur elsewhere in GI tract. |
| Incidence of cancer | Markedly increased risk of colon cancer in longstanding cases. | Incidence of secondary malignancy is present but is much lower than in ulcerative colitis. |

bad news). Abdominal films may show gallstones, a "sentinel loop," and the "colon cutoff sign." An abdominal ultrasound can evaluate gallbladder and biliary tract disease. An abdominal CT scan may show an enlarged pancreas with pseudocysts.

**Lore has it that meperidine causes less sphincter of Oddi spasm than morphine.**

### Treatment

Because acute pancreatitis usually resolves on its own, initial treatment is usually supportive, consisting of NPO (nothing by mouth), IV hydration, and pain control with meperidine. As pain resolves, the patient's diet is slowly advanced. In severe pancreatitis, volume loss and/or shock must be aggressively treated with normal saline, blood transfusion, and pressor drugs. A surgeon should be consulted. Consider antibiotics if cholecystitis or cholangitis is also present.

### Complications

The complications of acute pancreatitis can develop quickly and can include renal failure, shock, pancreatic necrosis with possible infection, ARDS, pancreatic abscess, pseudocysts, and chronic pancreatitis.

## PULMONARY TUBERCULOSIS

After years of decline, TB is making a big comeback. This reversal has been blamed on the explosion of AIDS in the 1980s as well as on immigration, urban crowding, and fewer dollars for TB monitoring and control. Most cases of active TB are due to reactivation rather than to primary disease. Risk factors for tuberculosis include immunosuppression (eg, HIV), alcoholism, pre-existing lung disease (eg, silicosis), diabetes, old age, homelessness, malnourishment, and crowded living conditions with poor ventilation (eg, military barracks). Immigrants from third-world nations and persons with known exposure to infected patients are also at risk.

### Signs and Symptoms

Signs and symptoms of active pulmonary tuberculosis include cough productive of purulent sputum, weakness, weight loss, malaise, anorexia, night sweats, fever, and hemoptysis. Symptoms of tuberculosis can resemble bacterial pneumonia. Tuberculosis is a common cause of fever of unknown origin (FUO—see below). The kidney is the most common extrapulmonary site of tuberculosis infection.

### Workup

Most cases of tuberculosis are presumptively diagnosed with a positive acid-fast stain of the sputum, since it may take several weeks to culture TB from sputum owing to its slow incubation period. Chest x-ray findings in active pulmonary tuberculosis include enlarged, calcified intrathoracic lymph nodes and calcified pulmonary granulomas (Ghon complex) in the apical and posterior areas of the upper lobes of the lungs bilaterally. A positive PPD test is indicative only of previous exposure to *Mycobacterium tuberculosis* and may not be present in immunocompromised individuals (eg, HIV-infected patients) who have tuberculosis.

### Treatment

The first step in the treatment of TB involves respiratory isolation. Once the patient has been presumptively diagnosed as having tuberculosis via a positive sputum AFB smear, the patient is started on multidrug therapy (usually isoniazid, pyrazinamide, rifampin, and ethambutol or streptomycin) to prevent acquired drug resistance. Vitamin $B_6$ (pyridoxine) is commonly given with isoniazid to prevent the common side effect of peripheral neuritis. The treatment for patients under 35 years of age who show conversion to a positive PPD but who have no symptoms of active pulmonary tuberculosis is prophylactic isoniazid therapy for 9 months.

### HIV

Since HIV infection is spread almost exclusively through the transmission of bodily fluids, risk factors for HIV infection include unprotected anal and vaginal sex, oral sex, and needle sharing. Infants of HIV-positive mothers, health-care workers accidentally stuck with a needle containing blood from an HIV-positive patient (also mucocutaneous exposure), and patients receiving multiple transfusions of blood and blood products are also at risk.

TB is the number one infectious disease killer in the world.

## Signs and Symptoms

Although many HIV-infected patients are initially asymptomatic, they may present with flu-like symptoms during acute seroconversion—eg, malaise, fever, and generalized lymphadenopathy. Later stages of HIV may present with night sweats, weight loss, and cachexia in addition to the symptoms listed above. Advanced stages of HIV infection are characterized by the presence of opportunistic infections such as esophageal candidiasis, hairy leukoplakia, HIV wasting syndrome, chronic diarrhea caused by *Cryptosporidium*, PCP, and *Mycobacterium avium-intracellulare* (MAI) tuberculosis.

## Workup

The HIV test is an ELISA test that detects the presence of anti-HIV antibodies in the bloodstream. The ELISA test has a high sensitivity but a lower specificity; thus, a small number of people can have a positive ELISA test but not be infected with HIV. Anyone who has a positive ELISA test must therefore undergo a Western blot test for the presence of anti-HIV antibodies. The Western blot test has a high specificity, making it the confirmatory test for HIV infection. If both the ELISA and Western blot are positive, then check a viral load (ie, the number of viral RNA copies/mL of blood) CD4 count, PPD with controls, VDRL, CMV antigen, and toxoplasmosis Ab.

## Treatment

The treatment of HIV-positive patients depends primarily on the patient's CD4 count, the viral load (the number of viral RNA copies/mL), and the presence of AIDS-defining complications. Treatment regimens for HIV are evolving rapidly. Currently, you may place an asymptomatic patient on two nucleoside analogs (eg, AZT, ddI, 3TC, D4T). If there is progression of disease such as falling CD4 counts, rising viral loads, or presentation of opportunistic infections, many physicians would add a protease inhibitor (eg, saquinavir, ritonavir, indinavir, nelfinivir).

In addition, prophylactic trimethoprim-sulfamethoxazole therapy is started in patients with CD4 counts of less than 200 for prevention of PCP. Clarithromycin or azithromycin is given for MAI prophylaxis in patients with CD4 counts less than 75. Opportunistic diseases are treated as they arise (see Table 8).

## FEVER OF UNKNOWN ORIGIN (FUO)

FUO is one of the more vexing dilemmas in internal medicine. It is defined as a fever of greater than 38.3°C that has been present for at least three weeks' duration and is undiagnosed after 1 week of study in the hospital.

## Etiology

In adults, infections and cancer account for over 60% of cases of FUO, while autoimmune diseases account for approximately 15% of FUOs.

FUO can be divided into 5 etiologic categories:

- **Infectious:** Tuberculosis and endocarditis are the most common systemic infections causing FUO, while an occult abscess is the most common localized infection causing FUO.

| TABLE 8. Opportunistic diseases in AIDS | |
|---|---|
| **Disease** | **Treatment Options** |
| CMV | Ganciclovir, foscarnet |
| Esophageal candidiasis | Fluconazole, ketoconazole |
| Cryptococcal meningitis | Amphotericin B, fluconazole |
| HSV | Acyclovir, foscarnet |
| Herpes zoster | Acyclovir, foscarnet |
| Kaposi's sarcoma | Cutaneous—observation, intralesional vinblastine<br>Severe cutaneous—systemic chemotherapy, alpha-interferon, radiation<br>Visceral disease—combination chemotherapy |
| Lymphoma | Combination chemotherapy, radiation therapy with dexamethasone (in CNS lymphoma) |
| *Mycobacterium avium-intracellulare* | Clarithromycin, ethambutol, clofazimine, rifabutin |
| *Mycobacterium tuberculosis* | See above |
| *Pneumocystis carinii* (PCP) | Trimethoprim-sulfamethoxazole, trimethoprim-dapsone, pentamidine, atovaquone, clindamycin, prednisone |
| Toxoplasmosis | Pyrimethamine, sulfadiazine, clindamycin |

- **Neoplastic:** Leukemias and lymphomas are the most common cancers that cause FUO.
- **Autoimmune:** Still's disease, SLE, rheumatoid arthritis, and polyarteritis nodosa are the most common causes.
- **Miscellaneous:** This category includes drug fever, temporal arteritis, sarcoidosis, Whipple's disease, recurrent pulmonary emboli, alcoholic hepatitis, factitious fever, and inflammatory bowel disease.
- **Undiagnosed** (10–15%).

## Workup

Workup of FUO should initially include CBC with differential, ESR, and multiple blood cultures. Depending on the clinical presentation, imaging studies may include CXR, sinus CT, upper GI series with small bowel follow-through, barium enema, proctosigmoidoscopy, gallbladder study, and abdominal and pelvic CT. Gallium scan is limited by a high rate of false positives. Antibody titers can be done if an infectious or autoimmune cause is suspected. The key to making a diagnosis is a detailed history and repeated physical examinations and tests.

## Treatment

Empiric broad-spectrum antibiotics are a reasonable treatment choice but should be discontinued if the fever does not respond. Avoid empiric steroids.

| TABLE 9. Causes of acute renal failure | | |
|---|---|---|
| **Prerenal** | **Renal (Intrinsic)** | **Postrenal** |
| Dehydration | Prolonged renal ischemia | Prostate disease |
| Acute blood loss | Acute glomerulonephritis | Kidney stones |
| Extensive burns with plasma loss | Nephrotoxic drugs (eg, NSAIDs, | Pelvic tumors |
| Low cardiac output | aminoglycosides) | Recent pelvic |
| Fluid retention with heart disease | Thromboembolism | surgery |
| | Hypercoagulable state | |

Adapted with permission from Stobo et al., *Principles and Practice of Medicine*, Twenty-third Edition, Stamford, CT: Appleton & Lange, 1996, page 383.

## ACUTE RENAL FAILURE

Acute renal failure is an abrupt decrease in renal function leading to the retention of creatinine and BUN. Learn this disease well because (1) the clinical manifestations are often nonspecific, (2) it can become rapidly fatal, and (3) it can usually be reversed if recognized early and managed properly.

### Etiology

Acute renal failure is conveniently classified as prerenal, intrinsic, or postrenal. Prerenal failure is caused by decreased renal plasma flow and decreased GFR. In intrinsic renal failure, the site of injury is within the nephron unit. Postrenal failure can result from anything that obstructs urinary outflow from the kidney (see Table 9).

### Signs and Symptoms

Patients may complain of malaise, anorexia, and nausea secondary to uremia. Physical examination may reveal a pericardial friction rub, asterixis, or hypertension. Hypovolemia suggests prerenal failure, whereas hypervolemia is consistent with renal or postrenal failure. Other signs and symptoms reflect the underlying cause (see Table 10).

| TABLE 10. Physical exam findings in acute renal failure | | |
|---|---|---|
| **Prerenal** | **Renal (Intrinsic)** | **Postrenal** |
| Weight loss, or weight gain in heart disease | Weight gain | Enlarged prostate |
| | Obtundation | Weight gain |
| Poor skin turgor | Hypotension changing to | Bladder distention |
| Orthostatic changes | hypertension | Pelvic mass |
| Ascites or edema | Increased jugular venous distention and pulmonary congestion | |
| | Muscle trauma and ischemia | |
| | Infected IV and arterial lines and surgical wounds | |

Stobo et al., *Principles and Practice of Medicine*, Twenty-third Edition, Stamford, CT: Appleton & Lange, 1996, page 383.

**TABLE 11.** A cast of casts

| Urine Sediment (UA) | Etiology |
|---|---|
| Hyaline casts | Prerenal |
| Red cell casts, red cells | Glomerulonephritis (intrinsic) |
| White cells, white cell casts, +/- eosinophils | Allergic tubulointerstitial nephritis (intrinsic) |
| Granular casts, renal tubular cells | Acute tubular necrosis (intrinsic) |

## Workup

Key labs include urinalysis (UA), serum electrolytes, urine electrolytes, and urine osmolality. Significant proteinuria suggests intrinsic renal failure. Cells and casts seen on urinalysis are useful in categorizing the etiology (see Table 11). Urine electrolytes are also useful in differentiating prerenal and intrinsic renal failure (Table 12). Renal ultrasound is useful in ruling out obstruction as evidenced by a dilated ureter and enlarged kidneys. Foley placement with postvoid residual measurement also helps rule out an obstructive etiology and facilitates easy tracking of urine output.

## Treatment

Initial treatment consists of loop diuretics, IV hydration, treatment of the underlying cause, and alkalinization of the urine. If acute renal failure persists or worsens despite initial measures, you must consider hemodialysis or peritoneal dialysis.

## GLOMERULONEPHRITIS

Glomerulonephritis can be defined as inflammation of the glomerulus, although the renal vasculature, interstitium, and tubular epithelium may also be involved. Glomerulonephritis usually presents as nephrotic or nephritic disease.

**Nephrotic syndrome** is characterized by severe proteinuria (> 3.5 g protein in the urine per 24-hour period), edema, hypoalbuminemia, and hyperlipid-

**TABLE 12.** Urine indices in prerenal and renal failure

| Index | Prerenal | Renal |
|---|---|---|
| BUN/Cr ratio | > 20 | 10–20 |
| Urine Na+ (mEq/L) | < 20 | > 40 |
| FE$_{Na}$* | < 1% | > 1% |
| Urine osmolality (mOsm/kg) | > 500 | < 350 |
| Urine specific gravity | > 1.040 | 1.010–1.016 |

*Memorize the calculation of FE$_{Na}$:

$$FE_{Na} = \frac{U_{Na} / P_{Na}}{U_{Cr} / P_{Cr}}$$

emia. Diseases typically presenting this way include minimal change disease, focal and segmental glomerulosclerosis, membranous glomerulonephritis, and membranoproliferative glomerulonephritis.

**Nephritic syndrome** is characterized by hypertension, edema, moderate proteinuria, and smoky-colored urine with the presence of red blood cell casts. Typical causes of nephritic syndrome include poststreptococcal glomerulonephritis, IgA nephropathy (Berger's disease and Henoch-Schönlein purpura), and rapidly progressive glomerulonephritis (RPGN).

### Sign and Symptoms

The clinical findings in glomerulonephritis are nonspecific, but edema is more consistent with nephrotic syndrome.

### Workup

Urinalysis with microscopic examination of the urine is usually significant for hematuria, proteinuria, and the presence of red cells, white cells, and red cell casts. A 24-hour urine collection for total protein excretion and creatinine clearance can establish the presence of nephrotic syndrome as well as the degree of renal failure. A low serum albumin and hypercholesterolemia are also suggestive of nephrotic syndrome. In addition, light and electron microscope histologic findings from renal biopsy can be used to diagnose renal disease.

### Treatment

In general, corticosteroid therapy with a high-protein, low-salt diet is used to treat most acute causes of nephrotic syndrome. Minimal change disease is usually self-limited and has an excellent prognosis. Treatment for other types of nephrotic and nephritic syndromes consist of treating the underlying cause (eg, corticosteroids for SLE nephropathy).

### DIABETES MELLITUS

Although diabetes mellitus (DM) is occasionally diagnosed on admission when it presents as diabetic ketoacidosis or nonketotic hyperglycemic hyperosmolar coma, you will see DM most often as a chronic medical issue in your patients. DM is a metabolic syndrome of abnormal hyperglycemia secondary to an absence of insulin and/or to an abnormality in insulin secretion and can be classified as two types.

**Type I.** Also known as insulin-dependent diabetes mellitus (IDDM), type I diabetes is most commonly diagnosed in juveniles and is characterized by a lack of insulin, thus requiring exogenous insulin. There is a strong association with HLA-DR3 or HLA-DR4 in type I diabetes.

**Type II.** Also known as non-insulin-dependent diabetes mellitus (NIDDM), type II diabetes usually occurs in obese patients over the age of 40. Most type II diabetes is due to insulin resistance.

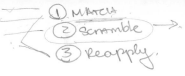

## Signs and Symptoms

The common presenting symptoms of type I and symptomatic type II diabetes mellitus include polydipsia, polyuria (including nocturia), and polyphagia. Type I diabetes is also commonly associated with rapid weight loss.

## Differential

Aside from spontaneous diabetes mellitus, other causes of hyperglycemia include pancreatic diseases (eg, chronic pancreatitis, hemachromatosis), hormonal abnormalities (eg, glucagonoma, Cushing's syndrome), medications (eg, corticosteroids, thiazide diuretics, phenytoin), and gestational diabetes.

## Workup

The National Diabetes Data Group (NDDG) and the World Health Organization (WHO) Criteria for the Clinical Diagnosis of Diabetes Mellitus suggest that a patient meet one of the three following criteria to be diagnosed with diabetes:

1. **A random plasma glucose** level greater than 200 mg/dL together with the presence of the classic symptoms of diabetes (eg, polydipsia, polyuria, weight loss), or
2. **A fasting plasma glucose** level of greater than 125 mg/dL, or
3. **An oral glucose tolerance test** (OGTT) (oral dose of 75 g glucose) showing a 2-hour postprandial plasma glucose level of greater than 200 mg/dL.

An elevated **hemoglobin A1C** (glycosylated hemoglobin) and the presence of urine glucose and urine ketones also support the diagnosis of diabetes.

## Treatment

Patients with type I diabetes mellitus require exogenous insulin to maintain blood glucose levels and to prevent diabetic ketoacidosis. Since obesity commonly results from and contributes to insulin resistance, patients with type II diabetes mellitus should initially be treated with a weight loss and exercise regimen, which may increase insulin sensitivity in the target tissues. If this fails to lower blood glucose levels, patients with type II diabetes mellitus should be given oral hypoglycemic agents (eg, glipizide, glyburide, metformin), which can stimulate the β-islet cells of the pancreas to produce insulin. If the patient's blood glucose levels remain high despite oral hypoglycemic therapy, exogenous insulin is required (see Figure 12).

## Complications

Acute complications in patients with type I diabetes include diabetic ketoacidosis (DKA), which may be precipitated by infections, myocardial in-

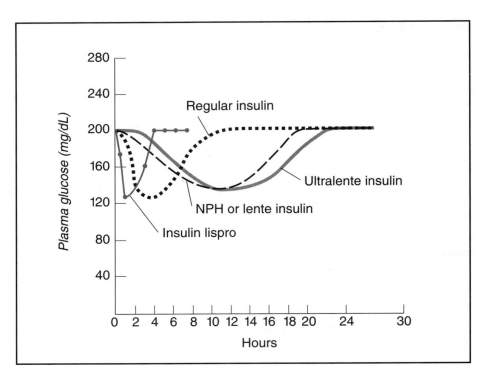

**FIGURE 12.** Effects of various insulins in a fasting diabetic patient. Tierney et al., *Current Medical Diagnosis & Treatment*, Stamford, CT: Appleton & Lange, 1997, page 1083.

farctions, alcohol, certain medications (eg, corticosteroids, thiazide diuretics), pancreatitis, and noncompliance with insulin therapy. Patients with DKA typically present with abdominal pain, vomiting, Kussmaul respirations (increased tidal volume), and a fruity, acetone odor. These patients are severely dehydrated with many electrolyte abnormalities (eg, hypokalemia, hyperglycemia, increased anion gap metabolic acidosis) and can develop mental status changes as a result. Since patients with type II diabetes mellitus have endogenous levels of insulin present, they are less prone to developing DKA. Acute complications in patients with type II diabetes mellitus include nonketotic hyperglycemic coma, which presents as profound dehydration, significant mental status changes, and an extremely high plasma glucose (plasma glucose > 600 mg/dL).

Chronic complications in type I and type II diabetes include microvascular as well as macrovascular disease, resulting in retinopathy (proliferative and nonproliferative), diabetic nephropathy, coronary artery disease, peripheral vascular disease, and stroke. Other complications include diabetic neuropathies (symmetric peripheral neuropathy, autonomic neuropathies, and mononeuropathies), foot ulcers (due to diabetic neuropathy and peripheral vascular disease), and an increased risk of infection (due to high plasma glucose levels).

## SYSTEMIC LUPUS ERYTHEMATOSUS

Systemic lupus erythematosus (SLE) is an inflammatory autoimmune disorder that primarily strikes younger women. SLE is a multisystem disease that is characterized by recurrent exacerbations and remissions.

## Signs and Symptoms

SLE is characterized by multiple systemic complaints such as fever, malaise, anorexia, and weight loss as well as multiple system derangements (see Figure 13). Classic cutaneous manifestations include photosensitivity and "butterfly" malar rash. In addition, over 90% of patients have joint symptoms.

## Differential

Drug-induced lupus erythematosus should be considered before a diagnosis of spontaneous SLE is made. Classic drug causes include isoniazid, hydralazine, procainamide, and quinidine.

## Workup

Patients are often anemic, leukopenic, and thrombocytopenic secondary to the presence of autoantibodies (eg, positive Coombs). Most patients have positive antinuclear antibodies (ANA). However, ANA is not specific for SLE. On the other hand, anti-double-stranded DNA and anti-Sm antibodies are much more specific but less sensitive for SLE (see Table 13).

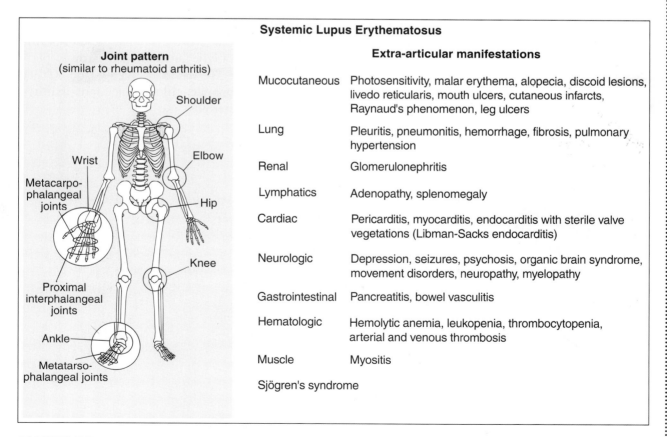

**Systemic Lupus Erythematosus**

| Joint pattern (similar to rheumatoid arthritis) | Extra-articular manifestations | |
|---|---|---|
| | Mucocutaneous | Photosensitivity, malar erythema, alopecia, discoid lesions, livedo reticularis, mouth ulcers, cutaneous infarcts, Raynaud's phenomenon, leg ulcers |
| | Lung | Pleuritis, pneumonitis, hemorrhage, fibrosis, pulmonary hypertension |
| | Renal | Glomerulonephritis |
| | Lymphatics | Adenopathy, splenomegaly |
| | Cardiac | Pericarditis, myocarditis, endocarditis with sterile valve vegetations (Libman-Sacks endocarditis) |
| | Neurologic | Depression, seizures, psychosis, organic brain syndrome, movement disorders, neuropathy, myelopathy |
| | Gastrointestinal | Pancreatitis, bowel vasculitis |
| | Hematologic | Hemolytic anemia, leukopenia, thrombocytopenia, arterial and venous thrombosis |
| | Muscle | Myositis |
| | Sjögren's syndrome | |

**FIGURE 13.** The many manifestations of SLE. Stobo et al., *Principles and Practice of Medicine*, Stamford, CT: Appleton & Lange, 1996, page 198.

**TABLE 13.** Associations of autoantibodies with SLE

| Test | Sensitivity, Specificity for SLE | Other Disease Associations | Comments |
|---|---|---|---|
| Antinuclear antibody (ANA) | > 95%, low | RA (30–50%), discoid lupus, scleroderma (60%), drug-induced lupus (100%), Sjögren's syndrome (80%), miscellaneous inflammatory disorders. | Often used as a screening test. A negative test virtually excludes SLE; a positive test, while non-specific, increases posttest probability. Titer does not correlate with disease activity. |
| Anti-double-stranded-DNA (anti-ds-DNA) | 60–70%, high | Lupus nephritis, rarely RA, CTD, usually in low titer. | Predictive value of a positive test is > 90% for SLE if present in high titer; a decreasing titer may correlate with worsening renal disease. Titer generally correlates with disease activity. |
| Anti-Smith antibody (anti-SM) | 30–40%, high | | SLE-specific. A positive test substantially increases posttest probability of SLE. Test rarely indicated. |

Reprinted with permission (from Nicoll et al., *Pocket Guide to Diagnostic Tests*, Second Edition, Stamford, CT: Appleton & Lange, 1997, page 316.

## Treatment

Initial measures of mild cases of SLE arthropathy include conservative measures such as joint rest and NSAIDs. Patients with severe manifestations, including thrombocytopenic purpura, hemolytic anemia, myocarditis, pericarditis, convulsions, and nephritis, are treated with prednisone. Other immunosuppressants, such as cyclophosphamide, chlorambucil, and azathioprine, are used in SLE that is resistant to steroids.

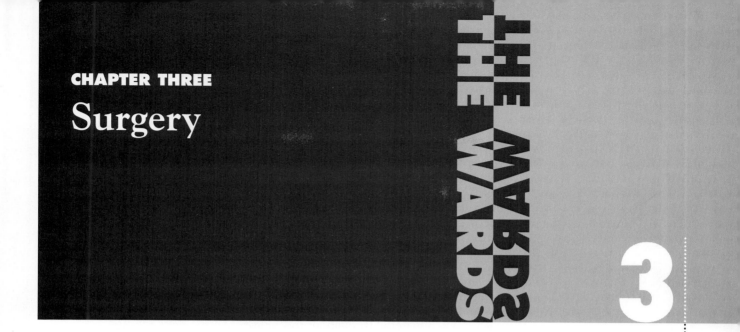

## CHAPTER THREE

# Surgery

**THE WARDS**

**3**

# WARD TIPS

The general surgery rotation is typically among the most rigorous, challenging, and exhausting experiences of medical school. The large volume of relevant subject matter, the demands made on time and energy, and the accelerated pace of work are generally considered to be unequaled among core or elective clerkships. Many students thus look forward to their surgery rotations with unbridled enthusiasm, extreme trepidation, or, more commonly, some combination of the two. Your experiences in surgery, like those of other services, will depend on your accumulation of knowledge, your performance of appropriate scut, and your interactions with the clinical team, nursing staff, and ancillary personnel. Of course, the culture of surgery can color your experiences and perceptions of the field, which is often regimental, inverse-pyramidal (big and important at the top, small and abusable at the bottom), and unforgiving. Most students, however, come away from their surgery rotations with a vastly increased fund of knowledge, confidence in their clinical skills, and, inevitably, a newfound appreciation for food and sleep.

In surgery, giants still roam the earth.

## WHAT IS THE ROTATION LIKE?

The surgery clerkship at most medical schools attempts to expose students to the principles of basic surgical management, including pre- and postoperative care of surgical patients, as well as to impart an understanding of the general principles of surgical disease. In addition, students gain some hands-on experience in basic bedside procedures, sterile technique, and operating room tasks (although this is often limited to cutting sutures, retracting tissue, and suctioning). The structure of the rotation will vary from school to school, from hospital to hospital, and even from service to service at the same hospital, depending on the patient population served, the nature of the surgical illnesses managed, and the specific clinical emphases of the attendings on a given service. As a rule, however, most core clerkships are structured to offer the student inpatient and ambulatory experience in general elective surgery, with additional experience on a trauma/emergency service and, possibly, some minimal exposure to some of the subspecialties of general surgery, including plastic/reconstructive, transplantation, and cardiothoracic. As with your other rotations, your experience in surgery will depend on the specific team of residents and attendings with whom you work.

In addition to clinical experience on the surgery service, students often receive formal didactic instruction in the form of conferences and lectures on basic principles of patient management and surgical diseases. These may include formal departmental grand rounds, weekly multidisciplinary conferences (eg, joint conferences with radiology, gastroenterology, and pathology), and lectures by the faculty specifically organized for the students. You may also participate in weekly service conferences in which the house staff presents details of the patient census, operative and perioperative complications, and patient cases illustrating interesting clinical issues. In addition to this allocated didactic instruction, you may receive informal teaching sessions from the house staff as time permits. Of course, as a student, you will be expected to read in what little time you have left when the workday is done, as you will be expected to learn much material throughout the course of your surgery rotation.

## WHO ARE THE PLAYERS?

**Balance your time between the OR and the wards.**

**Attendings**. Each service is usually staffed by several attendings, each of whom has senior responsibility for the management of patients. These patients may be private patients followed by the attending in his or her private clinic or patients admitted to the service by the ward team (eg, from the emergency room or from other services from which patients may be referred for management of surgical problems). In these latter cases, the attending who is "on call" for new admissions (ie, for patients who are not admitted electively by their own attendings) will be responsible for patient management. The various attendings on a given service will usually rotate call with one another on a weekly or monthly basis. Of course, call is from home.

In addition to having chief responsibility for the perioperative management of their patients, the attendings on a surgical service have ultimate control during the surgeries themselves. At most teaching institutions, much of the actual operating is done by the chief and senior residents under the guidance of the attending. The extent to which this is true, however, depends on the nature of the service—eg, on whether it is an elective general surgery service at a private hospital, a trauma/general surgery service at a county hospital, or a vascular service at a VA—as well as on the nature of the surgical disease in question and the complexity of the surgery itself. Simple procedures such as hernia repairs and appendectomies, for example, are frequently done by interns and junior residents, while complicated operations like the Whipple procedure (pancreaticoduodenectomy for pancreatic cancer) are generally done by the chief resident and attending. There is always an attending for every surgery, although some procedures are done entirely by the residents under the attending's umbrella of guidance and responsibility.

**Chief resident**. If the attending acts as "chairman of the board" of the service, the chief resident functions as chief executive officer, assuming responsibility for the management of the entire service as well as for the day-to-day running of the ward team. The chief is usually on call every night for admissions or patient emergencies. All the patients on the service are managed by the chief resident, regardless of who their individual attendings are. Hence, the chief resident must be aware of every important issue affecting each patient on the service, including lab and x-ray results, plans for wound/dressing/line care, plans for advancing patients' diets, and dispositions. Because each attending on a service may have specific preferences for certain management issues (eg, staples out on day 5, advance from NPO to clear liquids versus soft diet), the chief must be well informed about these issues, as he or she must answer to the attendings if things go wrong.

Because culpability tends to roll downhill, it is in the best interests of all the residents and students to ensure that things function as smoothly as possible and that the chief is kept abreast of any problems. Chiefs, of course, do the majority of operating on the more complex cases. In addition to clinical work, chief residents often have significant administrative and didactic responsibilities. They are typically in charge of arranging patient presentations for conferences and may schedule teaching sessions for the students on their service. They also arrange for admissions and oversee consultations to other services. Moreover, as a student, you may find that the chief resident has major responsibility for your evaluation. The onus is therefore on you to make sure your efforts do not go unnoticed by your chief.

**Senior resident(s).** On any given surgery service, there may be one or two senior residents—ie, residents in their third or fourth clinical year—who assist the chief resident in the management of the service. Typically, the senior resident is responsible for running rounds in the morning and updating the service for the chief (since the chief may or may not walk on rounds with the team each morning). Also, when issues come up during the day which are not easily managed by the interns and junior residents, the senior resident may be called upon to take care of the task, since the chief may be busy operating. Of course, senior residents do their fair share of operating as well, handling cases of lesser complexity than chief cases (eg, bowel resections for cancer, mastectomies). You can expect to work much more closely with your senior than with your chief on a daily basis. Be aware, however, that seniors may be watching you very carefully, as their input to the chief plays a significant role in your ultimate evaluation for your several weeks of hard work.

**Interns and junior residents.** These are the scut monkeys of the surgery service (as is the case on other services, only on surgery there's usually significantly more scut to be done). Interns and second-year residents have responsibility for the minutiae of patient care—writing notes, checking labs, writing and dictating discharge summaries, checking wounds and changing dressings, etc. They respond to pages from the nursing staff when patients are crashing. They are harried, get little sleep, and have no lives, so part of your job is to make their jobs easier.

**Subinterns.** This includes acting interns, senior clerks, and fourth-year med students. As a general rule, if there are subinterns (sub-I's) on your team, their goal will be to go into surgery. This means that sub-I's will be working their hardest to function at an intern level and to shine before their chiefs and attendings. As a third-year student, you may initially be intimidated by the specter of working on a service with machines like these. Bear in mind, however, that expectations of a third-year's performance differ from those of a sub-I. Also keep in mind that you are probably capable of performing most of the tasks that the sub-I's do; you're just on a steeper portion of the learning curve. A typical sub-I will be expected to take call on a schedule approximately comparable to an intern's (again, services vary in their expectations), will assume some responsibility for evaluating patients on consults or

**Surgery fosters a more formal pecking order.**

in the ER, will take on a fair amount of daily scut, and will try to squeeze into the OR whenever possible. As acting interns, though, they should also assume some responsibility for the education of the service, particularly the third-year students. So use your sub-I's as a resource—they may have valuable advice to give you about performing well on surgery (and they are a reasonable source of knowledge about surgical disease).

## HOW IS THE DAY SET UP?

Typically, there are 2–3 OR days per week, when the residents and attendings will spend most of the day in surgery. Although some of the surgical cases may be simple outpatient "come-and-go" procedures such as breast biopsies and hernia repairs, most will be "come-and-stay" surgeries in which patients are admitted for postoperative care lasting one to several days. The remainder of the work week will usually be clinic days in which new patients are seen for their referred problems, established patients are worked up for their preoperative evaluation, and postoperative patients are seen for follow-up after discharge. On both operative and clinic days, the entire inpatient service will need to be rounded on, and most teams will try to write all the progress notes on morning rounds before heading off to the OR or clinic. This, of course, means that the workday starts especially early on a surgery service—usually anywhere from 5:00 to 6:00 AM. Here's the overall structure of a typical OR day on an elective general surgery service:

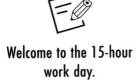

**Welcome to the 15-hour work day.**

| 5:00–6:00 AM | Prerounds |
|---|---|
| 6:00–7:30 AM | Morning rounds |
| 7:30–8:00 AM | OR preop preparation of patients |
| 8:00 AM–12:00 NOON | Surgery or work time |
| 12:00 NOON–1:00 PM | Noon conference |
| 1:00–6:00 PM | Surgery or work time |
| 6:00–7:30 PM | "Afternoon" rounds |
| 7:30 PM–? | Postrounds scut time |

This is just a sample schedule; times may vary depending on the number of patients on the service and the number and length of operative cases. On clinic days, the morning schedule is usually similar, as rounds must be completed before the start of clinic. The evening schedule may be lighter depending on whether there is clinic scheduled in the afternoon and on how many patients need to be worked up or admitted for surgery the next day.

On operative days, the senior and chief residents will usually be tied up in the OR, so the responsibility for scut, consults, procedures, and the like falls to the junior resident(s), intern(s), and students. You may thus find yourself shuttling around from the OR to the ward between cases to assist the interns in writing orders, checking labs, changing dressings, calling consults, reading films, etc. Because your role in the OR is usually minimal, you may be expected to spend the bulk of your time doing scut, especially if you are on a scut-heavy service with a high census. In the OR, you may be able to actively participate in a case or you may be relegated to observing from outside the surgical field, depending on the attendings' and residents' preferences, your own interest in getting hands-on surgical experience, and the need for your help in taking care of patient issues on the floor. Overall, you should strive to create a balanced experience—one in which you spend enough time in the OR to understand sterile technique and get a basic handle on issues of intraoperative care while devoting most of your time to helping residents take care of patients and reading relevant material.

## WHAT DO I DO DURING PREROUNDS?

The daily tasks on a surgery service begin with prerounding. The team may expect you to preround on your handful of patients before the beginning of walk (run) rounds. On other services, the team may simply round as a group on everybody and write the notes (see Key Notes, page 97) in transit from room to room. As a rule, each patient should be seen in the morning and the following information updated:

- Hospital day number, postop day number, antibiotic day number(s), etc.
- **Events overnight:** Any episodes of respiratory distress? Any fever? Problems with pain management? Emesis? Op-site bleeding?
- **Subjective data:** How is the patient's pain control? Has he or she passed gas or had a bowel movement? (Relevant for postoperative feeding.) Is the patient tolerating POs, or is there nausea or emesis? Any shortness of breath?
- **Vitals:** Maximum temp, current temp, BP and HR, RR, $O_2$ saturation, weight.
- **I/Os:** Record the total intake, total output, PO intake (is the patient NPO, on clear liquids, or on solid food?), IV fluids (type and rate of fluid repletion, any boluses given), urine output (including Foley status), stool output, emesis and NG output, and output of indwelling drains.
- **Other data:** What kind and amount of pain medication is the patient getting? Is the patient on a PCA (patient-controlled analgesia device) or receiving boluses of pain meds from the nurses? What antibiotics is the patient on and for how many days (and how many days remain)? Are any other significant medications being given (eg, steroid taper, antiemetics, promotility agents, etc)? Is the patient diabetic, and if so, how high has the blood glucose been running and how much insulin is the patient requiring?
- **Physical exam:** You should perform a focused, directed exam based on the patient's overall well-being and presenting problem. In general, all patients should receive a brief respiratory, cardiac, and abdominal exam in addition to a global assessment of mental status every morning. In addition, postop patients will require assessment of urinary status (look at the Foley bag), drain output, and wound healing. (Look at the dressings; is there wound drainage? Any purulent exudate? Any excessive peri-incisional tenderness or erythema? Do the sutures or staples need to come out? Is there any sign of wound dehiscence?)
- **Assessment/plan:** You should construct an assessment and plan for rounds, even if it is incorrect. It shows that you have been thinking.

## HOW DO I DO WELL IN THIS ROTATION?

Your role on the surgery service will be a hodgepodge of scut, reading, and simply being there with the team. *You should always show up on time.* This may sound simple, but it is often difficult to remember where and when you were expected to meet with your team or attending, especially on postcall days. Expect to stay late for evening rounds (unless excused by your chief), and make yourself visible to the residents and attendings. Your residents may expect you to follow two to three patients very closely and take primary responsibility for their management, or there may be a "team approach" wherein the entire team shares responsibility for every patient (obviously in this case, you won't be expected to know as much detail about every patient, but you may have more information to track).

As is the case on most rotations, your primary role on the surgery rotation is that of "Highly Absorbent Information Sponge." Reading about perioperative care, the pathophysiology of surgical illness, the basics of trauma evaluation, etc, will occupy a significant amount of your time, but necessarily so. The field of surgery is relevant to practitioners in all specialties, whether you want to go into primary care medicine, psychiatry, pathology, anesthesiology, or whatever.

**Work your butt off.
Work your butt off.
Work your butt off.**

As stated above, you may be expected to participate in many intern-level tasks, including performing preop H&Ps in clinic, checking labs and x-rays, following patients' intake and output in the perioperative period, taking out sutures and staples postoperatively, writing discharge paperwork, evaluating patients in the ER, placing and changing arterial and venous lines, assisting in the operating room, writing medication orders, and giving presentations on rounds and in conferences. The balance of these activities will depend on your own initiative and on the demands of your service. Be willing to do a little extra scut on other patients for some *quid pro quo* teaching from the interns. It will be well worth your while. In general, show interest, be generous of your effort, accept responsibility eagerly and fulfill it competently, make your interns' lives easier, follow your patients closely, be a team player, give crisp and succinct oral presentations, and make a little extra effort at reading and presenting interesting issues to the rest of the team, and you will have a successful surgery experience. Do anything less and you will almost certainly pass the rotation, but you may get stepped on by over-enthusiastic classmates or by solicitous sub-I's. So protect yourself by working hard. Hard work, after all, is what surgery is all about.

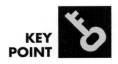

**KEY POINT**

---

**TIPS FOR SUCCESS**

The blueprint for survival and success on surgery focuses on several key points:

- Enthusiasm
- Assertiveness
- Voracious reading
- Efficiency on rounds
- Efficiency at paperwork
- Efficiency in clinic
- Efficiency at eating
- Efficiency at sleeping
- Respect for authority
- Appropriate humility

## KEY NOTES

After prerounds, you will need to complete brief SOAP progress notes on each patient. These will follow the typical format but will usually be significantly shorter on a surgery service, as seen below.

Other types of chart notes you may encounter on the surgery rotation include the following:

**Admission H&P.** If this is a preop H&P for an elective surgery, you should include a succinct HPI, a brief PMH with particular attention to illnesses

---

**SOAP Note**

Surgery PN: HD#3, POD#2, Abx = Ceftizox D#1 Flagyl D#1, Central Line Day #2

**S:** Pt. ambulating, pain well controlled on PCA. c/o peri-incisional pain, no drainage. No flatus or bowel movements. Good use of incentive spirometer ($\uparrow$ 1500 cc).

**O:** VS $T_m$ 38³ / $T_c$ 38¹ BP 110/63 P 86 R 16 $O_2$ sat 99% 2 L NC; GCS 14–15 (if ICU pt)

24 hr. I/O 2100/2000 (3000/2800—yesterday's I/O); UO 1500 (24 hr. tot)

$D_5$1/2 NS @ 80 cc/hr, JP output → 15 cc—12 hr. total (if patient in ICU—also document pulmonary artery catheter readings)

PE: Chest CTA with BS equal bilaterally; right chest tube suction intact with no air bubbles and moderate (30 cc) serosanguineous drainage

CV: RRR, nl S1/S2, no M/R/G

Abd: dressing C/D/I, staples intact, no induration/erythema. + hypoactive BS

JP w/ mod. serosanguineous drainage (> 15 cc drainage—12 hr. total)

Labs:

| 136 | 101 | 14 |  |
|---|---|---|---|
| 4.2 | 22 | 0.9 | Hb/Hct 9.2/29 (10.1/30—ie, yesterday's Hb/Hct) |

Wound Cx pending

CT scan, x-rays, etc

**A/P:** 55 yo WM POD#2 s/p exp lap for SBO, doing well

Low-grade temperature most likely secondary to atelectasis.

→ Cont Abx

→ Encourage OOB, ambulation, and incentive spirometry

→ Consider D/C PCA; switch to PO analgesics

→ Keep NPO for now, will advance to clear fluids when flatus passed

→ D/C JP drain, D/C Foley

---

PN = Progress note

HD = Hospital day

POD = Postop day

PCA = Patient-controlled analgesic

$T_m$ = Maximum temperature

$T_c$ = Current temperature

NC = Nasal cannula

GCS = Glasgow Coma Scale

UO = Urine output

JP = Jackson-Pratt

CTA = Clear to auscultation

BS = Breath sounds

RRR = Regular rate and rhythm

M/R/G = Murmurs/rubs/gallops

C/D/I = Clean/dry/intact

SBO = Small bowel obstruction

OOB = Out of bed

D/C = Discontinue

NPO = Nothing by mouth

**Don't forget to get and document consent.**

that have significance for perioperative management (eg, history of atrial fibrillation, COPD, diabetes, etc), and information on meds and allergies. Your exam should be comprehensive but more focused on the particular organ system in question (eg, a thorough abdominal exam for GI cases, a detailed peripheral vascular exam for vascular cases) and should always include a rectal exam as well as a breast exam for women. In addition, your admit note should document that you discussed the risks, benefits, alternatives, and expectations of the surgical procedure and that the patient understands these and gives consent.

**Operative note.** This is a note entered into the chart at the completion of a surgical procedure documenting the findings and events of the case. It is usually a brief summary and should include pertinent data regarding the participants, the pre- and postoperative diagnoses (usually the same but sometimes different, particularly in exploratory cases), total fluid exchange, disposition, and any complications. A sample operative note is shown below.

CRNA = Certified registered nurse anesthetist

LR = Ringer's lactate

EBL = Estimated blood loss

GB = Gallbladder

CBD = Common bile duct

IOC = Intraoperative cholangiogram

---

**Brief Op Note: Blue Surgery Team**

**Preop dx:** Biliary colic

**Postop dx:** Cholelithiasis

**Procedure:** Laparoscopic cholecystectomy + intraoperative cholangiography

**Surgeons:** Attending

**Assistants:** Resident (PGY-5), Intern (PGY-1), Med Student (MS-3)

**Anesthesia:** General endotracheal

**Anesthesiologist:** Attending/CRNA

**Fluids:** 1400 cc LR

**Blood transfusions:** None (no cell saver)

**EBL:** 200 cc

**Findings:** Distended gallbladder w/ sl. thickened wall, multiple stones w/in GB, no CBD stones by IOC

**Specimens:** GB to path    Cultures taken: None

**Drains:** None

**Complications:** None apparent

**Disposition:** To recovery room in stable condition, awake and extubated

---

**Postop check.** Generally, any patient undergoing surgery will need to be seen several hours postop to be evaluated for immediate complications (eg, hypotension, hemorrhage, dyspnea), adequacy of urine output, level of comfort, etc. A brief postop note, again in the standard SOAP format, should then be written. The subjective section should mainly address the patient's postoperative pain control, and the objective portion should include vital signs, intraoperative and postoperative blood loss and fluid intake, urinary output, wound drainage, appearance of incision and dressings, postop lab results from the recovery room, and any significant abnormalities on physical exam.

**Procedure note.** Frequently, surgical patients will undergo various minor procedures, including central line insertion, chest tube placement/removal, extubation, I&D of abscesses, thoracocentesis, paracentesis, lumbar puncture, and suturing of lacerations. When these are done as bedside procedures, they should be documented in the medical chart with an appropriate procedure note. The procedure note should follow the standard format. Remember to get informed consent and to document it in the chart.

## KEY PROCEDURES

Because surgery is principally an intervention-oriented specialty, you should attempt to gain some hands-on experience with certain types of procedures that may be relevant to you in other specialties. These include suturing lacerations (including learning techniques of local anesthesia), knot tying and suture cutting, gowning and gloving in sterile fashion, arterial line placement, IV starting, ABGs, paracentesis, thoracocentesis, chest tube placement, incision and drainage of abscesses, staple and suture removal, dressing

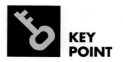

**KEY POINT**

---

**TUBES AND DRAINS**

- **JP drain, or Jackson-Pratt drain:** Used to drain surgical wounds in the event of contamination; to keep bacteria and blood coming out, they are attached to suction. You will see the resident "strip" or milk these, which means pulling along the length of the clear tube filled with blood to prevent clotting.

- **Penrose drain:** No suction; just a yellow tube stuck in a wound to drain away bacteria and blood like a plastic wick.

- **Levine or NG tube:** An orogastric or nasogastric tube leading from the nasopharynx or oropharynx to the stomach; used preoperatively to drain the stomach of fluids (gastric decompression) and for the same purpose postoperatively. Also used for feeding when the patient's gut starts working after surgery.

- **G-tube or gastrostomy tube:** Goes right from the stomach to the outside; resembles a permanent NG tube used for feeding patients with an obstruction above the stomach or for decompression in patients with pyloric outlet obstruction. Frequently used in older patients who are at risk for aspiration pneumonia from inhaling gastric contents.

- **J-tube or jejunostomy tube:** Primarily used for feeding.

- **GJ-tube/Moss tube:** Has 2 ports, both entering the stomach; one stops there and the other goes to the jejunum. Acts like one G-tube and one J-tube.

- **T-tube:** Biliary tube shaped like a "T."

changing, Foley catheterization, nasogastric tube insertion, central venous cannulation, and drain pulling (see Tubes and Drains). You should also become familiar with the process of patient preparation and transfer to and from the operating suite. Surgical ties are best learned from a resident and then practiced diligently at home. Of course, you'll get plenty of practice at retraction in the OR.

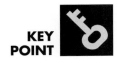

**KEY POINT**

## OPERATING ROOM ETIQUETTE

Interestingly enough, one of the most difficult (and sometimes among the most frustrating) concepts that a student must learn during his or her surgical ward rotations is the maintenance of a sterile field in the operating room. This includes not only making sure you are not contaminating the operating field (or yourself) but also staying out of the way while the other team members in the operating room (eg, surgeons, scrub nurse, circulating nurse, x-ray technicians) work. Since you will probably be the most inexperienced member of the group in the operating room, it is important to know some of the points of etiquette associated with working in the operating room. These include the following:

- When you first enter the operating room, before you scrub in, introduce yourself both to the OR circulating nurse and to the scrub nurse, and tell them that you will be scrubbing in on the case. Tell the circulating nurse what size gown and gloves you will need. If you don't know your glove size, follow this general guideline:

    Size 6 = small
    Size 7 = medium
    Size 8 = large

- Remember to double-glove to protect yourself against needlesticks. When double-gloving, many people prefer that the outer set of gloves be one-half size larger than the inner set so that they aren't too tight.

- Ask the circulating nurse or resident if he or she needs any help in moving or positioning the patient on the operating table or prepping the patient for surgery.

- Before scrubbing, place your beeper on one of the nonsterile side tables with a piece of paper attached to the beeper with your name on it. This not only will allow the circulating nurse to return your pages but will also help you find the beeper if you accidentally leave it in the operating room after the case is over.

- Remember to take off any jewelry (eg, rings, bracelets, watches) and put on your mask, cap, and safety eyewear before you start scrubbing.

- Although there is no specific rule on how long to scrub, a good rule of thumb is to always scrub 1–2 minutes longer than your attending surgeon so that he or she won't be able to criticize you for not scrubbing thoroughly enough.

- Offer to help with the draping of the patient after you are gowned. If no help is needed, quietly stand out of the way of others who are draping the patient.

- Do not reach over or pass any instrument unless specifically instructed to do so.

- When the surgeon is using the bovie (electrocautery device) to incise through fat, muscle tissue, and fascia, use the suction device to suck up the smoke and noxious odor associated with it.

- Always announce out loud to the scrub nurse the presence of any sharps on the field that are returned to the instrument tray (eg, "needle down," "knife back"). It is also helpful to announce to the anesthesiologist when the initial incision is made so that he or she knows when the surgery has started and can document the time of incision.

- Try to make yourself helpful by paying attention to minor details such as providing adequate retraction, adjusting the overhead lights, and suctioning excess blood from the area of dissection. These measures will allow the surgeon to have good visualization of the anatomic structures in the operating field.

- Try to learn the names of the surgical instruments so that you can help the scrub nurse and allow the case to proceed in an efficient manner.

- Those of you who wear glasses should be aware that possibly the easiest way to contaminate yourself is to accidentally reach to adjust your glasses with your sterile glove. Work to avoid that habit in the operating room.

- If you do end up contaminating your gown, glove, or sleeve, step out of the operating field and let the scrub nurse know so that he or she can replace the contaminated parts and help ensure that you don't end up contaminating anything else.

If you follow these basic principles of operating room etiquette, you are likely to find your OR experience to be far more enjoyable and less stressful. One last thing: don't forget to carry a pen in the pocket of your scrubs so that you can write the postop note and postop orders when the case is completed.

## QUICK SURVIVAL TIPS

**Things to remember on postop orders:**

- Strict I/Os.
- DVT prophylaxis.
- Incentive spirometer 10 times every hour when awake.
- Meds: Preop meds, antibiotics, ulcer prophylaxis.
- PRN meds: Sleeper, pain, antipyretic, and stool softener.
- AM labs.
- NPO until flatus after GI surgery.

**Maintenance IV fluids:**

- 4 cc/kg/hour for first 10 kg, plus 2 cc/kg/hour for second 10 kg, plus 1 cc/kg/hour beyond 20 kg (4-2-1 rule).
- Shortcut: Weight in kg plus 40 cc/hour (for adults).

- Typical postop maintenance fluids for 70-kg adult: D5 1/2 NS + 20 mEq KCl at 110 cc/hour; increased fluid requirement for fever, NG suction, wound drain, diarrhea.

### Transfusions:

- Premedicate with Tylenol 650 mg PO and Benadryl 25 mg PO.
- Watch for volume overload, consider diuresis between units (furosemide 20 mg IV).
- Transfuse each unit RBC over 3–4 hours if not acutely bleeding.

### Postop fever etiology—the "5 W's":

- **Wind:** Atelectasis (most common cause on POD #1), pneumonia.
- **Water:** UTI.
- **Wound:** Infection.
- **Walking:** Pulmonary embolus and DVT.
- **Wonder drug:** Drug fever.

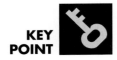

**KEY POINT**

## HOW TO SUTURE LIKE A PRO

One way to get more out of your operating room experience during your surgical rotations is to learn to be proficient at suturing and surgical knot tying. Unfortunately, the only way to become proficient at these skills is to practice, practice, practice! The best way to sharpen your suturing technique is to go to the emergency room and obtain the following:

- **Sutures of different types and sizes.** The most common suture with which to practice surgical knot tying is 3–0 silk suture ties. Ideally, however, you should try to become proficient in suturing with many different types of sutures, such as 5–0 nylon (most commonly used when suturing up the skin), 1–0 Vicryl (most commonly used when suturing up deep fascia and muscle layers), and 4–0 Vicryl (most commonly used when closing up the subcutaneous layer). It is also helpful to remember which sutures are absorbable (eg, Vicryl, PDS, Dexon, chromic catgut) as opposed to nonabsorbable (eg, nylon and silk); which are natural (eg, silk, catgut) as opposed to synthetic (eg, nylon, PDS); and which are monofilament (eg, nylon) as opposed to braided (eg, silk, Dexon, Vicryl).

- **A "laceration tray" from the ER.** Specific instruments you will need include a needle holder, a pair of pickups, and a pair of suture scissors. Laceration trays usually have many of these instruments in varying sizes.

- **A box of gloves.** Remember that when suturing on a patient, you should be double-gloved to protect against needlesticks. Thus, it would make sense to practice suturing and surgical knot tying with two sets of gloves on so it won't prove to be too awkward when you work on a real patient.

- **A suture removal kit.** This should include a pair of forceps as well as a fine-pointed pair of scissors for taking out sutures.

The next step is to find a fourth-year medical student (eg, a subintern) or an intern (ideally one who is not very busy) who is willing to show you how to suture and tie surgical knots. The types of suture methods that you should learn include:

- Simple interrupted sutures (most commonly used to close up skin lacerations).

- Vertical mattress sutures (used to close skin that is under tension).

- Horizontal mattress sutures (also used to close skin that is under tension).

- "Buried" (subcutaneous) sutures.

- Figure-of-eight sutures (used to tie off a bleeding vessel).

- Running sutures (often used to quickly close deep fascial layers).

As for surgical knot tying, focus on learning how to tie surgical knots by the "instrument tie" and the two-handed free knot tie before progressing to the "slicker," more advanced one-handed surgical knot tie. Good material to practice suturing on include pigs' feet (for the classic die-hard surgeon-to-be!), orange peels, and two-sided sponges.

## WHAT DO I CARRY IN MY POCKETS?

Like any rotation, surgery has its necessary gear. Unlike most residents, however, surgery residents try to carry little extraneous material with them, as they tend to shift rapidly from OR to clinic to ward to cafeteria and thus want to be as unencumbered as possible. As a student, you, too, are usually allowed to adopt this minimalist posture. This means not carrying around too many handbooks and not wearing a fanny pack laden with tuning forks, otoscopes, etc. The main requirements for the surgery rotation include:

### Checklist

- ❑ **White coat:** Always wear one on the first day. Figure out if you're expected to wear it daily or just in clinic, etc.
- ❑ **Stethoscope:** Essential on any rotation. But beware of the fact that many surgeons frown on wearing the stethoscope as a necklace ("dog collar"), as this is a sign of an internal medicine doctor or resident. To be safe, carry it in the pocket of your white coat.
- ❑ **Penlight:** Critical for its common uses (checking pupils) and for examining wounds, etc.
- ❑ **Trauma scissors:** "Trauma scissors" or surgical shears are a pair of heavy-duty scissors used primarily to cut through a patient's clothing during an acute trauma situation or to cut through bulky dressings on rounds. These handy, all-purpose scissors will prove useful during both your general surgery and inpatient OB/GYN rotations.
- ❑ **Index cards/clipboard/patient data sheets:** You will need something easily portable to manage the reams of information (eg, lab data) on each patient. Figure out which method works most effec-

tively and efficiently for you; then stick with it and abandon extraneous gear.

❑ **Drug guide:** A must-have throughout your medical training (until you get to the level where you don't have to look up drug doses—which won't come for several years, if ever).

❑ **Antimicrobial guide:** *Sanford's Guide to Antimicrobial Therapy* is an excellent pocket resource for bacterial susceptibilities and drug dosing for common scenarios.

❑ **Surgery handbook:** There are a number of useful, concise pocket guidebooks for surgery students and residents. It is advisable to spend some time evaluating these books before purchasing one, as they differ markedly in style and organization (but are mostly consistent in content). Some of the more popular handbooks are reviewed in this chapter.

You should probably purchase the above items if you don't already own them. Most will come in handy for other rotations anyway, and a good pocket handbook is great to have as a quick reference before conferences or teaching (pimping) rounds. Sometimes it is also helpful to carry spare gauze (Kerlex rolls and 4 ✕ 4 cotton gauze pads), surgical tape, and other wound care accessories for rapid dispensing at the request of your chief resident on rounds. Many students use a "bucket" stocked full of the items the team conceivably may need for wound checks and dressing changes on morning rounds.

# Top-Rated Books

## HANDBOOK/POCKETBOOK

### Mont Reid Surgical Handbook
Koutlas
Mosby, 1994, 715 pages, ISBN 0815151489, $39.95

Great pocketbook designed for interns and junior surgical residents, but useful for motivated junior students. Rapid reading with quick, easily memorized facts for last-minute cramming before pimping sessions or entering the OR. Outline format. New edition now available.

### Surgical Intern Pocket Survival Guide
Chamberlain
International Medical Publishing, 1993, 74 pages, ISBN 0963406353, $7.50

Extremely practical pocketbook detailing the nuts and bolts of day-to-day surgical life. Written for the intern, but serves as an excellent guide for subinterns. Easily outlines an approach to the medical management of surgical patients, including sample orders and notes. Some parts may be too specific for beginning students, but most sections are quite useful. An excellent buy.

### Handbook of Surgery
Schrock
Mosby, 1994, 1013 pages, ISBN 0801676371, $39.95

A lengthy pocketbook with comprehensive coverage of surgical topics. The text is somewhat cumbersome for quick reading on the wards, and is often lacking in its discussion of differential diagnoses and pathophysiology. Sparse tables, illustrations, and diagrams. Best used by students who prefer the expanded outline/paragraph format.

### Current Clinical Strategies: Surgery
Wilson
Current Clinical Strategies, 1995, 61 pages, ISBN 188152812X, $12.75

A mini-pocket handbook in outline format that addresses key issues in history and physical, workup, and treatment of the most common surgical diseases. Includes descriptions of procedures and samples of surgical chart notes as well as order guidelines for specific diseases. Very bare bones and not nearly detailed enough for a reference; best used as a quick refresher on the wards.

### Manual of Surgical Therapeutics
Condon
Little, Brown, 1996, 439 pages, ISBN 0316154024, $34.95

Practical handbook presented in a style similar to that of the *Washington Manual*. Too big to fit in a pocket.

**B+** **The Washington Manual of Surgery**
Doherty
Little, Brown, 1997, 632 pages, ISBN 0316924466, $34.95

Worthy counterpart to the *Washington Manual* for medicine. Good coverage of basic general surgery topics as well as common problems in the surgical subspecialties. Practical chapters on day-to-day care of the surgical patient. Tends to gloss over signs and symptoms, making it more appropriate for interns.

**B** **Principles of Surgery, Companion Handbook**
Schwartz
McGraw-Hill, 1994, 771 pages, ISBN 0070560552, $32.00

Fair pocketbook, occasionally weak on differential diagnosis and treatment. The book's limited index compromises quick on-the-wards referencing. Chapters are nonstandardized in style and presentation; some are outline format, others are in paragraph form. Few tables or illustrations.

**B** **Surgery on Call**
Gomella
Appleton & Lange, 1996, 536 pages, ISBN 0838587461, $23.95

Practical, quick coverage of commonly encountered problems seen while on call. Includes section on lab test interpretation, procedures, and commonly used medications. No discussion of pathophysiology, but includes differential diagnoses and essentials of patient workup. Presented in an easy-to-read outline format. More useful for the subintern than for the third-year student.

**B-** **Handbook of General Surgery**
Bevan
Blackwell Scientific, 1992, 576 pages, ISBN 0632011114, $38.95

Concise introductory softcover surgical text geared toward students and written by British authors. Contains few statistics and lacks depth in many areas but is easy reading. No coverage of surgical subspecialties. Quite bulky as a pocketbook.

## REVIEW/MINI-REFERENCE

**A-** **Cope's Early Diagnosis of the Acute Abdomen**
Silen
Oxford University Press, 1996, 313 pages, ISBN 0195097599, $26.50

A classic brief surgical textbook that every serious student of surgery should read. Readable, personable approach to this critical surgical problem. Ideally, needs to be read before the surgical rotation. This text deals only with the acute surgical abdomen.

## Current Surgical Diagnosis and Treatment
Way
Appleton & Lange, 1994, 1428 pages, ISBN 0838514391, $45.00

**A-**

Remarkably comprehensive for a student reference book. Although it tends to be wordy, it is useful for prepping for lectures, rounds, and the OR. Includes chapters on most subspecialties of surgery. New edition expected in January 1998.

## Surgical Recall
Blackbourne
Williams & Wilkins, 1994, 367 pages, ISBN 0683008358, $27.00

**A-**

Practical and useful adjunct to a reference text. Presented in a two-column format with questions on one side of the page and answers on the other. Excellent for ward pimping prep. It coveres a wide breadth of topics and includes many surgical pearls. Quick, easy one-night read, although it covers most topics superficially. Very appropriate for junior students. Overall, a more cohesive, systematic approach than *Surgical Secrets*.

## Abernathy's Surgical Secrets
Harken
Mosby, 1991, 312 pages, ISBN 1560530138, $35.95

**B+**

Q & A format with current references after each section. Comparable to *Surgical Recall*. A quick source for the answers to the most commonly asked questions. Contains more illustrations than *Surgical Recall*. Tends to be esoteric, but so can pimping on the wards. New edition not yet reviewed.

## Essentials of General Surgery
Lawrence
Williams & Wilkins, 1992, 432 pages, ISBN 0683048694, $39.95

**B+**

Basic introductory text to surgery that is written at the third-year-student level. Definitely an easy read with adequate coverage of pathophysiology, but lacks detail and depth in many areas. Weak in its discussion of treatment and management. May be adequate if you're not considering surgery as a career choice. Some stand by this book.

## NMS Surgery
Jarrell
Williams & Wilkins, 1996, 647 pages, ISBN 0683062719, $30.00

**B+**

Cursory overview of surgery presented in outline format. Falls between a true reference and a handbook. Includes questions following each chapter and a comprehensive exam at the end. Good for pre-exam preparation, but not as useful as a primary source. More appropriate for USMLE Step 2.

**C+** **Oklahoma Notes General Surgery**
Jacocks
Springer-Verlag, 1996, 189 pages, ISBN 0387946373, $17.95

An overly simplistic outline-format review book. Includes 168 multiple-choice and true/false questions, but no explanations to answers. Not useful for the wards and not detailed enough for end-of-service or USMLE Step 2 exams.

**C** **Student's Textbook of Surgery**
Rambo
Churchill-Livingstone, 1996, 379 pages, ISBN 0865424853, $39.95

A somewhat simplistic, cursory treatment of surgical topics. Emphasizes a minimalist approach—that is, minimal coverage of anatomy, pathophysiology, diagnosis, and treatment. Save your money.

## TEXTBOOK/REFERENCE

**A-** **Principles of Surgery**
Schwartz
McGraw-Hill, 1994, 2075 pages, ISBN 0070559287, $105.00

A reference textbook for the serious surgery student. Good discussion of surgical disease processes. Expensive and requires considerable reading time.

**B** **General Surgery**
Ritchie
Lippincott, 1995, 978 pages, ISBN 0397511140, $154.00

A textbook focusing on the clinical aspects of the most commonly encountered problems in general surgery. Lacks pathophysiology or laboratory diagnosis. Focuses on procedure-oriented discussions. Most appropriate for general surgery residents and practicing general surgeons.

# HIGH-YIELD TOPICS

## ROTATION OBJECTIVES

The third-year clerkship in general surgery often involves time not only in general surgery but also in some of the surgical specialties. The following three questions can help you best focus in on the specific topics at hand:

- What is the natural history and appropriate evaluation of the surgical problem at hand?
- How do surgeons make the decision to intervene and prioritize the various therapeutic options?
- How do surgeons evaluate the risks and benefits of those therapeutic options in the context of a patient's problems, overall status, and life expectancy?

Given these considerations, the following list outlines common diseases and key topics that you are likely to encounter in the course of your surgery rotation. Disease entities that are further discussed in this chapter are listed in italics.

### Gastroenterology
- *Acute abdomen (acute appendicitis, acute pancreatitis)*
- *Gallstone disease (cholelithiasis, acute cholecystitis, acute cholangitis)*
- *Gastroesophageal reflux disease*
- *Peptic ulcer disease*
- *Inflammatory bowel disease*
- *GI bleeding (UGIB, LGIB)*
- *Small bowel obstruction*
- *Hernias*
- *Splenic rupture*
- *Diverticular disease (diverticulitis, Meckel's diverticulum)*
- Constipation, impaction
- Hemorrhoids, fistulas, fissures, perianal infection
- Achalasia
- Pancreatic pseudocysts
- Portal hypertension, ascites

### Shock
- *Hypovolemic*
- *Cardiogenic*
- *Septic*
- *Neurogenic*

### Oncology
- *Breast cancer*
- *Colorectal cancer*
- Other GI and GU cancers
- Skin cancer

### Urology/Nephrology
- Renal stones
- Ureteral obstruction
- Testicular torsion
- Benign prostatic hypertrophy

### Endocrinology
- Thyroid nodules
- Hyperthyroidism
- Hyperparathyroidism
- Cushing's syndrome

### Cardiovascular
- Cardiac revascularization
- Aneurysms
- Cerebrovascular insufficiency
- Pulmonary emboli
- Potentially life-threatening injuries and their treatment (pneumothorax, tamponade, etc.)

### Other
- Anesthesiology (intubation)
- Fluids and acid-base balance
- Wounds and wound healing
- Surgical infection
- Trauma
- Burns

# ACUTE ABDOMEN

The workup of a patient with acute abdominal pain is one of the most interesting and challenging diagnostic encounters you will face and is a key goal of the surgical rotation. Early diagnosis of the acute abdomen is critical, as many of the disease processes involved require early intervention to prevent significant morbidity or death.

## Signs and Symptoms

Differential diagnosis of the acute abdomen is usually made after assessing the following history:

- Onset, duration, and progression of pain (ie, maximal at onset, intermittent, constant, worsening).
- Location and distribution of pain, both at onset and at present.
- Nature of pain (burning, cramping, sharp, aching).
- Exacerbating and palliative factors.
- Associated nausea, vomiting, anorexia, or change in bowel habits.
- Associated hematemesis, hematochezia, or melena.
- Associated gynecologic complaints, last menstrual period.
- Any similar episodes in the past.
- Underlying metabolic or endocrine disease processes (diabetes, Addison's, porphyria, etc).
- Other past medical history (CAD, CHF, abdominal surgery, hernia, gallstones, EtOH, PUD).
- Medication history.

**All female patients with acute abdomen need a pelvic exam.**

Physical exam is indispensable in aiding the diagnosis. Findings to elicit on exam include:

- Evaluate vital signs for hypotension, orthostatic changes, fever, tachycardia, tachypnea, or other signs indicating infection, inflammatory process, or sepsis.
- On abdominal exam:
  - **Inspect:** Distention, scars, trauma, obesity; ask patient to point to location of maximal pain.
  - **Auscultate:** Absent bowel sounds (ileus), high-pitched sounds or tinkles (obstruction), bruits (aneurysm).
  - **Palpate:** Start at quadrant furthest from maximal pain. First lightly touch, then tap, gradually increase to deep palpation. Tenderness (rebound, referred), involuntary guarding, hepatosplenomegaly, masses, hernia (inguinal, femoral, incisional).
  - **Percuss:** Shifting dullness or fluid wave (ascites), liver and spleen span.
- Look for flank tenderness (renal inflammatory diseases or retrocecal appendix).
- Perform rectal exam for occult blood, mass lesions, tenderness, and presence or absence of rectal stool.
- Perform pelvic exam for adnexal tenderness, masses, cervical discharge, cervical motion tenderness, and uterine size and consistency.

SURGERY

110

- Assorted additional findings, including jaundice, urinary tract abnormalities, and signs of dehydration (dry mucous membranes, sunken eyes).

## Differential

The differential diagnosis for the acute abdomen is broad, so it is helpful to divide the causes into abdominal quadrants (see Figure 1).

Most disease processes may present atypically in terms of both the location and the nature of the abdominal complaints, but Figure 1 is a rough guideline to aid in formulating differentials (also see Figures 2 and 3). Additional processes to consider in the differential of acute abdomen but that are often difficult to localize include:

- Small bowel obstruction
- Paralytic ileus
- Diabetic ketoacidosis
- Addisonian crisis
- Acute intermittent porphyria
- Ischemic bowel

- Uremic crisis
- Sickle cell crisis
- Toxins (lead, venom)
- Pericarditis
- Obstructive uropathy

---

**Right Upper Quadrant (RUQ)**
Acute cholecystitis/biliary colic
Peptic ulcer disease (PUD)
Gastritis
Cholangitis
Hepatitis
Pneumonia

**Left Upper Quadrant (LUQ)**
Acute pancreatitis
Perforated viscus
MI
Splenic rupture/infarction
GERD/gastritis
PUD

**Epigastrium**

GERD
Peptic ulcer disease
Gastroenteritis
Esophagitis
Gastritis

Pancreatitis (acute/chronic)
Angina, MI
Perforated viscus
Aortic aneurysm

**Right Lower Quadrant (RLQ)**
Acute appendicitis
Inflammatory bowel disease
Meckel's diverticulum
Acute cholecystitis
Pyelonephritis, nephrolithiasis
Diverticulitis
Ovarian torsion, cyst, ruptured
  ectopic, PID
Intussusception
Ruptured carcinoma

**Left Lower Quadrant (LLQ)**
Diverticulitis
Sigmoid volvulus
Colorectal carcinoma
Mesenteric ischemia
Colitis
Pyelonephritis, nephrolithiasis
Ovarian torsion, cyst, ruptured
  ectopic, PID

---

**FIGURE 1.** Quick differential of acute abdomen by quadrant.

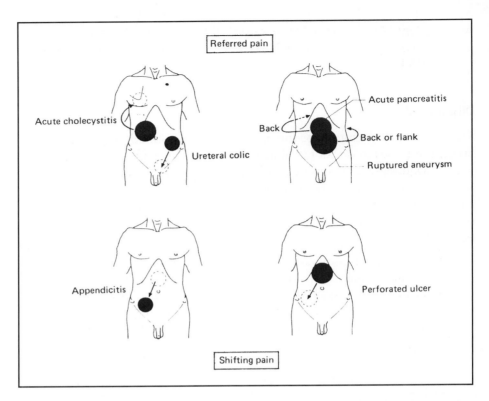

**FIGURE 2.** Referred pain and shifting pain in the acute abdomen. Solid circles indicate the site of maximum pain; broken lines indicate sites of lesser pain. Way, *Current Surgical Diagnosis & Treatment,* Tenth Edition, Stamford, CT: Appleton & Lange, 1994, page 443.

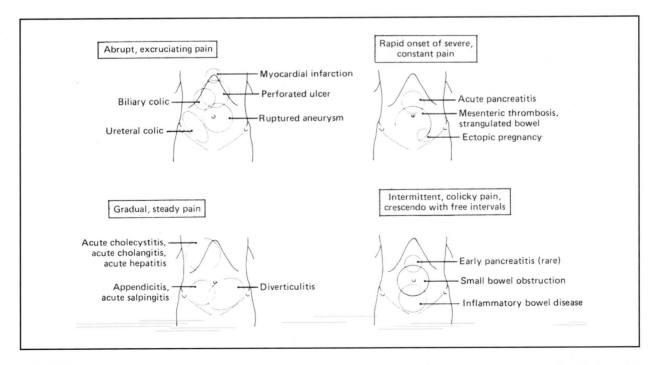

**FIGURE 3.** The location and characterization of pain is helpful in the differential diagnosis of the acute abdomen. Way, *Current Surgical Diagnosis & Treatment,* Tenth Edition, Stamford, CT: Appleton & Lange, 1994, page 444.

An excellent review source for discussion of the workup and basic management of the acute abdomen is *Cope's Early Diagnosis of the Acute Abdomen* (this is *the* classic text).

## Workup

Standard initial studies include CBC, chem 7, LFTs, amylase, lipase, lactic dehydrogenase, and three-way abdominal films. Further workup, including additional imaging, will be driven by the history, physical, and clinical symptoms.

## Treatment

The essence of managing an acute abdomen is operative intervention at the appropriate juncture, if necessary. Not all processes are properly managed by exploratory laparotomy, but it should be employed whenever a surgically correctible or identifiable disease is suspected. A thorough history and evaluation will allow you to decide whether to operate or merely to observe the patient. Mainstays of expectant (preoperative) management include:

- NPO.
- NG suction (for N/V, hematemesis, suspected obstruction).
- Aggressive IV fluid hydration and correction of electrolyte abnormalities.
- Monitoring of vital signs every hour.
- Serial abdominal exams (evaluate for progression of signs and symptoms of peritonitis versus resolution).
- Foley catheterization to evaluate fluid status and response to rehydration.
- Serial laboratory exams, including CBC and electrolytes.
- Operative intervention for acutely life-threatening processes.

## ACUTE APPENDICITIS

Acute appendicitis should *always* be near the top of your differential for an acute abdomen. Peak incidence is in the teens to mid-20s; appendicitis presenting at the extremes of age may have uncommon manifestations and hence may be difficult to diagnose. Acute appendicitis in infants and the elderly is also more likely to progress to perforation (as many as 75% of elderly patients) owing not only to delay in seeking treatment but also to delays in diagnosis. Appendicitis may also present quite atypically in patients with retrocecal/retrocolic appendices or during pregnancy. If untreated, appendicitis can progress to perforation and peritonitis or to abscess formation, with the former bearing a 5% mortality rate (versus a 0.1% rate in uncomplicated disease).

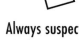

Always suspect acute appendicitis in abdominal pain.

## Etiology

Luminal obstruction of the appendix by hyperplasia of lymphoid tissue (55–65%), a fecalith (35%), a foreign body, a carcinoid tumor, a parasite, or other process results in distention of the viscus, hypersecretion of fluid and mucus behind the obstruction, mural inflammation, and, often, secondary postobstructive bacterial overgrowth. As this process continues, overdistention of the appendix can result in high intraluminal pressure that leads to compression of the capillary blood supply, resulting in appendiceal gangrene. Alternatively, the inflammatory process can become contained and walled off by omentum or peritoneum, resulting in a periappendiceal abscess. Both of these processes can result in perforation of the appendix with subsequent peritonitis from leaked colonic contents. The worst-case-scenario complication is pylephlebitis, a septic thrombophlebitis of the portal vein that presents with high fever, chills, and jaundice. The mainstay of acute appendicitis management is therefore early diagnosis and operative intervention before perforation has occurred.

## Signs and Symptoms

A classic description of the progression of acute appendicitis is as follows:

- Pain beginning in the epigastric area manifests as dull, vague discomfort, dyspepsia from irritation of visceral peritoneum (sensitive to stretch, becomes irritated as the appendix becomes distended). Pain may last 1–12 hours.
- Nausea, vomiting, and anorexia are seen following pain (presence of hunger is uncommon).
- Pain may wane slightly for a brief period; a low-grade fever (approximately 99–100°F) may be seen.
- Pain localizes to the right lower quadrant (RLQ) at McBurney's point (two-thirds of the distance from the umbilicus to the right anterior superior iliac spine). Pain is now sharper owing to irritation of parietal peritoneum from the progressively distended appendix.
- With perforation, there may be a transient decrease in pain, changing to diffuse tenderness with rebound, guarding, high fever, hypotension, and a very high WBC. The patient wants to remain very still, and there may have been pain on the drive to the ER from "bumps" in the car.
- RLQ tenderness is maximal at McBurney's point with rebound and guarding.
- **Rovsing's sign:** Referred pain in the RLQ is elicited by deep palpation in the LLQ; insensitive but fairly specific.
- **Psoas sign:** RLQ pain is elicited by passive extension of the hip (puts stretch on iliopsoas tendon, which overlies the location of the appendix); insensitive (see Figure 4).
- **Obturator sign:** RLQ pain is elicited by passive internal rotation of the hip; insensitive (see Figure 4).
- Palpable RLQ mass is found (may indicate an abscess); rectal exam elicits pain on right side.

## Differential

- Gastroenteritis (N/V *before* pain, viral syndrome, poorly localized pain, no leukocytosis)
- Mesenteric lymphadenitis
- Intussusception
- Pelvic inflammatory disease (CMT, discharge, bilateral lower abdominal tenderness, high fever)

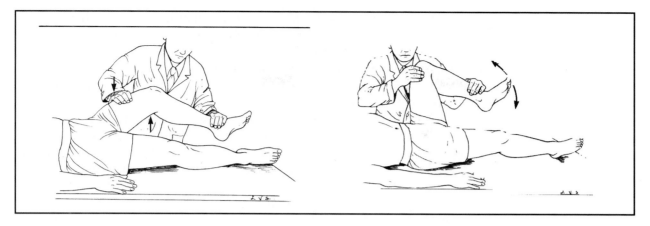

**FIGURE 4.** Psoas test and obturator test. Saunders, *Current Emergency Diagnosis & Treatment,* Fourth Edition, Stamford, CT: Appleton & Lange, 1992, page 114.

- Inflammatory bowel disease
- Ovarian cyst torsion; ectopic pregnancy
- Diverticulitis
- Small bowel obstruction
- Mesenteric ischemia
- Abdominal aortic aneurysm (AAA)
- Pancreatitis (atypical presentation)
- Acute cholecystitis (atypical presentation)
- Perforated peptic ulcer
- Pyelonephritis, nephrolithiasis
- Mittelschmerz (ruptured ovarian follicle: sudden-onset pain, middle of menstrual cycle, no N/V)
- DKA

## Workup

The diagnosis of acute appendicitis is based on the history and physical exam. Nonspecific laboratory and radiographic findings may be of some use in corroborating the suspicion, but their absence does not rule out appendicitis. Those patients in whom you strongly suspect the diagnosis should be taken urgently/emergently to the OR for exploratory laparotomy and appendectomy.

Laboratory and radiographic findings are as follows:

- Mild leukocytosis (11,000–15,000) with a left shift (> 75% PMNs in 75% of patients).
- UA may show few RBCs or WBCs.
- **KUB:** Fecalith; absent bowel gas pattern in RLQ with otherwise normal gas pattern (nonspecific); loss of psoas shadow; splinting; "sentinel loop"; free gas (perforation).
- **Ultrasound:** May see enlarged appendix or appendiceal abscess; helps rule out gynecologic abnormality (but studies show that U/S is less reliable in female patients).

## Treatment

The treatment of suspected acute appendicitis is early appendectomy (also NPO, IV fluids, and NG suction if indicated). Open appendectomy via RLQ incision is standard, but laparoscopic procedures are becoming more common, in part as a result of shorter hospital stays and decreased postoperative complication rates. Laparoscopy has the additional benefit of allowing definitive diagnosis to rule out gynecologic diseases or other processes before the appendix is resected ("diagnostic laparoscopy"). Normal appendices are removed approximately 20% of the time (this rate is higher in women due to gynecologic disease); it is classically accepted that negative "appy" rates below 20% mean that the surgeon is missing cases of true appendicitis. Given the lack of reliable diagnostic criteria in this potentially life-threatening disease, a high rate of "unnecessary" interventions is deemed acceptable.

Treatment of a walled-off periappendiceal abscess may be achieved through conservative therapy that includes broad-spectrum antibiotics, expectant management, and U/S- or CT-guided percutaneous abscess drainage. An elective appendectomy should be done 6–8 weeks after the acute episode has resolved ("interval appendectomy").

## ACUTE PANCREATITIS

Acute pancreatitis is an acute eruption of pancreatic inflammation that is characterized by severe abdominal pain, nausea and vomiting, electrolyte and acid–base abnormalities, and, in some fulminant cases, hemorrhage, sepsis, and respiratory failure. Recurrent alcoholic pancreatitis has a predilection for progressing to chronic pancreatitis associated with chronic pancreatic exocrine and endocrine insufficiency, which are manifested as malabsorption and diabetes, respectively.

### Etiology

- **Alcohol (40%):** Possible etiologies include increased pancreatic ductal pressure or ethanol-induced increased ductal permeability via toxic metabolites.
- **Gallstones (40%):** Obstruction of the pancreatic ductal system by an impacted stone (see Figure 5).
- Trauma (including iatrogenic trauma from ERCP).
- Drugs (eg, didanosine, steroids, estrogens, thiazides, azathioprine).
- Hypercalcemia.

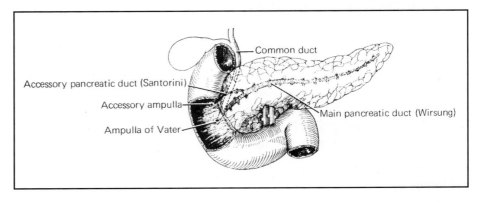

**FIGURE 5.** Anatomy of pancreatic ductal system. Way, *Current Surgical Diagnosis & Treatment*, Tenth Edition, Stamford, CT: Appleton & Lange, 1994, page 568.

- Hyperlipidemia.
- Familial pancreatitis.
- Idiopathic.

## Signs and Symptoms

- **Abdominal pain:** Acute, severe "boring" epigastric pain, often radiating to the back (90%).
- Nausea/vomiting.
- **Dehydration:** Severe hypovolemia with tachycardia, hypotension, shock.
- Fever.
- Abdominal tenderness, epigastric mass (pseudocyst, abscess, phlegmon).
- **Grey-Turner's sign:** Ecchymotic discoloration of flank from pancreatic hemorrhage (1–2%).
- **Cullen's sign:** Ecchymosis of the periumbilical area from hemorrhage (1–3%).
- **Chvostek's sign:** Facial spasm from tapping cheek over facial nerve (hypocalcemia).
- **Dullness over left lower lung:** Pleural effusion.

## Differential

Ruptured abdominal aortic aneurysm, perforated peptic ulcer, acute appendicitis, acute cholecystitis, myocardial infarction, mesenteric ischemia, small bowel obstruction, nephrolithiasis, pyelonephritis, hepatitis.

## Workup

- Amylase (increased in > 90%), lipase (increased; more specific but less sensitive), CBC (moderate leukocytosis), electrolytes, glucose, BUN, Cr, $Ca^{2+}$ (decreased if severe), LFTs, PT/PTT, ABG (may see respiratory failure in severe cases).
- **CXR:** May show basilar atelectasis, left pleural effusion.
- **Three-way abdominal x-rays:** May see "sentinel loop" or "colon cutoff" signs suggestive of peripancreatic inflammation; ileus may be present; pancreatic calcifications (chronic pancreatitis).
- **Abdominal CT (study of choice):** Evaluate for peripancreatic fluid, phlegmon, pancreatic calcifications, pseudocysts (see Figure 6). Up to 15% of CTs may appear normal despite the correct diagnosis of pancreatitis.

## Treatment

The treatment of acute pancreatitis may be operative or nonoperative depending on the severity of disease and on the presence of operable complications such as hemorrhage, pancreatic necrosis, or pseudocyst formation.

**Nonoperative management:**

- Fluid and electrolyte repletion; monitor $Ca^{++}$ and $Mg^{++}$.
- NPO; consider nasogastric intubation for emesis.

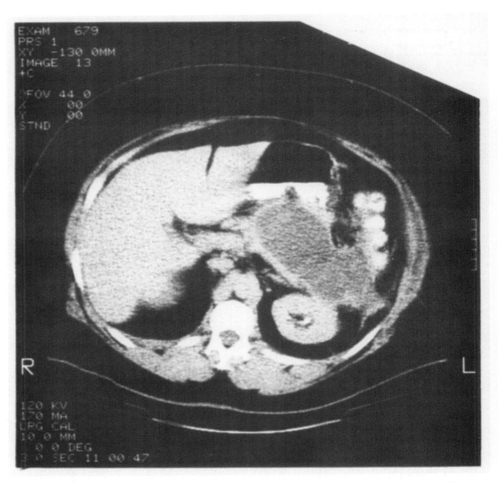

**FIGURE 6.** Pancreatic pseudocyst, shown here on CT scan, is a possible complication of acute pancreatitis. Way, *Current Surgical Diagnosis & Treatment,* Tenth Edition, Stamford, CT: Appleton & Lange, 1994, page 578.

- **Pain control:** Classical teaching—use Demerol to minimize sphincter of Oddi spasm.
- Respiratory monitoring and support as necessary.
- **Nutrition:** May require TPN if patient is to be NPO for more than several days.
- Alcohol-withdrawal prophylaxis.
- No benefit of antibiotics except in cases of pancreatic sepsis/abscess.

**Operative management:**

- Surgical debridement of pancreatic necrosis.
- Operative internal drainage of pseudocysts via cystogastrostomy, cystojejunostomy, or cystoduodenostomy (not usually performed in the acute setting).
- Operation to control pancreatic hemorrhage.
- Diagnostic laparotomy in cases of uncertainty.
- Cholecystectomy for gallstone pancreatitis (usually after pancreatitis has resolved; done with an evaluation of the biliary tree).

## Complications

The death rate for acute pancreatitis is 10–15%, with a worsening prognosis for increasing Ranson's criteria or coexistent hemorrhage, respiratory failure,

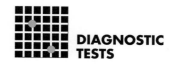

## RANSON'S CRITERIA

Risk of mortality is 20% with 3–4 signs; 40% with 5–6 signs; 100% with 7 or more signs.

| **On admission:** | **Developing during initial 24–48 hours:** |
|---|---|
| Age > 55 years | Hematocrit fall > 10% |
| WBC > 16,000/mL | BUN rise > 5 mg/dL |
| SGOT (AST) > 250 IU/dL | Serum $Ca^{2+}$ < 8 mg/dL |
| Serum LDH > 350 IU/L | Arterial $pO_2$ < 60 mmHg |
| Blood glucose > 200 mg/dL | Estimated fluid sequestration > 6 L |
| Base deficit > 4 mEq/L | |

or severe persistent hypocalcemia. Pseudocysts develop in about 2–4% of cases and are initially managed nonoperatively (expectant therapy), since 40% resolve spontaneously. Pseudocysts that are drained surgically have about a 10% recurrence.

You will be pimped on Ranson's criteria.

## GALLSTONE DISEASE

The three major processes you should be aware of are:

1. **Biliary colic:** Transient obstruction of the cystic duct without acute inflammation or infection, causing recurrent bouts of postprandial abdominal pain (see Figure 7).

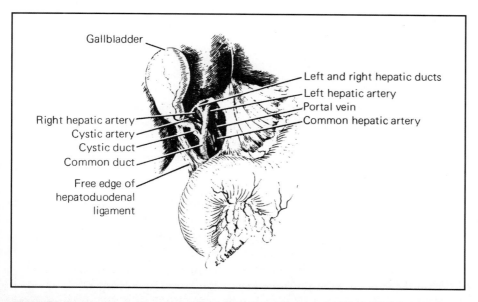

**FIGURE 7.** Anatomy of a gallbladder. Way, *Current Surgical Diagnosis & Treatment*, Tenth Edition, Stamford, CT: Appleton & Lange, 1994, page 539.

2. **Acute cholecystitis:** Acute inflammatory eruption of the gallbladder caused by protracted stone impaction in the cystic duct, which may be accompanied by sepsis, gallbladder necrosis, or abscess formation.

3. **Acute cholangitis:** A severe life-threatening disease caused by gallstone or biliary sludge blockage of the common bile duct, often resulting in severe septic shock if not treated early.

Gallstone pancreatitis is also of extreme importance but is covered in the section on acute pancreatitis.

## CHOLELITHIASIS AND BILIARY COLIC

Gallstones may be asymptomatic in up to 80% of patients. Symptoms are due to transient cystic duct blockage from impacted stones.

### Signs and Symptoms

- Postprandial abdominal pain (usually RUQ) radiating to right subscapular area or epigastrium, abrupt onset with gradual relief.
- Nausea and vomiting.
- Fatty food intolerance, dyspepsia, flatulence.
- May have RUQ tenderness and palpable gallbladder.

### Differential

Acute cholecystitis, peptic ulcer disease, myocardial infarction, acute pancreatitis, gastroesophageal reflux disease, and hepatitis.

### Workup

- RUQ ultrasound may show gallstones (95% sensitive): Has replaced oral cholecystography—radiopaque substance concentrated in biliary system.
- EKG and CXR to rule out cardiopulmonary processes.
- Consider upper GI series to rule out hiatal hernia or ulcer.

### Treatment

- Dietary modification (avoid triggering substances like fatty foods).
- Pharmacologic dissolution of cholesterol stones with ursodiol (desat-

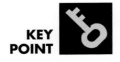
**KEY POINT**

### ESSENTIALS OF GALLSTONES

- Stone formation requires (1) imbalance of the ratio of cholesterol/lecithin/bile salts; (2) nucleating nidus; and (3) stasis.
- Cholesterol stones (75% stones) risk factors: Female, overweight, fertile, forty years old, flatulent. Radiolucent.
- Pigmented stones: Hyperbilirubinemia due to hemolysis, also parasites. May have gram-negative bacteria in core. Radiopaque.
- Only approximately 15% of gallstones are visible on KUB.

urates the bile-impairing nidus formation); effective in only approximately 50% of patients; frequent recurrence.
- Lithotripsy and dissolution: Extracorporeal shock waves to break up stones, followed by dissolution therapy on the small fragments.
- Cholecystectomy (usually laparoscopic): Definitive and curative.

## ACUTE CHOLECYSTITIS

Acute cholecystitis is usually caused by prolonged blockage of the cystic duct by an impacted stone, resulting in postobstructive distention, inflammation, superinfection, and, in extreme cases, gangrene of the gallbladder. Some cases of acute cholecystitis occur in the absence of cholelithiasis (known as acalculous cholecystitis; often seen in chronically debilitated patients, those on TPN, trauma or burn victims, etc).

### Signs and Symptoms

- RUQ pain, nausea and vomiting similar to biliary colic but typically more severe and of longer duration.
- Fever.
- RUQ tenderness; Murphy's sign (inspiratory arrest during deep palpation of RUQ); may have guarding or rebound.
- May have mild icterus.

### Differential

Biliary colic, cholangitis, gastroesophageal reflux disease, hepatitis, acute pancreatitis, myocardial infarction, acute appendicitis, renal colic, Fitz-Hugh-Curtis syndrome (acute gonococcal perihepatitis), peptic ulcer disease, pneumonia, and hepatitis.

### Workup

- Leukocytosis (12,000–15,000).
- Mild hyperbilirubinemia (2–4 mg/dL) or hyperamylasemia is common; mild increase in alkaline phosphatase.
- Ultrasound shows stones, bile sludge, pericholecystic fluid, and/or thickened gallbladder wall.
- HIDA scan when ultrasound equivocal; failure of the gallbladder to image *implies* acute cholecystitis.

Ultrasound is the gold standard for gallstones; HIDA scan is the gold standard for cholecystitis.

### Treatment

- IV antibiotics, IV fluids with electrolyte correction.
- Early cholecystectomy (within 72 hours of onset of symptoms) in patients without significant operative risk factors. Should be accompanied by intraoperative cholangiogram to rule out common bile duct stones.
- Expectant approach for patients with significant medical problems. Since 50% of cases resolve spontaneously, these patients can be

treated medically (as long as there is no deterioration of condition) until resolution of acute inflammation, with a 4- to 6-week delay of operation.

## Complications

Progression of acute cholecystitis may result in gallbladder gangrene, empyema, perforation, fistulization, sepsis, or abscess formation (seen in 15–20%).

## ACUTE CHOLANGITIS

Acute cholangitis is a bacterial infection of the biliary duct system that is caused by obstruction of the common bile duct by stones, strictures, or neoplasms.

### Signs and Symptoms

- **Charcot's triad:** RUQ pain, fever/chills, jaundice (complete triad present in 70% of patients).
- **Reynold's pentad:** Charcot's triad plus shock and altered mental status.

### Differential

Acute cholecystitis, acute pancreatitis/pancreatic sepsis, and acute hepatitis.

### Workup

- Ultrasound may show dilated ducts or stones.
- Blood cultures: Positive in about 50% of cases.
- May have elevated WBC, hyperamylasemia, elevated alkaline phosphatase, elevated transaminases, or increased GGT.

### Treatment

- IV antibiotics and aggressive IV fluid management. Most patients require admission to an ICU or step-down unit.
- Patients with acute toxic cholangitis require emergent bile duct decompression via endoscopic sphincterotomy, percutaneous transhepatic drainage, or operative decompression.
- After acute episode has been managed in routine cases, PTC (percutaneous transhepatic cholangiography) or ERCP (endoscopic retrograde cholangiopancreatography) should be performed to locate the cause of obstruction and possibly treat with stone extraction, stent placement, or sphincterotomy.

## GASTROESOPHAGEAL REFLUX DISEASE

Hiatal hernia is present in 80% of patients with gastroesophageal reflux disease (GERD). There are two types of hiatal hernias:

- **Type I:** Sliding hiatal hernia (90%). The gastroesophageal junction and fundus of the stomach are displaced into the posterior mediastinum.
- **Type II:** Paraesophageal hernia (< 10%). The fundus herniates alongside the esophagus, while the gastroesophageal junction remains in normal position. Incarceration and strangulation are common complications, so surgical repair should be performed.

## Signs and Symptoms

- **Heartburn:** Retrosternal and epigastric burning pain; usually postprandial, especially on recumbency; may be relieved with fluids, antacids, sitting, or standing.
- **Water brash:** Sour-tasting, rancid fluid regurgitated into the throat and mouth.
- **Dyspepsia, eructation:** Secondary to weakened sphincter and impaired motility.
- **Wheezing (especially nocturnal):** Due to aspiration of refluxed material.
- Little clinical evidence on exam.

## Differential

Myocardial infarction, angina pectoris, gallstone disease, acute pancreatitis, peptic ulcer disease, asthma, achalasia, and esophageal carcinoma.

## Workup

- **Barium swallow:** Demonstrates herniation and filling defects of esophagitis as well as stricture.
- **Esophageal manometry:** Measures mean LES pressure (decreased) and patterns of esophageal peristaltic contractions.
- **Esophageal pH monitoring:** Best method for diagnosing reflux and assessing severity; can measure percentage of total time with low esophageal pH, number of episodes of reflux, duration of episodes, etc.
- **EGD:** Demonstrates esophagitis, allows tissue biopsy (to rule out Barrett's).

## Treatment

- **Behavioral and dietary modifications:** Head-of-bed elevation, avoiding food before sleeping, frequent small meals, and avoiding substances which decrease LES pressure (EtOH, tobacco, tranquilizers, anticholinergics).
- **Pharmacotherapy:** Empiric therapy with over-the-counter antacids, H$_2$ blockers (ranitidine, famotidine) used for 8–10 weeks, followed by omeprazole if refractory. Prokinetic drugs (cisapride, metoclopramide) may be useful as well.
- **Surgery:** Indications include failure of medical therapy, severe esophagitis (ulceration, strictures, hemorrhage), and aspiration. Goal is to restore LES pressure and reduce hernia.

GERD can masquerade as angina or asthma.

- **Nissen fundoplication:** Gastric fundus is wrapped concentrically around GE junction. Can be done laparoscopically.
- **Hill procedure:** Posterior cardia is anchored to median arcuate ligament overlying aorta.
- **Belsey procedure:** Exaggerated gastroesophageal angle in stomach is anchored below diaphragm.
- **Angelchick prosthesis:** A prosthetic ring is wrapped around the esophagus below the diaphragm (no longer used due to ring migration).

## Complications

- Esophagitis leading to stricture formation.
- Aspiration pneumonia.
- Barrett's esophagus: Leads to adenocarcinoma in 15% of cases.

## PEPTIC ULCER DISEASE

**Duodenal ulcer essentials:**

- Usually within 2 cm of pylorus, ages 20–45.
- *Helicobacter pylori* colonization in 95% of cases.
- Risk factors: Tobacco, EtOH, NSAIDs, steroids, caffeine.
- Epigastric pain (gnawing, burning) occurring 1.5–3 hours after eating and late at night; relieved by antacids, food, and milk.
- Variable nausea, vomiting, and anorexia.
- Epigastric tenderness on exam.

**Gastric ulcer essentials:**

- Ninety percent on lesser curvature, ages 40–60.
- *H. pylori* colonization in 65% of cases, about one-third caused by NSAIDs, same risk factors.
- Epigastric pain may be worsened by food; commonly asymptomatic.
- Nausea and vomiting common.

## Differential

Gastroesophageal reflux disease, gallstone disease, acute/chronic pancreatitis, gastric adenocarcinoma, and angina.

## Workup

- **Stool occult blood.**
- **Endoscopy:** EGD has an accuracy exceeding 96% in the diagnosis of ulcers and allows for the biopsy of gastric lesions to rule out malignancy (5–10% gastric ulcers) and *H. pylori* infection.
- **Upper GI series:** May show filling defects characteristic of duodenal ulcer, evidence of duodenal bulb deformity, or radiographic signs of gastric lesions.
- **Gastric analysis:** Measures baseline acid output and maximal output after stimulation (pentagastrin or histamine); abnormal levels indicate hypersecretory state (40% of duodenal ulcers).

- **Serum gastrin:** If elevated in the setting of a hypersecretory state, suggestive of Zollinger-Ellison syndrome (gastrinoma).

## Treatment

**Medical management:**

- Eliminate tobacco, EtOH, caffeine, NSAIDs, steroids.
- Antacids, H$_2$ blockers, proton-pump inhibitor (if refractory to H$_2$ blocker).
- *H. pylori* eradication with triple therapy (bismuth, metronidazole, tetracycline).

**Surgical indications:**
- Perforation (acute-onset abdominal pain, peritoneal signs, free air under diaphragm on x-ray).
- Obstruction (postprandial emesis and increased pain, succussion splash, metabolic alkalosis).
- Hemorrhage.
- Intractable pain.
- Medical failure (after 12 weeks of compliance with treatment).

**Surgical management (see Figure 8):**
- **Duodenal ulcer:**
  - Vagotomy
    - Truncal vagotomy requires drainage procedure to prevent delayed gastric emptying via pyloroplasty or gastrojejunostomy (Billroth II); 10% recurrence.
    - Selective vagotomy spares biliary tree innervation to prevent stasis but requires drainage procedure.
    - Highly selective vagotomy (parietal cell vagotomy) does not require drainage procedure; 15% recurrence.
  - Antrectomy and vagotomy with Billroth I (gastroduodenostomy) or Billroth II; 2% recurrence.
- **Gastric ulcer:** Excision of ulcer with drainage procedure; 5% recurrence.

## Complications

Recurrent (marginal) ulcer at distal side of new anastomosis; dumping syndrome (recurrent postprandial episodes of sympathetic overload, nausea/vomiting, abdominal cramping, diarrhea); fistulization; diarrhea; alkaline reflux/bile gastritis; gastric remnant carcinoma; postsurgical gastroparesis; and afferent loop syndrome.

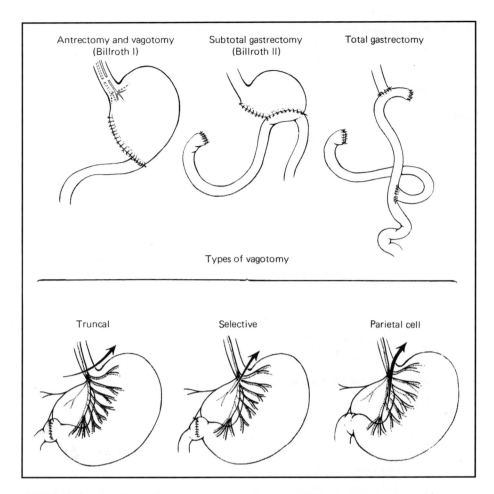

**FIGURE 8.** Surgical options for peptic ulcer disease. Total gastrectomy is reserved for Zollinger-Ellison syndrome. Do not attempt this at home. Way, *Current Surgical Diagnosis & Treatment,* Tenth Edition, Stamford, CT: Appleton & Lange, 1994, page 480.

## INFLAMMATORY BOWEL DISEASE

Inflammatory bowel disease (IBD) is a catchphrase for several chronic, often progressive inflammatory disease processes that affect the small bowel, colon, and rectum to varying degrees. The two principal disorders, Crohn's disease and ulcerative colitis, differ in their histologic and clinical manifestations, their natural course, and their modes of therapy.

### CROHN'S DISEASE (REGIONAL ENTERITIS)

Crohn's disease is a chronic, progressive granulomatous disease of the GI tract. Its peak incidence occurs between the ages of 20 and 40. Crohn's disease is characterized by:

- *Segmental* involvement ("skip lesions") from the mouth to the anus, most commonly at the distal ileum and cecum.
- *Transmural* involvement of the bowel wall with stricture formation.
- Cobblestone mucosa, creeping mesenteric fat, fissures, linear ulcers, and granulomas.

## Signs and Symptoms

- Diarrhea (usually nonbloody).
- Recurrent abdominal pain.
- Anorectal lesions (fissures, fistulae).
- Malnutrition, weight loss.
- Extraintestinal manifestations: polyarticular arthritis, uveitis, stomatitis, erythema nodosum, pyoderma, cutaneous ulcers, and hepatobiliary disease.

## Differential

Ulcerative colitis, acute appendicitis, TB, lymphoma, and diverticular disease.

## Workup

- **Lab studies:** Anemia (B$_{12}$, folate, iron deficiency), hypoalbuminemia, abnormal D-xylose test.
- **Barium enema:** Strictures ("string sign"), cobblestones, transverse fissures (see Figure 9).
- **Sigmoidoscopy:** Patchy involvement, mucosal ulceration, cobblestoning, fissures.

## Treatment

**Medical management:** Supportive care, including NPO, IV fluids, and TPN for severe flareups. Steroids, sulfasalazine (for acute flareups), azathioprine, 6-mercaptopurine, and metronidazole are also useful.

> Look for extraintestinal manifestations in suspected IBD.

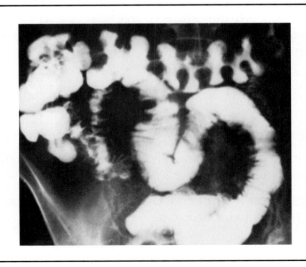

**FIGURE 9.** Crohn's disease on barium x-ray showing spicules, edema, and ulcers. Way, *Current Surgical Diagnosis & Treatment*, Tenth Edition, Stamford, CT: Appleton & Lange, 1994, page 630.

**Operative management**: Multiple surgeries are often required, and resections are *noncurative* (50% recurrence rate); therefore, surgery should be avoided at all costs.

- Indications include obstruction, fistula, abscess, and intractable disease.
- Consider stricturoplasty or bypass when possible.

## ULCERATIVE COLITIS

Ulcerative colitis is a chronic inflammatory disease of the rectum and colon. It exhibits a bimodal age distribution—15–30 and 50–70—and is more prevalent in Ashkenazi Jews. It generally begins in the rectum with *continuous* proximal progression, nontransmural inflammation, and pseudopolyps.

### Signs and Symptoms

- Diarrhea (usually bloody).
- Abdominal pain, tenesmus, and rectal urgency.
- Fever, weight loss, and growth retardation.
- Extraintestinal manifestations similar to Crohn's.
- Complications include toxic megacolon, increased risk of colon cancer, and primary sclerosing cholangitis.

### Differential

Crohn's disease, colorectal carcinoma, diverticulitis, infectious enterocolitis, and ischemic colitis.

### Workup

- Anemia, leukocytosis, increased ESR, hypoalbuminemia, and fluid/electrolyte abnormalities.
- Bacterial stool cultures to rule out infectious etiology.
- **Barium enema:** Contiguous mucosal irregularity, multiple small ulcers, pseudopolyp filling defects, and "lead pipe" colon.
- **Sigmoidoscopy:** Friable, edematous, and hyperemic mucosa in a contiguous pattern.

### Treatment

**Medical management:** Maintenance on sulfasalazine (prolongs remission).

- Supportive care, including NPO, IV fluids, NG suction, IV steroids, antibiotics, and TPN.

**Surgical management:** Indications include massive hemorrhage, toxic megacolon, colorectal CA, and obstruction.

- Colectomy with ileoanal anastomosis and ileal pouch.
- Proctocolectomy with ileostomy is *curative* (but patients with ileostomy have a high incidence of impotence and bladder dysfunction).

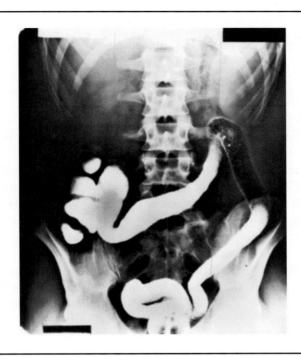

**FIGURE 10.** Ulcerative colitis on barium enema x-ray of colon. Note shortened colon, "lead pipe" appearance due to loss of haustral markings, and fine serrations at the edge of the bowel wall that represent multiple small ulcers. Way, *Current Surgical Diagnosis & Treatment,* Tenth Edition, Stamford, CT: Appleton & Lange, 1994, page 679.

## UPPER GASTROINTESTINAL BLEEDING (UGIB)

### Signs and Symptoms

- History of PUD, prior GI bleeds, NSAID use, EtOH use, liver disease, varices, severe vomiting/retching, anticoagulants, bleeding disorder, and steroids.
- **Hematemesis:** Vomiting bright red blood or coffee-ground emesis (blood exposed to gastric acid); usually from a source proximal to the ligament of Treitz.
- **Hematochezia:** Bright red blood per rectum (BRBPR); 80% from a source distal to the ligament of Treitz, 20% proximal.
- **Melena:** From an upper GI source. Black, tarry stools; usually from a source proximal to the ligament of Treitz.
- Dehydration (pallor, tachycardia, orthostasis) or hypovolemic shock.

### Differential

- Ninety percent of cases are caused by one of the following: peptic ulcer disease, gastritis, esophageal varices, esophagitis, or Mallory-Weiss tear (gastroesophageal junction tear following violent vomiting or retching).
- Also consider cancer, splenic vein thrombosis, nasopharyngeal bleeding, and hemoptysis.

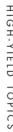

### Workup

Because of the potential acuity of GI bleeding, the workup occurs with treatment.

### Treatment

**Resuscitation:**
- **Two large-bore IVs:** First resuscitate with lactated Ringer's (2 L) and follow by PRBC until stable.
- **Type and cross** 6 units of blood, HCT, chem 7, LFTs, PT/PTT (initial HCT lags behind actual blood loss in the acute setting).
- **Assess magnitude of hemorrhage:** Vitals, serial HCTs, determine if patient is actively bleeding.
- Correct coagulopathy with FFP/vitamin K if necessary.

**Bleeding site:** Is it above or below the ligament of Treitz?
- **NG tube:** If bright red blood or coffee grounds, then saline lavage to remove blood clots until clear fluid returns. Bilious fluid without blood indicates that the source is likely distal to the ligament of Treitz.

**Localize bleeding source (after hemodynamic stabilization):**
- **Endoscopy:** Identify site; sclerotherapy of varices; coagulation of bleeding vessels.
- **Angiography:** Requires brisk bleeding (> 0.5 cc/min); selective sclerotherapy or embolization.

**Control bleeding:**
- **Sclerotherapy** or **embolization** during localization procedure.
- **Vasopressin** with nitroglycerin to reduce risk of MI (vasopressin decreases cardiac output and causes coronary constriction). Somatostatin/octreotide are as efficacious but have fewer side effects.
- **Balloon tamponade** for refractory variceal hemorrhage (Sengstaken-Blakemore tube).

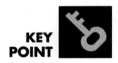

**KEY POINT**

---

### SURGICAL INDICATIONS

- **PUD:** Patients who require 6 or more units of blood in first 24 hours, or who rebleed on maximal medical therapy.
- **Esophageal varices:** Primary therapy is sclerosis with vasopressin or octreotide. If bleeding continues despite medical measures, consider:
  - TIPS (transjugular intrahepatic portosystemic shunt): Interventional radiology procedure in which a stent is passed via the jugular vein and IVC to bridge the liver into the portal venous system and decompress portal hypertension.
- Selective and nonselective portosystemic shunts.

---

## LOWER GASTROINTESTINAL BLEEDING

### Signs and Symptoms

- History of change in bowel habits, change in stool caliber, abdominal pain.

- History of hemorrhoids, PUD, prior bleeds, diverticulosis, IBD, liver disease, NSAID use, anticoagulants, and steroids.
- Hematochezia or melena.

## Differential

- **Acute:** Angiodysplasia (AVM), diverticular disease, inflammatory bowel disease, upper GI bleed (20%), ischemic colitis.
- **Chronic:** Colorectal cancer, hemorrhoids, and fissures.

## Workup

The workup occurs with treatment.

## Treatment

**Resuscitation:** Same as UGIB.

- Bleeding stops *spontaneously* after 2 units transfusion in 90% of cases.

**Bleeding site**: Is it above or below the ligament of Treitz?

- NG tube to look for blood vs. bile. If bloody, then go to endoscopy.
- Digital rectal exam, anoscopy, sigmoidoscopy to rule out hemorrhoids or polyps.

**Localize bleeding source (may be difficult):**

- Colonoscopy.
- Technetium-labeled RBC scan: Sensitive for slow bleeds, but less specific than angiography.
- Angiography: Requires brisk bleeding (> 0.5 cc/min).

**Control bleeding:**

- Diverticulosis and angiodysplasia usually stop spontaneously with transfusions and supportive therapy.
- Vasopressin injection during angiography.

**Surgical indications:**

- Persistent bleeding despite angiographic or endoscopic therapy.
- Segmental colectomy if bleeding site is well localized.
- If unable to localize site, consider total colectomy with ileorectal anastomosis, or a temporary ileostomy and a Hartmann pouch (distal rectal stump sutured closed).

## SMALL BOWEL OBSTRUCTION

### Etiology

- Adhesions (60%) from prior surgery
- Neoplasm (10–20%)
- External hernia (10–20%)
- Stricture from IBD
- Intussusception
- Gallstone ileus
- Foreign body

### Signs and Symptoms

- **Cramping abdominal pain:** Recurrent crescendo-decrescendo pattern at intervals of 5–10 minutes (see Figure 11).
- **Vomiting:** Early and nonfeculent in proximal obstruction. Follows

pain and becomes feculent in distal obstruction (feculence is from secondary bacterial overgrowth, not emesis of feces).
- Obstipation
  - **Complete obstruction:** No flatus or stool passed.
  - **Partial obstruction:** Continued passage of flatus.
- Fever (especially in strangulation), hypotension, and tachycardia (dehydration).
- Shock = strangulation.
- Abdominal distention, tenderness, prior surgical scars, hernias.
- **Bowel sounds:** High-pitched tinkles and peristaltic rushes.

### Differential

- Adynamic ileus.
- Large bowel obstruction: Cancer (65%), diverticulitis (20%), and volvulus (5%).
- Acute appendicitis (*always* near the top of your differential for an acute abdomen).
- Inflammatory bowel disease.
- Mesenteric ischemia.
- Renal colic/pyelonephritis.
- Metabolic causes of acute abdomen.

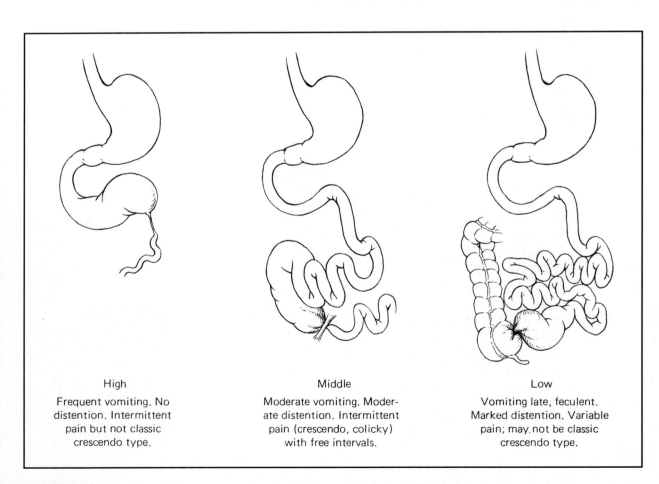

| High | Middle | Low |
|---|---|---|
| Frequent vomiting. No distention. Intermittent pain but not classic crescendo type. | Moderate vomiting. Moderate distention. Intermittent pain (crescendo, colicky) with free intervals. | Vomiting late, feculent. Marked distention. Variable pain; may not be classic crescendo type. |

**FIGURE 11.** Small bowel obstruction. Signs and symptoms vary with the level of blockage. Way, *Current Surgical Diagnosis & Treatment,* Tenth Edition, Stamford, CT: Appleton & Lange, 1994, page 625.

## Workup

- CBC (leukocytosis = strangulation), electrolytes (reflect dehydration [decreased K⁺ and Na⁺] and metabolic alkalosis due to vomiting), and increased amylase.
- Abdominal films: Stepladder pattern of dilated small-bowel loops and air/fluid levels (see Figure 12); may see absent colon gas pattern; gallstones sometimes visible; can distinguish large bowel obstruction (volvulus).

## Treatment

**Medical management:** Supportive care may be sufficient to treat partial SBO.

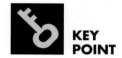

**KEY POINT**

---

### STRANGULATED VS. NONSTRANGULATED SBO

Nonstrangulated SBO carries a total mortality of about 2%, while the risk of death from strangulated SBO increases in proportion to time from diagnosis to operative therapy, with a peak of about 25%. A second-look laparotomy or laparoscopy may be performed 18–36 hours later for reevaluation of bowel viability.

---

- NPO, NG suction (decompression), IV hydration, correction of electrolyte abnormalities.

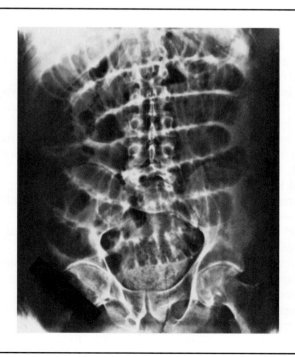

**FIGURE 12.** Small bowel obstruction of supine abdominal x-ray. Note dilated loops of small bowel in a ladder-like pattern. You might see air-fluid levels if upright x-ray done. Way, *Current Surgical Diagnosis & Treatment,* Tenth Edition, Stamford, CT: Appleton & Lange, 1994, page 626.

"Never let the sun rise or set on a bowel obstruction."

**Surgical management:**

- Exploratory laparotomy with lysis of adhesions and resection of necrotic bowel (if any) as well as a bowel run with evaluation for stricture, inflammatory bowel, and hernial sac.
- Perioperative antibiotics.

## HERNIAS

Hernia is the leading surgical disease in men and is 8–9 times more common in males than in females. A hernia is defined as an abnormal protrusion of a structure through the tissues that normally contain it.

**CLINICAL ANATOMY**

---

### KEY ANATOMY AND DEFINITIONS FOR HERNIAS

- **Layers of abdominal wall:** Skin, subcutaneous fat, Scarpa's fascia, external oblique, internal oblique, transversus abdominis, transversalis fascia, and peritoneum.
- **Inguinal (Poupart's) ligament:** Thickened lower border of the aponeurosis of the external oblique; runs from the anterior superior iliac spine to the pubic tubercle.
- **Inferior epigastric artery:** Branch of the external iliac; supplies lower part of abdominal wall.
- **Hesselbach's triangle:** Formed by the inguinal ligament inferiorly, the lateral border of rectus abdominis medially, and the inferior epigastric vessels laterally.
- **Superficial (external) inguinal ring:** Hole in the external oblique through which the spermatic cord or round ligament passes en route to the scrotum/labia majora; direct hernias pass directly through the transversalis fascia.
- **Deep (internal) inguinal ring:** Defect in the transversalis fascia lateral to Hesselbach's triangle through which the spermatic cord emerges from the peritoneal cavity; indirect hernias pass through both rings en route to the scrotum.
- **Direct inguinal hernia:** Acquired defect in the floor of Hesselbach's triangle (transversalis fascia).
- **Indirect inguinal hernia:** Congenital patent processus vaginalis with passage of the hernial sac through the internal inguinal ring (most common hernia in either sex).
- **Femoral hernia:** Protrusion through the femoral canal medial to the femoral vein (85% in women, highest risk of incarceration and strangulation).
- **Umbilical hernia:** Usually congenital patent umbilical ring that obliterates spontaneously before age 2. Risk factors in adults include multiple pregnancies, ascites, obesity, and abdominal trauma.
- **Incisional hernia:** Risk factors include poor surgical technique, wound infection, age, and obesity.
- **Incarceration:** Hernia cannot be reduced by external manipulation.
- **Strangulation:** Compromise of blood supply to contents of an incarcerated hernia.
- **Sliding hernia:** One wall of the hernia sac is formed by a viscus (cecum or sigmoid).
- **Pantaloon hernia:** Combination of a direct and an indirect hernia.
- **Richter's hernia:** Only one wall of the viscus lies within the hernial sac.
- **Spigelian hernia:** Ventral hernia occurring at the semilunar line at the lateral edge of the rectus muscle.

## Treatment

The repair of an inguinal hernia involves correcting the defect in the transversalis fascia that allowed protrusion of the herniated bowel loop or omental segment. Many strategies exist; they differ in the structures sutured, the number of abdominal wall layers involved in closure, etc. In addition, hernias can be repaired laparoscopically. Some common open anterior repair techniques are:

- **High ligation of the hernia sac:** Repair of persistent processus vaginalis in indirect hernias (mostly in children); the hernia sac is sutured closed at its superior pole near the deep inguinal ring.
- **Bassini repair:** The conjoined tendon (transversalis abdominis and internal oblique) is approximated to the inguinal ligament. The Shouldice repair is a variant.
- **McVay repair:** The conjoined tendon is approximated to Cooper's ligament; requires a relaxing incision in the anterior rectus abdominis fascia to release excess tension on the closure.
- **Mesh (Lichtenstein) repair:** Marlex mesh is used to reinforce abdominal wall strength, often for ventral hernias.

Recurrence after repair of inguinal hernia occurs in 1–3% of patients; risk factors for recurrence include excessive suture line tension, use of absorbable suture, failure to properly identify the hernia sac, postop wound infection, and chronic conditions that increase intra-abdominal pressure, including constipation, morbid obesity, prostatism, and chronic cough.

# SHOCK

Shock is defined as a physiologic state of circulatory failure resulting in inadequate tissue perfusion and tissue hypoxia. Shock can be a consequence of pump failure, insufficient circulating blood volume, hypotension from inappropriately low systemic resistance, anaphylaxis, or overwhelming sepsis. The evaluation and management of the patient in acute shock involves assessment of volume status, systemic vascular resistance, and cardiac output (see Table 1).

## HYPOVOLEMIC SHOCK

Secondary to intravascular volume depletion, the most common cause of shock.

### Etiology

- Acute blood loss.
- Protracted diarrhea, vomiting.
- Third spacing (interstitial, intraperitoneal): Burns, trauma, and acute pancreatitis.

**Emergency maneuvers in shock:**
1. Trendelenburg position
2. Oxygen
3. IV fluid boluses
4. IV pressors

| Condition | Skin | Neck Veins |
|---|---|---|
| Hypovolemia | Cold, clammy | Flat |
| Cardiac compression | Cold, clammy | Distended[1] |
| Cardiogenic | Cold, clammy | Distended |
| Neurogenic | Warm[2] | Flat |
| High output sepsis | Warm | Flat to normal |
| Low output sepsis | Cold, clammy | Flat |
| Hypoglycemia | Cold, clammy | Flat to normal |
| Inebriation[3] | Warm | Normal |

**TABLE 1.** Clinical presentations of shock

[1]May be flat if patient is also hypovolemic.

[2]In denervated areas.

[3]Listed only to emphasize that alcohol can mask signs of other conditions.

## Signs and Symptoms

- **Mild** (10–20% volume loss): Patient feels cold, orthostatic hypotension, flat neck veins, pale and cool skin.
- **Moderate** (20–40% volume loss): Patient is thirsty, tachycardic/hypotensive, and oliguric.
- **Severe** (> 40% volume loss): Altered mental status (agitation leading to obtundation), severe hypotension, tachycardia, and tachypnea.
- Decreased CVP; increased systemic vascular resistance.

## Treatment

Restore intravascular volume (crystalloid/blood products via large-bore IVs) and treat the underlying cause.

## CARDIOGENIC SHOCK

Secondary to pump failure (decreased cardiac output).

## Etiology

- Arrhythmia.
- Myocardial infarction.
- Vascular disease.
- Obstructive: Pericardial tamponade, tension pneumothorax, positive pressure ventilation.
- Myocarditis/cardiomyopathy.

## Signs and Symptoms

- Tachycardia, hypotension, tachypnea.
- Distended neck veins, peripheral edema, third heart sound with rales.
- In tamponade, also see muffled heart sounds with pulsus paradoxus, hypotension, and JVD.
- In tension pneumothorax, also see decreased breath sounds, hyperresonant chest, and/or tracheal deviation.
- Increased CVP; increased pulmonary capillary wedge pressure; EKG abnormalities.

## Treatment

Further therapy should be directed at the underlying cause and toward maintaining adequate blood pressure. Start with fluid resuscitation. Consider inotropes (to increase contractility), chronotropes, vasodilators (to decrease preload and to decrease afterload, which leads to decreased myocardial work), and diuretics (to decrease preload). Other possible interventions include pericardiocentesis (tamponade), chest tube (tension pneumothorax), ventilator adjustment, intra-aortic balloon pump (increases CO, decreases afterload, and increases myocardial perfusion), and antiarrhythmics.

## SEPTIC SHOCK

Secondary to systemic effects of infection. Toxins from both gram-positive and gram-negative sepsis cause shock by vasodilation of the peripheral circulation and increased capillary permeability, leading to massive fluid loss into the tissue.

## Signs and Symptoms

- Early (hyperdynamic): Fever, tachycardia, hypotension in a warm and pink patient (vasodilation).
- Late (hypodynamic): Mimics hypovolemic shock (increased capillary permeability and impaired cellular $O_2$ utilization).
- Leukocytosis with left shift and lactic acidosis.

## Treatment

Identify and treat source of infection with IV antibiotics, surgical drainage, and central line changes. As in other forms of shock, the patient will require IV fluid resuscitation, monitoring of cardiac function, pressors, and/or intubation to maintain adequate oxygenation.

## NEUROGENIC SHOCK

Secondary to loss of vascular sympathetic tone.

## Etiology

- Spinal cord injury
- Spinal anesthesia

### Signs and Symptoms

- Hypotension, normal or slow pulse (no reflex tachycardia), warm, dry skin, and flat neck veins.
- Inability to wiggle toes, decreased rectal tone.
- Cardiac output and systemic vascular resistance are low.

### Treatment

- Rule out other etiologies of shock first.
- IV fluids, Trendelenburg, and vasoconstrictors.
- Steroids, if seen in association with spinal cord injury.

---

## BREAST CANCER

Risk factors include previous cancer in the contralateral breast; family history; age, nulliparity, or first pregnancy after age 35; early menarche (< age 12) or late menopause (> age 50); history of atypical hyperplasia; oral contraceptive use; and history of endometrial cancer.

### Signs and Symptoms

Presence of breast mass (usually does not change in size with menstrual cycle), tenderness, nipple discharge or retraction, changes in breast appearence/contour/symmetry.

Reinforce the importance of the breast self-exam to the patient.

### Differential

**Benign mass.** Regular, well circumscribed, mobile, changes in size with cycle, tender.

- **Fibrocystic change (most frequent breast lesion):** Painful (increased before menses), fluctuation in size, often multiple/bilateral.
- **Fibroadenoma:** Firm, round, mobile, nontender.
- **Intraductal papilloma:** Bloody nipple discharge.
- Lipoma.
- Breast abscess.
- Fat necrosis.

**Malignant mass.** Hard, irregular, fixed, nipple retraction, dimpling of skin, edema, lymphadenopathy (see Figure 13).

- **Ductal carcinoma:** Most common breast malignancy (80%).
- **Lobar carcinoma** (8–10%).
- **Paget's carcinoma:** Infiltrating ductal CA in nipple. Symptoms include itching/burning of nipple with superficial ulceration or erosion.
- **Inflammatory carcinoma:** Most malignant, poorly differentiated, rapidly lethal. Symptoms include diffuse induration, warmth, erythema, edema, axillary lymphadenopathy.

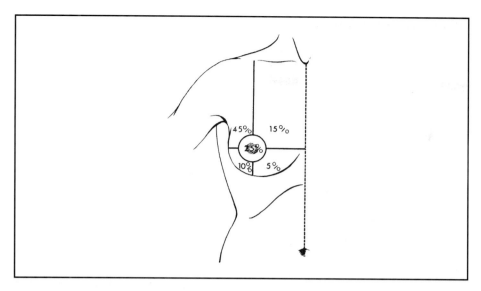

**FIGURE 13.** Frequency of breast cancer at various anatomic sites. Way, *Current Surgical Diagnosis & Treatment,* Tenth Edition, Stamford, CT: Appleton & Lange, 1994, page 297.

## Workup

- Fine needle aspiration (FNA) of palpable lump (10% false negative) and mammogram.
- Needle aspiration of palpable cystic lesion (with or without U/S guidance).
- Core needle biopsy for nondiagnostic FNA.
- Open excisional biopsy (with or without needle wire localization): Definitive, but most invasive.
- Ductography and cytology for nipple discharge.

Breast cancer is by far the most common type of cancer in women.

## Treatment

- **Modified radical mastectomy:** Total mastectomy with axillary node dissection (spares pectoralis).
- **Wide local excision (lumpectomy):** Complete excision of tumor with margins and axillary node dissection, followed by radiotherapy.
- **Adjuvant therapy** to eliminate micrometastases responsible for late recurrence.
  - **Pre- vs. postmenopausal:** Chemotherapy if premenopausal with nodes and estrogen-receptor positive.
  - **Estrogen-receptor positive versus negative:** Positive—use tamoxifen; negative—chemotherapy.
  - **Nodal involvement:** Positive nodes—use combination chemotherapy.

## COLORECTAL CANCER

Colorectal cancer is the second leading cause of cancer mortality in the U.S. after lung cancer, affecting approximately 150,000 new patients per year and

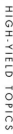

with an incidence increasing with age (peak incidence 70–80 years of age). Colorectal cancer accounts for 50,000–60,000 deaths per year.

## Signs and Symptoms

In the absence of screening, colorectal cancer typically presents symptomatically only after a prolonged period of silent growth (see Figure 14). Abdominal pain is the most common presenting complaint for all lesions.

**Right-sided lesions**: Often bulky, fungating, and ulcerating masses.
- Most commonly present as anemia from chronic occult blood loss.
- Patients may complain of weight loss, anorexia, weakness, or vague abdominal pain.
- Obstructive symptoms are rare (right colonic feces are fluid and cecal wall is distensible).

- **Left-sided lesions:** Typically "apple-core" or "napkin-ring" obstructing masses.
  - Typically present with alterations of bowel habits (decreasing stool caliber, constipation, or obstipation).
  - Blood-streaked stools (mild).
  - Obstruction (left colonic feces are more solid and the wall less distensible).

- **Rectal lesions:**
  - Usually present with bright red blood per rectum (BRBPR).
  - May have tenesmus, rectal pain.
  - Can coexist with hemorrhoids (must rule out rectal cancer in patients with rectal bleeding).

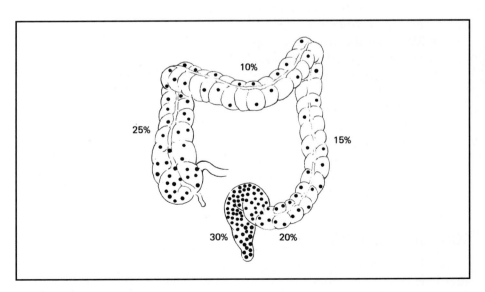

**FIGURE 14.** Distribution of cancer of the colon and rectum. Way, *Current Surgical Diagnosis & Treatment*, Tenth Edition, Stamford, CT: Appleton & Lange, 1994, page 654.

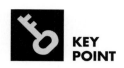
## RISK FACTORS AND SCREENING FOR COLORECTAL CANCER

**Risk Factors**

- Hereditary syndromes: Familial polyposis (100% risk), Gardner's, non-polyposis syndrome.
- Family history.
- Inflammatory bowel disease: Ulcerative colitis much more than Crohn's.
- Adenomatous polyps: Villous more than tubular; sessile more than pedunculated; greater than 2 cm increases risk.
- Past h/o colorectal cancer.
- High-fat, low-fiber diet.

**Screening**

- Digital rectal exam (DRE): Up to 10% of lesions are palpable with finger.
- Stool guaiac for occult blood (every year for patients age 55 and above): Up to 50% of positive guaiacs due to colorectal CA.
- Sigmoidoscopy: Can visualize and biopsy 50–75% of lesions.

## Differential

Inflammatory bowel disease, diverticulitis, ischemic colitis, hemorrhoids, peptic ulcer disease, and other intra-abdominal malignancies.

## Workup

- CBC (microcytic anemia), stool occult blood, carcinoembryonic antigen (CEA) baseline (nonspecific, but useful for follow-up after treatment and to screen for recurrence).
- **Sigmoidoscopy:** Biopsy all suspicious lesions.
- **Colonoscopy:** Visualize entire colon to rule out synchronous proximal lesions.
- **Barium enema (air contrast):** Rule out missed lesions after incomplete colonoscopy (see Figure 15).
- **Abdominal CT/MRI:** Staging.
- **Metastatic workup:** CXR, LFTs, and abdominal CT.
  - Hematogenous spread: Liver (40–50% of all patients), lungs, bone, brain.
  - Lymphatic spread: Pelvic lymph nodes (primary way for extension).
  - Direct extension: Local viscera.
  - Peritoneal spread.

## Treatment

- **Preoperative bowel prep:** Mechanical cleaning (eg, GoLytely), oral antibiotics.
- **Colonic lesions:** Surgical resection of lesion with bowel margins of 3–5 cm, along with lymphatic drainage and mesentery at origin of arterial supply. Primary anastamosis of bowel can usually be performed.

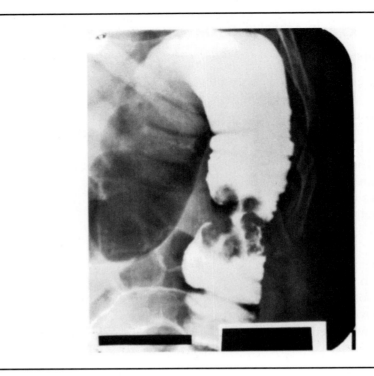

**FIGURE 15.** Barium enema x-ray showing classic "apple core" lesion of an encircling carcinoma in the descending colon. Note the loss of mucosal pattern, the "hooks" at the margins of the lesion due to undermining. Way, *Current Surgical Diagnosis & Treatment*, Tenth Edition, Stamford, CT: Appleton & Lange, 1994, page 658.

- Consider adjuvant chemo or radiotherapy, depending on stage.
- **Follow-up:** Serial carcinoembryonic antigen levels, colonoscopy, LFTs.
- **Rectal lesions:** Choice of resection depends on proximity to anal verge.
  - **Abdominoperineal resection:** For low-lying lesions near anal verge (remove rectum and anus; permanent colostomy).

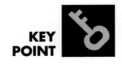

**KEY POINT**

| DUKES' STAGING (ASTLER-COLLER MODIFICATION) | | |
|---|---|---|
| | | **5-year survival** |
| A | Tumor limited to submucosa | >90% |
| B1 | Tumor invades into muscularis propria | 70–80% |
| B2 | Tumor invades **through** muscularis propria | 50–65% |
| C1 | B1 plus nodes | 40–55% |
| C2 | B2 plus nodes | 20–30% |
| D | Distant metastasis/unresectable local spread | Less than 5% |

- **Low anterior resection:** For proximal lesions (primary anastamosis of colon to rectum).
- **Wide local excision:** For small, low-stage, well-differentiated tumors in lower one-third of rectum.
- Ileoanal anastamosis (spares patient from having an abdominal ileostomy) and pouch procedures ("continent ileostomy") provide a reservoir to maintain fecal continence.

# Notes

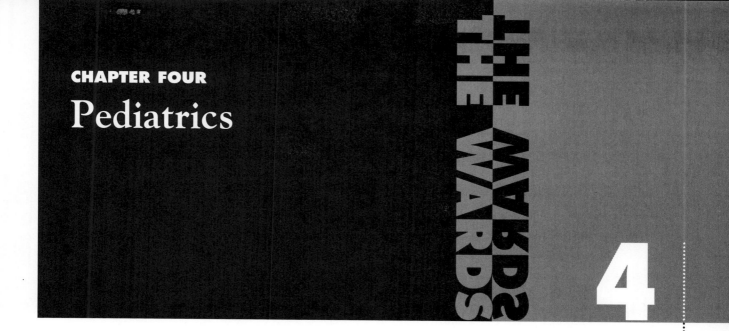

**CHAPTER FOUR**

# Pediatrics

**4**

# WARD TIPS

Welcome to pediatrics! The pediatric rotation is a 6- to 8-week block at most medical schools. This time is split between the inpatient ward and the outpatient setting. Traditionally, more time has been devoted to the inpatient service, but this may change with current reductions in hospital-based care. The outpatient portion of the rotation may be completed in a community pediatrician's office or in the outpatient service of the hospital. In addition, usually a week or less is devoted to the newborn service. The pediatric rotation emphasizes the care of the ill child as well as that of the healthy child.

## WHO ARE THE PLAYERS?

The ward team typically consists of an attending, 1–2 upper-level residents, 2–4 interns, and 1–4 medical students.

**Attendings.** The attending of a pediatric ward team may be a member of the general pediatric faculty or a member of one of the pediatric subspecialties. The attending is ultimately responsible for the patients. The attending generally rounds on a daily basis. This is your opportunity to formally present patients to someone who will be responsible for a large portion of your evaluation.

There is usually time devoted to didactics, so know your attending's area of interest, as he or she is likely to focus on that aspect during rounds.

**Residents.** The role of residents is to supervise the interns and the medical students. They are the ones who are responsible for most of the day-to-day teaching you will get on the service. Ask them to give you informal lectures and to show you interesting findings on the ward. Demonstrate your interest in doing procedures. Note that residents are also a good source of articles.

**Interns.** Interns are responsible for monitoring the daily progress of patients and for doing the grunt work. Needless to say, these people are busy—but you can help them along by following patients with them. Your daily progress note is a blessing to them. Discuss the patient's assessment and plan

**Your daily progress note is a blessing to the intern.**

with them, and make sure you understand the rationale behind all the orders you have written and tests you have ordered; this will also make you look more informed when you present to the residents and attending.

**Nurses, social workers, child life specialist, etc.** As on other services, these specialists are an invaluable source of information about your patients.

## HOW IS THE DAY SET UP?

The schedule of a typical day on the ward is as follows:

| | |
|---|---|
| 7:00–8:00 AM | Prerounds: check labs, check vitals, examine the patient |
| 8:00–9:00 AM | Team rounds |
| 9:00–10:00 AM | Attending rounds |
| 10:00 AM–12:00 NOON | Write progress note, order labs, etc |
| 12:00–1:00 PM | Lunch or lunch conference |
| 1:00–5:00 PM | Check afternoon labs, check out to the team members, etc |

## WHAT DO I DO DURING PREROUNDS?

Prerounding in pediatrics is similar to medicine except for a few variations. In general, children are not examined during prerounds if they are still sleeping. You may still wake the parents up to ask how their child is doing. Allow yourself some extra time for prerounds, as there are often calculations that need to be done prior to rounds. Most numbers are reported on a per-kilogram basis. For example, input is reported as cc/kg/day and kcal/kg/day.

## HOW DO I DO WELL IN THIS ROTATION?

As you have realized or will soon realize, your grades during the clinical years are more subjective than was the case during your preclinical period. Nevertheless, there are some basic rules that you can follow to help improve your evaluations.

**Know your patient.** You've probably heard this at least a thousand times, but this advice is a constant. You have the time to investigate patients thoroughly so that your busy interns, residents, and attendings can turn to you for detailed information they did not obtain during their workups. Often important but not thoroughly investigated aspects of the admission H&P are the diet, immunization history, development, and social history.

**Communicate with your patient.** Earning the trust of your pediatric patient and parents is no small task but is a necessity in effectively caring for your patient. You must take every step to ensure that patients know why they are here and what you are doing for them. Take your time in explaining concepts and procedures, and do so at a level that is appropriate to the patient. That may mean using very concrete terms and humor, so try practicing on yourself or on a fellow student, and remember to be very, very patient.

**Communicate with parents.** This rotation is unique in that you will need to interact with concerned (and, unfortunately, sometimes unconcerned) parents who will be in the room with you. In all likelihood, you will be the one with the most time to speak with a child's family, so you may enjoy the closest relationship with them. It is therefore critical that you maintain an open and direct line of communication with parents regarding a child's condition, his or her prognosis, and any planned procedures. Nobody knows the patient better than the primary caregiver, so listen carefully. At times this can prove exceedingly difficult, as parents will often ask many questions that lie beyond your current medical knowledge, placing you in the awkward position of potentially undermining their trust in you.

Despite these concerns, you should never give an answer if you are unsure of its validity (this holds true for medicine as a whole, but especially for concerned and frustrated parents). It is okay to say, "I do not know, but I will find out from the resident for you." In this way, you are acting as a liaison for your team and helping alleviate family worries while simultaneously showing your genuine concern for the child. Be especially wary of discussing prognosis given your limited experience. You will not lose face in the eyes of a child's parents for not having all the answers; to the contrary, they will end up trusting and respecting you for caring about their child and helping them understand what is happening.

**Show genuine interest in patients.** Make sure any interest you show is genuine, as there is nothing worse than insincerity. Remember how frightened you were of doctors as a child? Try to alleviate some of the patient's fears. On the flip side, you can't make a better impression than having your patients praise you to the attendings.

**Read about the patients you admitted on a given day as soon as you get the chance.** The sooner you read about a patient's problem, the more likely it is that you will remember the topic and the presentation of that patient—and the more knowledgeable you will be the next day, when you present to your team. During your reading, you will discover questions that you should have asked the patients, new labs to order, etc. These inputs will allow you to make valuable contributions and to ask intelligent questions.

**Practice your presentation.** The only time your attending (who, by the way, makes a large contribution to your evaluation) has the chance to see you at work is during rounds—so use this time to your advantage. Don't stutter and mumble your presentations; instead, make sure they are organized, precise, and accurate. Also make sure that the assessment-and-plan sections are well thought out. Discuss them beforehand with the resident. Handing out a review article about the topic may not hurt either.

**Ask for feedback.** The attendings and residents will usually schedule a time for feedback halfway through the rotation. If they don't schedule such time, ask for it. Then, when you meet with them, ask them to give you a detailed evaluation of your performance, emphasizing areas where you can improve. Never accept the answer that you are "doing fine." "Fine" may be average or better—who knows?

**Never put down your colleagues.** Nothing looks worse than team members criticizing each other, especially in front of a patient. This undermines a patient's trust and can compromise their care. So if you need to say something, save it until you leave the patient's room, and then say it tactfully. Remember the importance of maintaining team morale so you can work as a cohesive unit. Derogatory remarks are never appropriate on the wards (or any-

Popular kid topics include Barney, the Power Rangers, and the Disney flick du jour.

where else, for that matter). They're also a sure-fire way for you to trash your own evaluation.

## KEY NOTES

The H&P and daily progress notes for pediatrics are similar to those of medicine, but there are a few variations.

Children are more than just "little adults."

1. **Past medical history:** Maternal history (mother's age, gravida, para, abortions); pregnancy (onset of prenatal care, weight gain, complications, blood type, Coombs, rubella immunity status, RPR/VDRL, HIV, PPD, hepatitis B, blood type, drug/alcohol/tobacco use); labor and delivery (spontaneous or induced, duration, complications, presentation, method of delivery, meconium); neonatal (birth weight, gestational age, complications in the nursery, length of stay).

2. **Nutrition:** Infants—breast or formula (what type), frequency, amount; toddlers—introduction of cereal and baby foods, milk intake; older children—appetite, type of food eaten.

3. **Immunization:** An often-overlooked section that is not to be missed in pediatrics. Ask to see the immunization record.

4. **Developmental history:** Ask the parents when the child first began to sit, walk, and talk and when he or she completed toilet training. Ask about school performance.

5. **Family history:** Focus on inherited diseases, miscarriages, early deaths, congenital anomalies, developmental delay, mental retardation, consanguinity (aka inbreeding), sickle cell, asthma, seizure disorders, atopy, and cardiovascular diseases.

6. **Social history:** This is a very important section in pediatrics and should include comments regarding the child's interaction with the family, the home environment (who lives there, smoking in the home, etc), the primary caregiver, attendance in day care or school, performance in school, the manner in which the parent can be reached, friends, sexual activity, and alcohol, tobacco, and/or drug use.

## TIPS FOR EXAMINING CHILDREN

Infants from the age of 6 months on often have anxiety toward strangers. Here are some tips:

Take time to play with the young patient before attempting a physical exam.

- Anxious children will search your eyes for good intentions. Kind eyes will get you far!

- Take off your white coat before entering the exam room (unless your attending prefers otherwise). Consider wearing a tie with cartoon characters on it—or wear a sticker on your shirt.

- Observe the child's interactions with the parents, primary caregiver, etc.

- For infants and toddlers, do as much of the exam as possible with the parents holding the child. If the patient is in respiratory distress, which may worsen with agitation (as would be the case with epiglottitis), then the child should be left in the parent's arms.

- It is best to perform the cardiac and pulmonary portion of the exam first, when the infant is still quiet. Once you have accomplished this sometimes-difficult task, move on to the other portions of the physical.

- Let the child touch the instruments and play with them. You may try examining the parents before the child to let him or her know that the procedure is not painful. Save the invasive and painful parts of the exam for the end.

- With newborns, infants, and toddlers—observe, auscultate, and then palpate.

- Use age-appropriate terms.

- Smile and speak in a soft tone. Tell the child how well he or she is doing. Demonstrate what you are about to do on yourself or on a parent. Be funny whenever possible.

Variations in the physical exam are as follows:

- **Vital signs:** Temperature should include the method by which it was obtained (axillary temperature is 2° below rectal; oral temperature is 1° below rectal). Include weight (kg and percentile), height (cm and percentile), and head circumference (cm and percentile). Plot these on graphs along with old values if available.
- **General appearance:** Comment on alertness, playfulness, consolability, hydration status (tearing, drooling), development, social interactions, responsiveness (eg, smiling), and nutritional status.
- **Skin:** Jaundice, acrocyanosis, mottling, birthmarks, cradle cap, rashes, and capillary refill.
- **Hair:** Lanugo and Tanner stage.
- **Head:** Circumference, sutures, fontanelles.
- **Eyes:** Red reflex in the newborn, strabismus (cover test in preschoolers), and scleral icterus.
- **Ears:** Use the largest speculum you can. For ease of examining the ear, have the child held facing you. Ask the parents to cross their legs over both of the child's legs. Also ask the parent to use one arm to wrap around the child's arm and body and to use the other arm to hold the child's head. In an infant, pull the auricle backward and downward. In an older child, pull the external ear backward and upward.
- **Nose:** Patent nares, nasal flaring (respiratory distress).
- **Mouth:** Teeth, palate (cleft), thrush.
- **Heart:** The average heart rate in an infant is 140–160 bpm; in an older child, it is less than 120 bpm. Always check for femoral pulses in infants to exclude coarctation.
- **Chest:** Expiration is more prolonged than in adults; in young infants, respiratory movements are produced by abdominal movements. Look for any skin retraction between the ribs (respiratory distress).
- **Abdomen:** Deep palpation should be performed on every infant. Check umbilicus (or stump).
- **Back:** Check for scoliosis and deep dimples.
- **Genitalia:** Circumcision, testes (descended bilaterally), labia (adhesion), hymenal opening, and Tanner stage.

Check the tympanic membranes last.

Report vital signs as ranges with a maximum value.

- **Musculoskeletal:** Barlow and Ortolani maneuvers.
- **Neurologic:** Tone, strength, primitive reflexes (root, suck, grasp, Moro, stepping, etc), development.

## KEY PROCEDURES

The key procedures in pediatrics are lumbar puncture, urine catheterization, and blood drawing. If the patient needs a painful procedure done, parents are usually asked to leave the room. Explain to the parents that the child should not watch the parents stand by while he or she may be experiencing pain. The parent can act as the "rescuer" when the procedure is over.

## WHAT DO I CARRY IN MY POCKETS?

The white coat is generally not used in pediatrics, so don't rely on those handy oversize pockets to store your peripheral brain and instruments of the trade. Try using a fanny pack or a small over-the-shoulder camera bag for these tasks.

### Checklist

- ❏ Toy for distraction
- ❏ Stethoscope
- ❏ Ophthalmoscope
- ❏ Otoscope with tips of different sizes and insufflator bulb
- ❏ Penlight
- ❏ Tongue blades
- ❏ Calculator (to figure out dosages for meds)
- ❏ Optional: stickers for a reward (dinosaurs, Power Rangers, and Barney are very popular), cartoon Band-Aids (Snoopy, Garfield, etc)

# TOP-RATED BOOKS

## HANDBOOK/POCKETBOOK

### Clinical Handbook of Pediatrics
Schwartz
Williams & Wilkins, 1995, 949 pages, ISBN 0683076248, $29.95

`A-`

A spiral-bound pocket reference focusing on the diagnostic approach to a broad range of pediatric problems. Contains an extensive differential diagnosis list followed by a discussion of the list items that includes a quick blurb on treatment and often algorithms for diagnosis. This book also includes a useful chapter outlining the H&P with many pearls.

### Current Clinical Strategies: Pediatrics
Chan
Current Clinical Strategies, 1997, 102 pages, ISBN 1881528243, $8.75

`A-`

Practical pocketbook detailing admit orders, specific pharmacologic treatment options, and management of common pediatric diseases. Includes useful charts on developmental milestones and immunization. An excellent value.

### Handbook of Pediatrics
Merenstein
Appleton & Lange, 1997, 1029 pages, ISBN 0838536255, $29.95

`A-`

A useful handbook with good coverage of a variety of diseases. Discusses etiology, clinical and lab findings, treatment, and prognosis, but sometimes lacking in practical wards information. Includes a limited drug formulary that is quite cumbersome. Makes excellent use of tables, charts, and algorithms. May be helpful for quick "downtime" reading on the wards, although it is a bit bulky to carry around.

### Pediatric Pearls—The Handbook of Practical Pediatrics
Rosenstein
Mosby, 1993, 368 pages, ISBN 080167171X, $34.95

`A-`

A very readable pocketbook organized by organ systems. Includes concise discussions of disease entities, treatment, and management. A useful supplement, but not a primary reference.

### The Harriet Lane Handbook
Barone
Mosby, 1996, 775 pages, ISBN 0815149441, $30.95

`B+`

Classic pocketbook designed for the house officer. Extensive drug formulary section and numerous tables and charts interspersed among outline-format, quick-read text. Roughly organized by systems, and includes sections on pediatric subspecialties. Gives practical, "how-to" information, but does not discuss pathophysiology or include differential diagnoses. Can be difficult to use as a junior student; better for a subintern. A must-have for the house officer.

**B+** Manual of Pediatric Therapeutics
Graef
Little, Brown, 1994, 691 pages, ISBN 0316138754, $34.95

Relatively comprehensive manual with adequate discussion of general principles, management, and treatment of common pediatric diseases. Presented in concise, outline format with good use of tables and charts. Equivalent to the *Washington Manual* for pediatrics.

**B+** Pocket Handbook of Pediatric Antimicrobial Therapy
Nelson
Williams & Wilkins, 1996, 106 pages, ISBN 0683180533, $14.95

A specialized version of *Sanford*, probably necessary only for house officers. Often available for free from drug reps.

**B** Pocket Paediatrics
O'Callaghan
Churchill Livingstone, 1992, 394 pages, ISBN 0443043604, $26.95

Limited coverage of pediatric disease with variable amount of information given per topic. Major weakness in drug formulary section and discussions of treatment options. Limited utility.

## REVIEW/MINI-REFERENCE

**A** Current Pediatric Diagnosis and Treatment
Hay
Appleton & Lange, 1997, 1217 pages, ISBN 0838514006, $45.00

Up-to-date, very readable, comprehensive reference book of pediatrics with excellent organization of disease entities. Includes chapter on HIV infection. Excellent use of tables, graphs, and illustrations. Overall, a useful book for home reference and a good value for serious pediatric students.

**A** Fundamentals of Pediatrics
Rudolph
Appleton & Lange, 1994, 701 pages, ISBN 0838582338, $39.95

Excellent, well-organized, and readable softcover reference book that contains sufficient information for the core rotation. Includes useful algorithms summarizing approaches to commonly encountered pediatric diseases. Certainly suffices as a general home reference book, but consider a more detailed textbook if you're going into pediatrics.

**A-** Nelson Essentials of Pediatrics
Behrman
Saunders, 1994, 795 pages, ISBN 0721637752, $43.95

Condensed softcover "baby" version of *Nelson's Textbook of Pediatrics* with concise explanations. Well organized into clinical diagnosis, differential diagnosis, and treatment and prevention. Worthy alternative to Rudolph's *Fundamentals of Pediatrics*, but not quite as good.

## Pediatrics
Bernstein
Williams & Wilkins, 1996, 665 pages, ISBN 0683006401, $37.95

**A-**

Introductory softcover text geared toward junior students during their clinical rotations. Divided into common primary care problems and pediatric subspecialty problems. Very readable, but not as comprehensive as similar texts.

## Oski's Essential Pediatrics
Johnson
Lippincott-Raven, 1997, 761 pages, ISBN 0397515146, $34.95

**B+**

Good reference text organized by problems. Includes illustrations and tables. Easy to read and gives a good, basic overview of treatment and management, but lacks detail and depth. Each section is variable in coverage. Useful for the time-limited student.

## NMS Pediatrics
Dworkin
Williams & Wilkins, 1996, 679 pages, ISBN 068306245X, $36.95

**B**

Consists of a comprehensive, detailed outline of pediatrics with questions. Geared more toward USLME Step 2.

## Pediatric Secrets
Polin
Hanley & Belfus, 1997, 447 pages, ISBN 1560531711, $36.95

**B**

Presented in question-and-answer format typical of *Secrets* series. Organized by organ systems and includes good use of tables, charts, and mnemonics. Designed to prepare for pimping sessions, although such sessions are infrequent in pediatrics. Best used as leisure reading material or to feed the attending's appetite for interesting facts and trivia.

## TEXTBOOK/REFERENCE

## Nelson Textbook of Pediatrics
Behrman
Saunders, 1996, 2200 pages, ISBN 0721655785, $97.00

**A**

An authoritative textbook of pediatrics that is well organized with clear explanations and comprehensive discussions on diagnosis and treatment of pediatric disorders. Worth the investment for someone going into pediatrics as a career; otherwise best borrowed from the library.

## Rudolph's Pediatrics
Rudolph
Appleton & Lange, 1996, 2337 pages, ISBN 0838584926, $95.00

**A**

Comprehensive hardcover reference book for serious pediatric students. Similar in price and scope to *Nelson Textbook of Pediatrics*. A worthy alternative that is worth examining.

**B+**

**Pediatric Medicine**
Avery
Williams & Wilkins, 1994, 1636 pages, ISBN 0683002937, $99.00

Hardcover reference text with in-depth explanations of disease entities. Easier reading than other major textbooks, but not as well organized. Discussions are clear and concise but a bit cursory on treatment options in some sections. Expensive; consider borrowing from the library if you're not pediatrics bound.

# HIGH-YIELD TOPICS

## ROTATION OBJECTIVES

The following is a list of core topics that you are likely to encounter in the course of your pediatrics rotation. Conditions and topics discussed in further detail in this chapter are italicized.

**Well-child care visits**
- Well-child visits from the newborn period to age 18
- *Developmental milestones*
- Counseling and anticipatory guidance
- *Immunization schedule*

**Behavioral pediatrics**
- Attention-deficit hyperactivity disorder (see p. 276)

**Chromosomal disorders**
- Trisomy 21
- Turner syndrome

**Infectious diseases**
- *Management of fever*
- *Meningitis*
- *Otitis media* and otitis externa
- Orbital and preorbital cellulitis
- Pharyngitis (bacterial and viral)
- *Pneumonia*
- Gastroenteritis
- *Urinary tract infection*
- Cellulitis
- Sexually transmitted diseases
- HIV

**Dermatology**
- Childhood exanthems
- Milia
- Neonatal acne
- Seborrheic dermatitis
- Diaper rash
- Impetigo
- Scabies
- Eczema

**Gastroenterology**
- Gastroesophageal reflux

- Pyloric stenosis
- Intussusception
- Appendicitis
- Constipation
- *Neonatal hyperbilirubinemia*
- Failure to thrive

**Hematology/oncology**
- Iron-deficiency anemia
- Sickle-cell anemia
- Acute lymphocytic leukemia
- Wilms' tumor

**Nephrology**
- Fluid and electrolyte imbalance
- Hemolytic–uremic syndrome
- Dehydration

**Cardiology**
- Ventricular septal defect
- Atrioventricular septal defect
- Tetralogy of Fallot
- Coarctation of the aorta
- Patent ductus arteriosus

**Pulmonology**
- Apnea
- *Asthma*
- *Cystic fibrosis*
- Bronchiolitis
- *Croup*
- *Epiglottitis*
- Bronchopulmonary dysplasia

**Endocrinology**
- Diabetes

**Neurology**
- *Febrile seizures*
- Epilepsy

**Trauma**
- Head injury

**Trauma** (*cont'd*)
- Child abuse
- Nursemaid's elbow

**Autoimmune**
- Henoch-Schönlein purpura

- Juvenile rheumatoid arthritis
- Kawasaki disease

**Neonatology**
- *Apgar score*
- Prematurity

## DEVELOPMENTAL MILESTONES

From birth to maturity, most children go through the same sequence of growth and development. Pediatricians use developmental milestones to monitor growth and to identify developmental delays. Table 1 summarizes the key milestones.

## IMMUNIZATION SCHEDULE

Table 2 outlines the immunization schedule for children from birth through 6 years of age.

## MANAGEMENT OF FEVER

During your weeks on the pediatric ward, you will be admitting a lot of children with fever. Be thankful that new management guidelines have decreased the number of hospitalizations for fever. To better understand the new guidelines, a few definitions have to be explained.

- Fever is defined as a rectal temperature higher than 38°C (100.4°F).
- In order for the acute febrile illness to qualify as a fever without source, the etiology of the fever must not be evident after a careful history and physical.
- A toxic-appearing patient describes a clinical picture that includes lethargy, signs of poor perfusion, marked hypoventilation, hyperventilation, and cyanosis.
- "Lethargy" is defined as a level of consciousness characterized by poor or absent eye contact or failure of the child to recognize the parents or to interact with persons or objects in the environment.
- Low-risk infants include previously healthy infants with no focal bacterial infection evident from the physical exam who are non-toxic-appearing, and with negative laboratory screening (WBC between 5000 and 15,000/mm³, less than 1500 bands/mm³, normal urinalysis, and, when diarrhea is present, stool with less than 5 WBC/high-power field).

The management of a young child with fever depends on the age group of the child. Children are divided into three groups for this purpose: younger than 28 days, 28–90 days, and 3–36 months.

**Management of an infant younger than 28 days of age.** All children less than 28 days of age who have fever need to be hospitalized. A sepsis evaluation that includes cultures of cerebrospinal fluid, blood, and urine; a complete blood count with differential; cerebrospinal fluid analysis for cells, glucose, and protein; chest x-ray; and a urinalysis must be performed. An

| TABLE 1. Key developmental milestones | |
|---|---|
| 4–5 months | Rolls over |
| 6 months | Sits without support |
| 9 months | Crawls |
| 12 months | Walks alone, two words other than "mama/dada" |
| 18 months | Runs, knows some body parts |
| 2 years | Walks up and down stairs without help, uses 2-word combinations, understands 2-step commands |
| 3 years | Pedals a tricycle, uses 3-word combinations |

| | Birth | 2 months | 4 months | 6 months | 12–15 months | 15–18 months | 4–6 years |
|---|---|---|---|---|---|---|---|
| **TABLE 2.** Simplified immunization schedule | | | | | | | |
| HBV | X | X | | X | | | |
| DTP | | X | X | X | | X | X |
| HIB | | X | X | X | X | | |
| Polio | | X | X | X | | | X |
| MMR | | | | | X | | X |

appropriate antibiotic regimen must be started; one popular choice is ampi-cillin and cefotaxime. Alternatively, if the infant is low risk, a full sepsis evaluation is performed and the infant is monitored closely without antibi-otics while awaiting laboratory results.

**Management of a febrile infant 28–90 days of age without a source.** All infants at this age who appear toxic as defined previously need to be hospi-talized, given a full sepsis workup, and started on parenteral antibiotics. For non-toxic-appearing infants, outpatient management is adequate. There are two options that can be used to approach this problem:

| Option 1 | Option 2 (less accepted) |
|---|---|
| CBC/blood culture | UA/urine culture only |
| UA/urine culture | Careful observation |
| Lumbar puncture | |
| Ceftriaxone 50 mg/kg/day IM | |
| Return for reevaluation in 24 hours. | |

**Management of a febrile child 3–36 months without a source.** The risk of bacteremia in this age group is small (4.3%). Again, if the child is toxic-appearing, he needs to be admitted to the hospital, given a complete sepsis workup, and started on parenteral antibiotics. If the child does not appear toxic and the temperature is less than 39.0°C, no diagnostic tests or antibi-otics are necessary. The parents should be instructed to give the child aceta-minophen 15 mg/kg/4 hours and to return to office if the fever persists for more than 48 hours or if the clinical condition deteriorates.

If the non-toxic-appearing child has a temperature higher than 39.0°C, he needs the following:

- Catherized urine culture for males less than 6 months of age or fe-males less than 2 years of age.
- Stool culture if there is evidence of blood or mucus in the stool or greater than 5 WBCs/HPF in the stool.
- Chest radiograph if there is evidence of dyspnea, tachypnea, rales, or decreased breath sounds.
- Blood culture and empiric antibiotics for a temperature higher than 39.0°C or, according to some, a temperature higher than 39.0°C with a WBC greater than 15,000.
- Acetaminophen 15 mg/kg/4 hours.
- Follow-up in 24–48 hours.

Prompt lumbar puncture is essential in any patient with possible CNS infection.

# MENINGITIS

Meningitis is an inflammation of the leptomeninges caused by viruses, bacteria, or fungi. The most common bacterial pathogens vary with age group (see Table 3). Viruses commonly causing meningitis include enteroviruses, mumps, herpes simplex virus, varicella–zoster virus, arbovirus, Epstein–Barr virus, rabies, and adenovirus.

## Signs and Symptoms

See Table 4 for meningitis signs and symptoms according to age.

## Differential and Workup

The differential diagnosis of meningitis (bacterial and aseptic) includes brain abscess, subdural empyema, mastoiditis, tumors, cysts, trauma, vasculitis, tuberculous or fungal meningitis, cysticercosis, Lyme disease, leptospirosis, and rickettsial diseases.

Helpful tests include:

- CT or MRI helps narrow the list of differential diagnoses. Get the CT before the LP if there are focal neurologic findings or papilledema.

- CSF by LP must be obtained for cell count with differential, glucose, protein, Gram stain, and culture. The CSF composition in acute meningitis depends on the etiology of the meningitis (see Table 5).

- Blood should be drawn for CBC, electrolytes, glucose, and culture. White blood cell counts are nonspecific and are often unremarkable in aseptic meningitis. For bacterial meningitis, the white blood cell counts are usually elevated.

- EEGs may be helpful in patients who present with seizures. Often the changes are nonspecific and characterized by generalized slowing. Focal slowing is characteristic of herpes simplex virus infections.

In aseptic meningitis, many patients feel better after the LP.

## Treatment

The therapy for meningitis consists of antibiotics and supportive care. The initial choice of antimicrobial is based on the most likely organisms involved

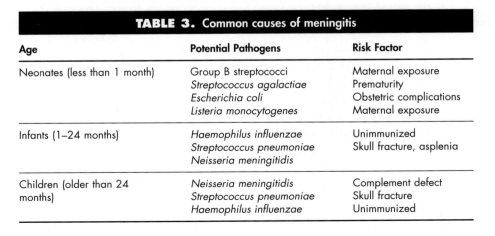

| Age | Potential Pathogens | Risk Factor |
| --- | --- | --- |
| Neonates (less than 1 month) | Group B streptococci<br>*Streptococcus agalactiae*<br>*Escherichia coli*<br>*Listeria monocytogenes* | Maternal exposure<br>Prematurity<br>Obstetric complications<br>Maternal exposure |
| Infants (1–24 months) | *Haemophilus influenzae*<br>*Streptococcus pneumoniae*<br>*Neisseria meningitidis* | Unimmunized<br>Skull fracture, asplenia |
| Children (older than 24 months) | *Neisseria meningitidis*<br>*Streptococcus pneumoniae*<br>*Haemophilus influenzae* | Complement defect<br>Skull fracture<br>Unimmunized |

TABLE 3. Common causes of meningitis

| TABLE 4. Age-related signs and symptoms of meningitis | | | |
|---|---|---|---|
| **Age** | **Symptoms** | **Early Signs** | **Late Signs** |
| 0–3 months | Paradoxical irritation (irritable when held and less irritable when not held) Altered sleep pattern Respiratory distress Vomiting, poor feeding Diarrhea Seizures | Lethargy Irritability Temperature instability | Bulging fontanelle Shock |
| 4–24 months | Altered sleep pattern Lethargy Seizures | Fever Irritability | Nuchal rigidity Coma Shock |
| Over 24 months | Headache Stiff neck Lethargy Photophobia Myalgia Seizures | Fever Nuchal rigidity Irritability Kernig's sign* Brudzinski's sign** | Coma Shock |

\* Kernig's sign: Flexion of the hip 90° with subsequent pain with extension of the leg.
\*\* Brudzinski's sign: Involuntary flexion of the knees and hip following flexion of the neck while supine.

given the patient's age group (see Table 3). Once the organism has been identified, the antibiotics can be adjusted.

Empiric antibiotic therapy for meningitis is shown in Table 6.

The supportive care of meningitis includes:

- Strict fluid balance
- Frequent urine-specific gravity assessment
- Seizure precautions
- Daily weights
- Daily measurement of head circumference in babies
- Neurologic assessment
- Isolation until causative organism is identified
- Rehydration with isotonic solutions until euvolemic; then switch to 2/3 maintenance fluids

## Complications

The acute complications of bacterial meningitis include seizures, subdural effusions, cerebral edema, subdural empyema, ventriculitis, and abscess.

| TABLE 5. CSF findings in meningitis | | | | | |
|---|---|---|---|---|---|
| **Component** | **Normal** | **Bacterial** | **Herpes** | **Viral** | **Spirochetal** |
| Glucose (mg/dL) | 40–80 | < 30 | > 30 | > 30 | 42–110 |
| Protein (mg/dL) | 20–50 | > 100 | > 75 | 50–100 | 13–150 |
| Leukocytes/µL | 0–6 | > 1000 | 10–1000 | 100–500 | 20–500 |
| Neutrophils (%) | 0 | > 50 | < 50 | < 20 | < 10 |
| Erythrocytes/µL | 0–2 | 0–10 | 10–500 | 0–2 | 0–2 |

| TABLE 6. Empiric antibiotic therapy for meningitis | | |
|---|---|---|
| Age | Antibiotics | Duration |
| Neonates | Ampicillin (200 mg/kg) and cefotaxime (100–150 mg/kg) Ampicillin and gentamicin (7.5 mg/kg) (alternative) | 14–21 days for group B streptococcus or *Listeria* At least 2 weeks after CSF sterilization for gram-negative enteric meningitis |
| Infants and children | Cefotaxime (200 mg/kg) or ceftriaxone (100 mg/kg) | 7–10 days for uncomplicated HIB or meningococcal disease 10–14 days for pneumococcal meningitis |

## OTITIS MEDIA

Otitis media is an acute suppurative infection of the middle ear cavity. Common pathogens include *Streptococcus pneumoniae*, *Haemophilus influenzae*, *Moraxella catarrhalis*, and viruses (influenza A, RSV, parainfluenza).

### Signs and Symptoms

The presenting symptoms of otitis media are ear pain, fever, crying, irritability, difficulty sleeping, difficulty feeding, vomiting, and diarrhea.

The four classic physical findings in otitis media are a bulging tympanic membrane, altered color (ie, red) or lucency of the tympanic membrane, decreased mobility of the tympanic membrane with an insufflator, and altered landmarks.

Otitis media is an extremely common outpatient diagnosis.

### Differential

The differential diagnosis of acute otitis media includes otitis externa, mastoiditis, foreign body in the ear, ear canal furuncle, ear canal trauma, hard cerumen, mumps, toothache, and temporomandibular joint dysfunction.

### Workup

The diagnosis is based on the physical exam and presenting complaints.

The conditions that predispose children to otitis media include viral upper respiratory tract infection, passive exposure to tobacco smoke, day care outside the home, trisomy 21, hypothyroidism, and cleft palate.

### Treatment

The drug of choice for the treatment of otitis media is amoxicillin 40 mg/kg/day for 10 days in 3 divided doses. Trimethoprim, 8 mg/kg/day, with sulfamethoxazole, 40 mg/kg/day, for 10 days in 2 divided doses is an alternative.

## PNEUMONIA

Pneumonia can be defined as inflammation of the lung parenchyma. It may be classified according to etiologic agent, patient age, host reaction, or anatomic distribution (eg, lobar, interstitial, bronchial pneumonia).

## Signs and Symptoms

**Children older than 6 years of age.** The child may present with mild upper respiratory tract symptoms such as cough and rhinitis followed by abrupt fever, tachypnea, chest pain, and chills. Physical examination is significant for decreased breath sounds and rales of the affected lung, retractions, and use of accessory muscle. The symptoms of viral pneumonia are less fulminant than those of bacterial pneumonia.

**Children younger than 6 years of age.** Younger children with pneumonia may present with nonspecific complaints such as abdominal pain, fever, malaise, gastrointestinal symptoms, restlessness, apprehension, and chills. Respiratory signs such as tachypnea, cough, grunting, and nasal flaring may be subtle. Even with a productive cough, children rarely expectorate.

**Newborns.** Infants usually present with signs of respiratory distress, including tachypnea, cyanosis, nasal flaring, and retractions. They may also show symptoms of systemic infection, including poor perfusion, hypotension, acidosis, and leukopenia or leukocytosis.

## Differential

The differential diagnosis of pneumonia includes the full spectrum of infectious organisms ranging from viruses to bacteria as well as gastric aspiration, foreign body aspiration, atelectasis, congenital malformation, congestive heart failure, malignant growth, chronic interstitial lung disease, collagen vascular disease, and pulmonary infarct.

## Workup

The diagnosis is usually made on the basis of history and clinical findings. It is important to obtain a CXR in ill-appearing infants and children, patients who need hospitalization, and those who worsen clinically on antibiotics.

Helpful laboratory tests include:

- With bacterial pneumonia, the white blood cell count is often greater than 15,000/mL. A white blood cell count of less than 5000/mL in the newborn period indicates sepsis.
- Blood culture and viral serology (good sputums are hard to get).

## Treatment

The therapy for pneumonia depends on the organisms responsible for the clinical picture. The initial antibiotic regimen should be based on Gram stain of the sputum, tracheobronchial secretions, or pleural fluid as well as age, on clinical and radiographic findings, and known or suspected immune-compromised status. See Table 7 for empiric antibiotic therapy by age group. Criteria for hospitalization include respiratory distress, hypoxia, and evidence of consolidation or empyema on chest x-ray. Hospitalized children should be treated with IV antibiotics until afebrile and then with oral antibiotics for a total of 10 days of treatment.

## URINARY TRACT INFECTION (UTI)

Urine should be sterile. The growth of an abnormal number of bacterial colonies from the urine is the simple definition of UTI. UTIs can be classi-

| **TABLE 7.** Common etiologies of and empiric therapy for pneumonia | | |
|---|---|---|
| **Age** | **Organisms** | **Empiric Coverage** |
| Infants younger than 6 weeks | Group B streptococcus<br>*Chlamydia trachomatis*<br>*Staphylococcus aureus* | Ampicillin and gentamicin |
| 6 weeks – 6 months | Respiratory syncytial virus<br>*Streptococcus pneumoniae*<br>*H. influenzae* type B<br>Group A streptococcus<br>*Chlamydia trachomatis*<br>*Staphylococcus aureus* | Supportive care for suspected cases of viral pneumonia<br>Mild to moderate illness: oral amoxicillin, oral cefuroxime<br>Severe illness: IV cefuroxime, ceftriaxone, ceftazidime, or oxacillin |
| 6 months – school age | Respiratory syncytial virus<br>Parainfluenza viruses<br>Influenza virus<br>Adenovirus<br>*Streptococcus pneumoniae* | Supportive care for suspected cases of viral pneumonia<br>Mild to moderate illness: oral amoxicillin, oral cefuroxime<br>Severe illness: IV cefuroxime, ceftriaxone, ceftazidime, or oxacillin |
| School age | Mycoplasma pneumonia<br>*Streptococcus pneumoniae*<br>Adenovirus | Mild to moderate illness: oral erythromycin if myco-plasma suspected<br>Severe illness: IV cefuroxime, ceftriaxone, ceftazidime, and gentamicin |

fied as lower (cystitis) or upper (pyelonephritis). Organisms usually infect the urinary tract from below except in neonates, where they can also reach the urinary tract via hematogenous spread. The incidence is slightly higher in males during the newborn period. During childhood, it becomes 10 times more common in females.

The predominant organisms responsible for urinary tract infection are *Escherichia coli, Proteus, Pseudomonas aeruginosa, Klebsiella, Staphylococcus saprophyticus,* and the enteric streptococci.

Vesicoureteral reflux, obstructive uropathy, renal calculi, bladder dysfunction, and intermittent catherization increase the risk of developing a urinary tract infection. Infection in a small child should make you consider the possibility of abnormal anatomy.

## Signs and Symptoms

The signs and symptoms of a urinary tract infection in the pediatric population are often different from those in the adult population (see Table 8). Upper UTIs are more likely to produce constitutional symptoms such as fever, chills, flank pain, nausea, vomiting, costovertebral tenderness, and dehydration.

## Differential and Workup

Although a urinalysis can suggest a UTI, the definitive diagnosis of a urinary tract infection is made by a positive urine culture. A urine sample may be obtained either as a clean-catch midstream specimen or as a catheter or suprapubic aspirated specimen. The method employed depends on the age of the child and on the clinical suspicion.

| **TABLE 8.** Signs and symptoms of urinary tract infections | | | |
|---|---|---|---|
| **Newborns** | **Infants** | **Preschool** | **School-age** |
| Fever | Fever of unknown origin | Fever | Fever/chills |
| Hypothermia | Poor feeding | Enuresis | Enuresis |
| Poor feeding | Failure to thrive | Dysuria | Dysuria |
| Vomiting | Strong-smelling urine | Urgency | Urgency |
| Jaundice | Irritability | Urinary frequency | Urinary frequency |
| Failure to thrive | | Abdominal pain | Costovertebral |
| Sepsis | | Vomiting |   tenderness |
| Apnea | | Strong-smelling urine | Hematuria |

The criteria for a positive urine culture depend on the method by which the urine was obtained. The urine culture is considered positive if:

- More than $10^3$ colonies/mL are obtained from an intermittent ("in and out") catheterization sample.
- More than $10^5$ colonies/mL are obtained from a midstream clean-catch sample.
- Any colonies are obtained from a suprapubic tap sample.

If diphtheroid bacilli, *Staphylococcus*, or multiple organisms are present in the sample, suspect a contaminated sample and repeat the urine culture. Finally, any toxic-appearing child should have blood cultures, CBC with differential, electrolytes, BUN, and creatinine to rule out pyelonephritis and sepsis.

## Treatment

Empiric antibiotic treatment, usually amoxicillin or trimethoprim-sulfamethoxazole, is begun while awaiting sensitivity results. A 10-day course of the appropriate antibiotic is usually adequate. A repeat urine culture at 48–72 hours of therapy is done to ensure adequate treatment. Urinary tract infection is managed on an outpatient basis unless a child is suspected of having pyelonephritis or looks ill. In these patients, IV antibiotics (eg, ampicillin asnd gentamicin) are indicated. Renal ultrasound (evaluates the anatomy of the urinary tract) and a voiding cystourethrogram (evaluates reflux) should be done in all boys with their first UTI, girls younger than 5 years old with their first febrile UTI, older girls with recurrent UTIs, and any child with suspected pyelonephritis. Children with UTIs do not need prophylactic therapy unless they have the following indications:

- Prior to undergoing a VCUG
- Reflux of any grade (grades I–V) in infancy and early childhood
- Reflux of grades III–V in children older than 5 years of age
- More than 3 UTIs per year
- Pyelonephritis

## NEONATAL HYPERBILIRUBINEMIA

Hyperbilirubinemia is a condition that is characterized by excessive concentration of bilirubin in the blood. It can be classified as **unconjugated,** which can be of physiologic or pathologic origin, or **conjugated,** which is always of pathologic origin. The causes of direct hyperbilirubinemia include **ToRCHeS** infections (**T**oxoplasmosis, **R**ubella, **C**MV, **H**erpes, and **S**yphilis), metabolic

An elevated conjugated bilirubin value is always pathologic.

TABLE 9. Physiologic versus nonphysiologic jaundice

| | Physiologic Jaundice | Nonphysiologic Jaundice |
|---|---|---|
| Clinical features | Jaundice not present until or after 72 hours after birth. Total bilirubin rises by less than 5 mg/dL/day, peaking to less than 14–15 mg/dL. Direct bilirubin less than 10% of total bilirubin. Jaundice resolves by 1 week in term infants and 2 weeks in preterm infants. | Jaundice present mostly by the first 24 hours of life. Total bilirubin rises by more than 0.5 mg/dL/hour, total bilirubin of greater than 15 mg/dL in formula-fed full-term infants and in preterm infants, or greater than 17 mg/dL in breast-fed full-term infants. Direct bilirubin greater than 10% of total bilirubin. Jaundice persists beyond 1 week in term infants and 2 weeks in preterm infants |
| Causes | Delayed activity of glucuronyl transferase. Increased bilirubin load on hepatocytes. Decreased bilirubin clearance from the plasma. Decreased enterohepatic circulation. | Hemolytic diseases. Extravascular blood loss and accumulation. Increased enterohepatic circulation. Breast feeding associated with poor intake. Disorders of bilirubin metabolism. Metabolic disorders. Bacterial sepsis. |
| Physical exam | Clinical jaundice appears at a bilirubin level of 5 mg/dL and starts at the head, progressing down the body as the level increases. | Same as with physiologic jaundice. |
| Laboratories | Determination of direct and indirect concentration of bilirubin. Determination of maternal and infant blood types. Coombs test. Complete blood count with peripheral smear and reticulocyte count. Pathologic causes of jaundice must be ruled out. | Complete blood count with peripheral smear and reticulocyte count. Determination of maternal and infant blood types. Coombs test. Determination of direct and indirect concentration of bilirubin. |
| Therapy | Phototherapy and/or exchange transfusion for levels > 20 mg/dL. | Same as with physiologic jaundice. |

disorders, bacterial sepsis, obstructive jaundice, prolonged administration of total parenteral nutrition (IV nutrition), and neonatal hepatitis.

The causes of unconjugated hyperbilirubinemia include excessive bilirubin production (hemolysis), defective clearance of bilirubin from the blood, and defective bilirubin conjugation by the liver. The primary concern with unconjugated hyperbilirubinemia is the development of kernicterus. During the neonatal period, the most common cause of hyperbilirubinemia is delayed clearance, metabolism, and excretion of bilirubin by the immature liver.

Unconjugated hyperbilirubinemia is classified as physiologic and pathologic or nonphysiologic (see Table 9).

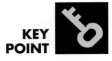

KEY POINT

## BREAST MILK VERSUS BREAST-FEEDING JAUNDICE

Breast milk jaundice is a syndrome of prolonged unconjugated hyperbilirubinemia that is thought to be due to an inhibitor to conjugation in the breast milk of some mothers. This hyperbilirubinemia is an extension of physiologic jaundice. It peaks at 10–15 days of age and declines slowly by 3–12 weeks of age. Breast-feeding jaundice appears to be due to decreased enteral intake as a result of poor feeding or failure to produce adequate milk supply, and increased enterohepatic circulation. It usually occurs during the first week of life.

## ASTHMA

Asthma is a bronchial disorder characterized by inflammation, reversible smooth muscle constriction, and mucus production. This leads to airway obstruction and difficulty breathing.

### Signs and Symptoms

Asthma may present suddenly or gradually. Those cases that present gradually are often associated with respiratory tract infection, whereas those with an acute onset are associated with allergens. Patients or parents may report chest congestion, prolonged cough, exercise intolerance, dyspnea, recurrent bronchitis, pneumonia, irritability, or feeding difficulties in younger children. Keep in mind that asthma can occur without overt wheezing. Key asthma triggers include airway irritants (eg, cigarettes, air pollution, ozone), allergies (eg, pollens, dust mites, pets, cockroaches), exercise, cold weather, respiratory infections, drugs (eg, aspirin, β blockers), stress, foods, and food additives. Try to elicit a history of past severity, frequency, emergency room visits, hospitalizations, ICU admissions, courses of steroids per year, and number of school days missed per year due to asthma. Don't forget to ask about family history of asthma, allergies, and atopic disease.

Signs of asthma include wheezing, tachypnea, tachycardia, prolonged expiration, intercostal and subcostal retraction, and nasal flaring. Cyanosis, diminished breath sounds (due to poor air exchange), and increasingly labored breathing should all raise red flags in your minds.

### Differential

The differential diagnosis of asthma includes aspiration, bronchiolitis, bronchopulmonary dysplasia, cystic fibrosis, gastroesophageal reflux, vascular rings, and pneumonia.

### Workup

The diagnosis of asthma is based on appropriate history; a physical exam with nasal flaring, retraction, decreased aeration, wheezing, prolonged expiration, inability to speak in full sentences, and tachypnea; chest x-ray findings of hyperinflation; and pulmonary function studies demonstrating decreased vital capacity, increased functional residual capacity, increased residual volume, and reversal of pulmonary abnormalities by inhalation of aerosolized albuterol.

Helpful laboratory tests include:

- Pulse oximetry.
- Arterial blood gas demonstrates hypoxia and respiratory acidosis.
- Spirometry demonstrates decreased 1-second forced expiratory volume ($FEV_1$) and peak expiratory flow rate (PEFR) in children 6 years or older.
- White blood cell count may demonstrate eosinophilia.
- Chest x-ray shows bilateral hyperinflation, bronchial thickening, peribronchial infiltration, prominent pulmonary arteries, or areas of increased density.

**Beware of asthma without wheezing.**

## Treatment

A suggested algorithm for the emergent management of asthma is outlined in Figure 1.

- **Acute therapy:** Bronchodilators are the drug of choice in an acute attack (albuterol 0.5 mL in 2 mL normal saline) as well as systemic steroids like PO prednisone and IV methylprednisolone. Treatment

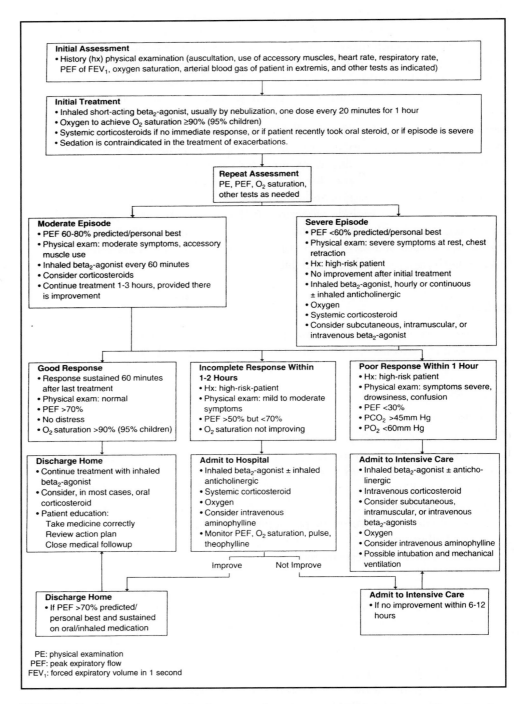

**FIGURE 1.** Management algorithm for acute asthma. *International Consensus Report on Diagnosis and Management of Asthma*, PHS #92-3091, 1992.

with corticosteroids for less than a 5-day duration does not require tapering.

- **Chronic therapy:** Avoid allergens; monitor peak flow. Inhaled corticosteroids and cromolyn sodium, a mast-cell stabilizer (Intal), should be used for prevention.

## CYSTIC FIBROSIS

Cystic fibrosis is a multisystem autosomal-recessive disorder that results from a mutation in the cystic fibrosis transmembrane conductance regulator (CFTR) gene. This is the most common lethal genetic disease affecting Caucasians.

### Signs and Symptoms

- **Respiratory:** Chronic respiratory tract infections, loss of pulmonary function, barrel chest, cyanosis, productive cough, dyspnea, pneumothorax, hemoptysis, nasal polyps, and chronic sinusitis.
- **Gastrointestinal:** Foul-smelling fatty stool, meconium ileus, fat-soluble vitamin deficiency, growth failure due to fat and protein malabsorption from pancreatic insufficiency, rectal prolapse, intestinal obstruction and esophageal varices due to biliary cirrhosis, and portal hypertension.
- **Reproductive:** Males are infertile due to obliteration of the vas deferens. Females have reduced fertility due to the thick, spermicidal cervical mucus.
- **Endocrine:** Abnormal glucose tolerance and type I diabetes.
- **Musculoskeletal:** Bone pain and joint effusion due to hypertrophic osteoarthropathy.
- **Fluid and electrolytes:** Hyponatremic, hypochloremic dehydration.

### Differential and Workup

The diagnosis of cystic fibrosis is made with the sweat chloride test. A sweat chloride value of > 60 mEq/L is considered positive. Indications for performing the test include:

- Respiratory signs and symptoms:
  - Infants diagnosed with asthma who have clubbed digits.
  - Children with nasal polyps and chronic pansinusitis
  - Patients with recurrent pneumonia (especially staphylococcal), chronic atelectasis, chronic pulmonary disease, bronchiectasis, or chronic cough.
  - Infants whose x-rays show persistent hyperaeration or atelectasis.
- Gastrointestinal signs and symptoms:
  - Late passage of the initial meconium.
  - Newborns with intestinal obstruction.
  - Failure to thrive in infancy and childhood.
  - Infants and children with steatorrhea or chronic diarrhea.
  - Patients with rectal prolapse.

- Patients who have disaccharide intolerance or celiac disease as part of their differential diagnosis.
- Children and young adults with cirrhosis of the liver and portal hypertension.
- Genetic risk factors:
  - The sibling has cystic fibrosis; and/or
  - The parent has cystic fibrosis.
- Miscellaneous signs and symptoms:
  - Hypoproteinemia.
  - Hypoprothrombinemia.
  - "Salty" taste to skin.
  - Unexplained hyponatremia.

### Treatment

The pulmonary manifestations of cystic fibrosis are managed with DNase, chest physiotherapy with postural drainage, bronchodilators, steroids, and antibiotics. The gastrointestinal manifestations of cystic fibrosis are managed with pancreatic enzyme supplements; $H_2$ blockers; antacids; a high-calorie, high-protein diet; and vitamin A, D, E, and K supplements.

Children should be monitored with pulmonary function tests (for > 6 years of age), sputum or throat cultures, chest x-rays, CBC, LFTs, BUN, creatinine, and urinalysis unless there are complications.

### CROUP

**Listen for a seal-like bark in croup.**

Viral croup is an acute inflammatory disease of the larynx, especially within the subglottic space. Parainfluenza virus is the most common cause of croup. Other organisms include respiratory syncytial virus, influenza virus, rubeola virus, adenovirus, and *Mycoplasma pneumoniae*.

### Signs and Symptoms

The clinical features of croup include low-grade fever, mild respiratory distress, stridor that worsens when the patient is agitated, a barking cough like that of a dog or a seal (usually at night), and a hoarse voice. The child prefers sitting upright, held by a parent in a calm, quiet atmosphere. Parents may note clinical improvement on the way to the hospital from the cool, crisp evening air.

### Differential

A number of conditions may present with clinical features similar to croup. These conditions include epiglottitis, foreign body aspiration, bacterial tracheitis, angioneurotic edema, and retropharyngeal abscess (see Table 10).

### Workup

**Croup has the "steeple sign."**

The physical exam should focus on the presence of inspiratory stridor, tachypnea, retractions, and breath sounds. Diminished breath sounds, restlessness, altered mental status, or cyanosis may indicate hypoxia. The PA radiograph will show subglottic narrowing that is often referred to as the "steeple sign."

| Croup | Epiglottitis | Tracheitis |
|---|---|---|
| **TABLE 10.** Characteristics of croup, epiglottitis, and tracheitis | | |
| Age: 3 mo to 5 y | Age: 2–7 y | Age: older child, but may affect any age |
| Usually viral etiology, commonly parainfluenza | Usually *Haemophilus influenzae* type B | Often *Staphylococcus aureus* |
| Develops over 2–3 days | Rapid onset over hours | Gradual onset over 2–3 days followed by acute decompensation |
| Usually low-grade fever | High fever | High fever |
| Usually only mild to moderate respiratory distress | Commonly severe respiratory distress | Commonly severe respiratory distress |
| Prefers sitting up, leaning against parent's chest | Prefers perched position with neck extended | May have position preference |
| Stridor improves with aerosolized racemic epinephrine | No response to racemic epinephrine | No response to racemic epinephrine |
| "Steeple sign" on AP neck films | "Thumb sign" on lateral neck films | Subglottic narrowing |

The white blood cell count is not very helpful in the workup of croup, and the blood draw may actually worsen the respiratory distress.

## Treatment

- Mild cases of croup (no stridor at rest) may be managed at home. Home therapy includes mist therapy, oral hydration, and minimal handling.
- More severe cases of croup (stridor at rest, hypoxia) require hospitalization. In addition to cool mist therapy, IV hydration, and minimal handling, oxygen is administered with careful monitoring using a pulse oximeter.
- Nebulized racemic epinephrine (0.5 mL of a 2.25% solution diluted with 2 mL sterile water) and dexamethasone (0.5–1.0 mg/kg PO, IM, or IV as a single dose or repeated every 12 hours) have been shown to be effective.
- Patients with impending respiratory failure will require intubation. Use an endotracheal tube with a slightly smaller diameter than usual.

## EPIGLOTTITIS

In comparison to viral croup, epiglottitis leads to inflammation and swelling of supraglottic structures (epiglottis and arytenoids). Epiglottitis can rapidly progress to life-threatening airway obstruction and is considered a true medical emergency. *Haemophilus influenzae* type B was once the most common organism responsible for epiglottitis. With immunization, however, other organisms are now more commonly found. These include *Streptococcus pneumoniae*, group A streptococci, *Corynebacterium diphtheriae*, and *Staphylococcus*.

### Signs and Symptoms

The clinical features of epiglottitis include sudden onset of high fever (39–40°C), dysphagia, drooling, muffled voice, inspiratory retractions, cyanosis, and stridor. The patient sits with the neck hyperextended and the chin protruding ("sniffing dog" position). Respiratory arrest is possible with progression to total airway obstruction.

### Differential

See the differential diagnosis for croup.

### Workup

As a medical emergency, epiglottitis requires prompt diagnosis based on clinical suspicion. Definitive diagnosis is made by direct fiberoptic visualization of the cherry-red and swollen epiglottis and arytenoids. This procedure must be done under a controlled situation (in the operating room in the presence of an anesthesiologist) in which the airway can be stabilized if needed. If the child is in little distress, the lateral neck x-ray may assist in definitive diagnosis. Again, this should be done under conditions in which airway stabilization is possible in the event of respiratory decompensation. The lateral x-ray demonstrates a swollen epiglottis obliterating the valleculae (classic "thumbprint" sign).

The white blood cell count is usually elevated with a predominance of neutrophils.

### Treatment

Once the diagnosis has been established, intubation should be performed immediately (remember your ABCs). Next, blood cultures, a CBC with differential, and standard chemistries should be obtained. The patient should be started on IV antibiotics that cover *H. influenzae*. An example of such an antibiotic is ceftriaxone (100 mg/kg/d).

The complications of epiglottitis are related to the organism responsible for the disease. *H. influenzae* can result in bacteremia, pneumonia, cervical adenitis, and septic arthritis. Because of this as well as the potential for airway obstruction, epiglottitis is a medical emergency.

## FEBRILE SEIZURES

Febrile seizures are simply seizures that occur in association with fever in children 6 months to 6 years of age. The incidence of febrile seizure is 3–4%.

### Signs and Symptoms

Febrile seizures are classified as simple and complex (see Table 11).

### Workup

**History.** When taking a history of a child who presents with a seizure, it is important to ask the parents to describe the seizure (focal vs. generalized), the

Never use a tongue blade on a child with epiglottitis.

Simple febrile seizure carries a better prognosis.

**TABLE 11.** Simple versus complex febrile seizures

| Simple Febrile Seizure | Complex Febrile Seizure |
|---|---|
| High fever (> 102°F) | Slight fever |
| Short duration (< 15 minutes) | Duration > 15 minutes |
| Generalized seizure | Focal seizure |
| One seizure in a 24-hour period | More than one seizure in a 24-hour period |
| Fever began within hours of the seizure | Febrile for a few days before the onset of the seizure |

duration of the seizure (keep in mind that parents often overestimate the duration), the number of seizures, the post-ictal state, events preceding the seizure, history of previous seizure, family history of febrile seizure and afebrile seizure, and the child's neurologic development, medication exposure, and trauma.

**Physical exam.** During the physical exam, special attention should be paid to rectal temperature, vital signs, mental status, nuchal rigidity (note that this is valid only for children older than 2 years of age), fullness of the fontanelle, and abnormalities or focal differences in muscle strength and tone.

The following laboratory tests are helpful:

- In younger children, calcium, magnesium, BUN, electrolytes, blood culture, and urinalysis.
- A lumbar puncture is necessary if CNS infection is suspected.
- A white blood cell count with differential is indicated in children who are suspected of having occult bacteremia.
- A serum glucose determination by Dextrostix is indicated.
- A head CT is indicated only if central nervous system disease is suspected.
- An EEG should be considered for complex febrile seizures.

## Treatment

The therapy for simple febrile seizures consists of control of the fever with antipyretics and appropriate treatment of the underlying illness. Reassurance and education of the parents about febrile seizures are essential. Thermometer use and antipyretic dosing should be reviewed.

For children who have complex febrile seizures, chronic anticonvulsant therapy may be necessary. The risk of recurrent febrile seizures or the development of epilepsy is greater if there is abnormal neurologic development or a history of afebrile seizure in the parent or sibling.

Anticonvulsants are infrequently used in the therapy of febrile seizures. They include diazepam, phenobarbital, and valproate sodium. Phenytoin and carbamazepine are ineffective.

## Complications

Approximately 30% of children who have one febrile seizure will have another episode, the majority of which will occur within 1 year of the initial one. For simple febrile seizures, there is no increased risk of developmental, intellectual, or growth abnormalities. The risk of developing epilepsy is 1%. The risk of developing epilepsy is higher (10%) if there is a neurologic or de-

**APGAR**

**A**ppearance
**P**ulse
**G**rimace
**A**ctivity
**R**espiratory effort

velopmental abnormality, complex seizure, an abnormal neurologic exam, or a family history of afebrile seizures.

## APGAR SCORE

The Apgar score is an objective method of evaluating a newborn's condition. The Apgar score is determined at 1 minute and 5 minutes after birth. However, assessment of the infant should begin immediately at birth, and the Apgar score should not be used in determining when to initiate resuscitation. Scores of 8–10 indicate no asphyxia; scores of 5–7 indicate mild asphyxia and that the baby needs stimulation and possibly ventilatory support; and scores of less than 5 indicate moderate to severe respiratory distress and that the baby needs assisted ventilation and possible cardiac support (see Table 12).

| **TABLE 12.** Apgar score | | | |
|---|---|---|---|
| | 0 | 1 | 2 |
| Color | Blue/pale | Body pink; extremities blue | Body and extremities pink |
| Heart rate | Absent | < 100/min | > 100/min |
| Reflex irritability | No response | Grimace | Cough or sneeze |
| Muscle tone | Limp | Some flexion | Full flexion |
| Respiratory effort | Absent | Weak cry | Strong cry |

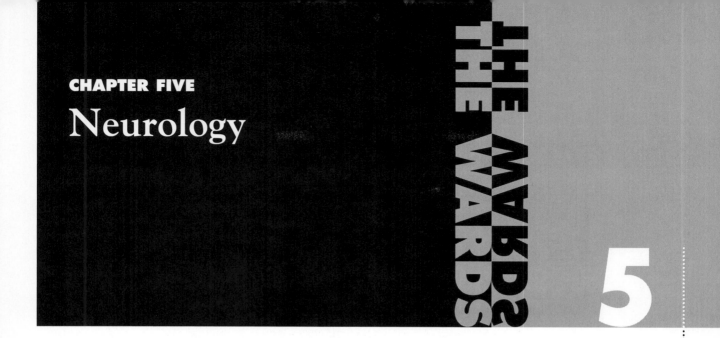

## CHAPTER FIVE
# Neurology

# WARD TIPS

Welcome to your neurology rotation! In the next few weeks, you will have the unique opportunity to focus your studies and patient interactions on the function and dysfunction of the nervous system. In this highly academic and scientific field, you will soon discover one of the things neurologists love to do: talk, talk, and talk about neurology. So get ready for lengthy rounds in which you'll discuss detailed differentials, neuroscience, and the latest research while attempting to answer the ever-present question, "Where's the lesion?" Naturally, you won't be expected to learn all of neurology in a few weeks—so, as in many other rotations, your questions will be more important than your answers. The more interested you are, the better you'll do in the neurology rotation.

## WHAT IS THE ROTATION LIKE?

Neurology rotations differ notably from site to site, so the first thing to do is find out how your responsibilities will be divided between inpatient wards, outpatient clinics, consult-liaison, and neurosurgery. Inpatient neurology tends to be like medicine but is typically less demanding. Student responsibilities center on admission H&Ps, working with the residents in acute management, developing differential diagnoses, and presenting to the team. The day-to-day activities include following labs and neuro exams, writing notes, and playing a supportive role in management. You should plan to read about your patients and understand a bit of the neuroanatomy, pathophysiology, and treatment involved. Always try to trace the neuroanatomic pathways that can cause your patient's symptoms so that you can localize the lesion. In addition to learning the basic neuro exam, this is often looked upon favorably by the attending. The workload tends to depend on the number of students per team, the presence of interns, the number of admissions, and the inpatient census. Don't hesitate to ask your residents/attendings on the first day: Who evaluates me? What are my responsibilities? Whom can I ask for help? What is the call schedule, and is it home call or in-house?

The patient population can be highly variable between hospitals. Patients tend to be admitted for ischemic strokes and hemorrhages, status

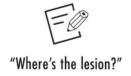

"Where's the lesion?"

epilepticus, meningitis and encephalitis, Guillain-Barré and other myasthenic crises, and acute changes in mental status of unknown etiology, to name just a few. Trauma and tumor patients are often managed by neurosurgery. Outpatient clinics are a great place to see a spectrum of common and uncommon nonacute diseases, such as peripheral neuropathies, multiple sclerosis, migraine, and movement disorders. If you have a particular area of interest, such as neuromuscular disorders, you may want to determine if you can spend a few afternoons each week seeing patients in clinic and observing electrophysiologic testing. In general, you are encouraged to seek out the variety of interesting experiences that neurology offers. Your residents and attendings will likely be impressed by your initiative, and you will benefit from the experience.

## WHO ARE THE PLAYERS?

Team Neuro often works like a medicine team, with a senior resident (R3 or R4) and at least one junior resident (R2). If there are interns, they tend to be from medicine or psychiatry; if there are none, the junior residents may function as "resi-terns." There may also be fourth-year medical students as subinterns and a handful of third-years. In addition, there is usually one ward attending, and there may be private attendings, subspecialty attendings (such as neurovascular or epilepsy), and various fellows. So you may end up presenting patients to a number of different attendings and teams. Other important players include the nursing staff, who among other things are trained to do neuro exams (ICU) and to report on seizures; the social worker, who is an indispensable resource in psychosocial issues and discharge planning; the pharmacist; and the technicians (who do EEGs, blood work, etc).

## HOW IS THE DAY SET UP?

A typical day might (or might not) consist of the following:

| | |
|---|---|
| 7:30–8:00 AM | Prerounds |
| 8:00–8:45 AM | Team work rounds |
| 9:00–10:30 AM | Attending rounds |
| 11:00 AM–12:00 NOON | Subspecialty rounds |
| 1:30–4:30 PM | Clinic |
| 5:00 PM–? | Go home (once you've finished your notes, checked labs, etc) |

Call days vary depending on how busy the service is, how many patients you are expected to carry, and how many admits are scheduled. When you are on call, you should find out who the admitting resident is. Often the consult resident will screen patients in the ER, decide whom to admit, and write the initial orders; you may want to ask this resident to page you so that you can see each patient's initial presentation and take part in forming the differential diagnosis. This is particularly important in patients with rapidly changing neuro exams.

Conferences can be long, overly theoretical, and difficult to follow. Don't be afraid to ask questions or to ask your residents to clarify points that you didn't understand. If most of the conferences are way over your head and you feel you aren't learning the basics, consider self-study using a basic clinical neurology handbook (such as Aminoff's *Clinical Neurology*). Ask your resident or attending if they'd be willing to improvise a few lectures on topics such as "Management of Acute Stroke," "Workup of Altered Mental Status," etc. Depending on the hospital, there may also be neuroradiology conferences to review films on the interesting patients on your team. The more CTs and MRIs you look at, the more familiar you will become with neuroanatomy. Anatomic localization is key in forming meaningful differentials.

## HOW DO I DO WELL IN THIS ROTATION?

Doing well in neurology is no different from any other rotation: be prompt and courteous, take good care of your patients, try to know them better than anyone else, read about their diseases, ask questions, and demonstrate your lifelong interest in the subject. Attendings and fellows love to teach students who are interested, so focus on the basics (reviewing neuroanatomy and studying disease presentation, workup, and treatment). You shouldn't be expected to understand obscure diseases or to track down unintelligible articles (unless your patient happens to have a rare and interesting condition). However, if you find yourself researching a case out of genuine interest, your residents and fellow students might appreciate a report or article that you find. At the very least, your residents will notice your effort and, quite possibly, may find the information useful and decide to add the article to their review files (a rare honor indeed). It is always appropriate to try to educate yourself and the other medical students on your team about something interesting, as long as you are not pompous or condescending about it. You may also want to develop a list of course objectives that fit your future aspirations—perhaps focusing on the execution of the neuro exam and on a basic understanding of the common neurologic diseases.

**Review your neuroanatomy and neuropathophysiology.**

## KEY NOTES

Neurology admission notes are like medicine notes with a few key distinctions:

- Indicate the handedness of the patient in ID. ("Patient is a 46-year-old, right-handed, African-American male.")
- Take a full medical history as well as a neurologic history.
- Remember to note the patient's risk factors, substance use, family history, and social situation.
- Don't forget to record the physical exam, noting vital signs, cardiac exam, jaundice, neck stiffness, etc.
- In documenting the neuro exam, the admission H&P should include the full exam; progress notes can be brief. An example of a brief physical/neuro exam with commonly used abbreviations is as follows:

NC/AT = Normocephalic, atraumatic

3FB = 3 finger breadths; refers to chin-to-chest distance

CTAB = Clear to auscultation bilaterally

RR = Rate regular

BS = Bowel sounds

HSM = Hepatosplenomegaly

C/C/E = Clubbing, cyanosis, edema

A&O×3 = Alert and oriented to person, place, and date

VFFTC = Visual fields full to confrontation

ERRLA = Equal, round, responsive to light/accommodation; refers to pupils

EOMI = Extraocular movements intact

T&P = Tongue and palate

4/5 = Strength 4 on a scale of 5

LT = Light touch

PP = Pin prick

T = Temperature

JPS = Joint position sense

FFM = Fast finger movements

RHM = Rapid hand movements

FTN = Finger to nose

HTS = Heel to shin

**There is no such thing as a "negative Babinski."**

---

**Gen:** Elderly Caucasian male in mild discomfort, moaning.

**VS:** T 37.2 P 59 BP 167/89 R 18 Sat 98% RA.

**HEENT:** NC/AT, sclera anicteric.

**Neck:** +Meningismus, 3FB.

**Lungs:** CTAB.

**Cardiac:** RR no murmurs.

**Abd:** Obese, +BS, soft without HSM/bruits/masses.

**Ext:** No C/C/E.

**MSE:** Pt A&O×3.
    Normal repetition, naming, follows commands.
    Able to attend and concentrate.
    Memory decreased, 0/3 → 2/3 with prompts at 5 min (pt recalls 0 of 3 objects at 5 min, 2 of 3 if given prompts).

**CN:** VFFTC, P 3 → 2 ERRLA.
    Fundi nl, no papilledema, exudates, hemorrhages.
    EOMI without nystagmus or diplopia.
    Face motion and sensation symmetric.
    T&P midline, nl tongue motion, no dysarthria.

**Motor:** Pyramidal weakness, 4/5 LUE = LLE.
    LUE spasticity; normal bulk without tremor or fasciculations.

**Sensory:** Grossly intact, symmetric to LT, PP, T, and JPS; Romberg absent.

**Coordination:** Slowed FFM LUE, LLE nl (also RHM). Normal FTN and HTS, no dysmetria/dysrhythmia.

**Reflexes:** Asymmetrically brisk on L 3+ on L biceps, brachioradialis, patellar and ankle, R 2+; plantar reflexes: plantar flexion on R, dorsiflexion on L (aka Babinski on L).

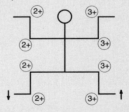

**Gait:** Stable, nl tandem, cannot heel walk.

- Don't forget to report imaging studies and lumbar puncture results.
- The assessment is a good place to organize and summarize; include the important symptoms and findings, localize the lesions to an anatomic location, and, lastly, give an organized differential diagnosis by likelihood.

## KEY PROCEDURES

The main procedure in inpatient neurology is the lumbar puncture (the dreaded "spinal tap," to your patients). Make sure your resident knows that you are interested in doing LPs; it's a good chance to practice. Check *Clinical Neurology*, *Clinician's Pocket Reference*, Ferri's *Care of the Medical Patient*, or similar guides for a description of the procedure. Contraindications include suspected intracranial mass lesion, local infection, spinal cord mass, or coagulopathy. Remember to get informed consent if possible (although this is not always possible in cases with altered mental status) and to write a procedure note documenting both the indications for that procedure and a summary of the procedure (see Chapter 1 for a sample). Find a good and enthusiastic teacher and ask for plenty of supervision early on. Attempting a difficult LP alone can be a nightmare for you and the patient.

Always rule out ↑ICP or focal neurologic deficit before attempting a lumbar puncture.

## WHAT DO I CARRY IN MY POCKETS?

**Checklist**

- ❑ Stethoscope
- ❑ Ophthalmoscope (optional)
- ❑ Eye chart
- ❑ Tuning fork (the big one)
- ❑ Penlight
- ❑ Reflex hammer (the larger the better)
- ❑ Safety pins (do not reuse them)
- ❑ Cotton swabs or clean tissues (for corneal reflex) and tongue blades

With the above items, you will be well equipped to perform a full neuro exam. Keep them within reach on attending rounds; providing your residents or attendings with these implements is a common courtesy.

# TOP-RATED BOOKS

## HANDBOOK/POCKETBOOK

**A-** **Handbook of Symptom-Oriented Neurology**
Olson
Mosby, 1994, 616 pages, ISBN 0801677793, $36.95

Clinically oriented pocket-size book in an outline format allowing fast access. Extensive detail, yet concise. Appropriate for students going into neuro or for those desiring an extensive knowledge base. Could double as both a pocketbook and a reference. Contains extensive references.

**A-** **Manual of Neurologic Therapeutics**
Samuels
Little, Brown, 1995, 451 pages, ISBN 0316770043, $33.95

Comprehensive coverage of major topics in an expanded outline format, with an excellent balance between concise, practical information and reference-level detail. Somewhat large for a pocketbook, but may be all you need for the rotation if not neurology bound.

**A-** **Neurology (House Officer Series)**
Weiner
Williams & Wilkins, 1994, 236 pages, ISBN 0683089064, $24.95

Clinically oriented pocketbook organized by signs/symptoms, with relevant and concise chapters. Lacking in tables and diagrams. Therapeutics sometimes out of date. Not a reference but rather an adjunct to the neuro exam to help you think like a neurologist. Aimed at the intern level.

**B** **Little Black Book of Neurology**
Lerner
Mosby, 1995, 447 pages, ISBN 0815154402, $36.00

Alphabetically organized pocketbook written in an essay format without an index, and thus not useful as a quick reference tool. Aimed at residents. Best used as a memory prod for those who already know the material. Has an eponym index in the back.

**C+** **Neurology**
Mumenthaler
Thieme, 1990, 574 pages, ISBN 0865773173, $29.50

Pathophysiologically oriented pocketbook with reference-like info, but lacking in sufficient detail to be a true reference book. Outdated with regard to treatment and new developments.

# REVIEW/MINI-REFERENCE

### Clinical Neurology
Aminoff
Appleton & Lange, 1996, 344 pages, ISBN 0838513832, $36.95

Clinically oriented with consistent, clear organization. Detailed enough to serve as a student reference. Emphasizes key clinical concepts. Excellent tables and diagrams to localize lesions. Very useful appendices (detailing a full neuro exam and screening motor/sensory exam similar to those found in handbooks).

### Neurological Exam Made Easy
Fuller
Churchill Livingstone, 1993, 220 pages, ISBN 0443042942, $20.95

A detailed review of the neuro exam with simple, easy-to-understand diagrams. Provides a framework for interpreting physical exam findings. For the non-neurologist interested in learning the neuro exam extremely well or for a neuro-bound student who wants to start with an excellent foundation.

### Four Minute Neurological Exam
Goldberg
MedMaster, 1992, 58 pages, ISBN 0940780054, $10.95

A unique and practical guide to a brief neurologic screening exam that may be too simplistic for use during neuro rotation (and is included in many other texts). Contains an interesting chapter on the principles of neuro localization.

### Neurology Secrets
Rolak
Mosby, 1993, 432 pages, ISBN 1560530561, $36.95

Q & A format typical of the *Secrets* series. Not as useful as a comprehensive text, but its value lies in preparing for pimping on the wards. Questions are clinically relevant and cover most topics, with excellent answers. Also includes references for controversial topics, clinical vignettes, and obscure info for extra butt kissing. Detailed index.

### Manter and Gantz's Essentials of Clinical Neuroanatomy and Neurophysiology
Gilman
F. A. Davis, 1996, 309 pages, ISBN 0803601441, $26.95

A fairly extensive review of neuroanatomy and neurophysiology. Too in-depth for those not interested in neuroscience. For those with a sincere interest, however, this classic covers neuroanatomy, blood supply, neurophysiology, and an approach to the neurology patient. Excellent pathway diagrams.

**Oklahoma Notes Neurology and Clinical Neuroscience**
Brumbac
Springer-Verlag, 1996, 186 pages, ISBN 0387946357, $17.95

Outline format, designed more as a boards review with bare-bones facts and key words in bold print. Not useful as a clinical reference and has no index. Includes a 100-question multiple-choice test.

**Clinical Neurology**
Hopkins
Oxford University Press, 1993, 486 pages, ISBN 0192622625, $42.50

Sizable reference that lacks clinical emphasis. Organized by disease process. Decent summaries of topics, but not detailed enough to serve as a reference. Notably lacking in tables, diagrams, and elements of the neurologic exam. Contains some British drug therapy and epidemiology, limiting its usefulness.

## TEXTBOOK/REFERENCE

**Principles of Neurology**
Adams
McGraw-Hill, 1997, 1618 pages, ISBN 0070674396, $83.95

Comprehensive reference text emphasizing the clinical aspects of neurologic disease. Consistent organization from chapter to chapter and very detailed, although tables and pictures are somewhat sparse. Most appropriate for students considering neurology.

**Merritt's Textbook of Neurology**
Rowland
Williams & Wilkins, 1995, 1058 pages, ISBN 0683074008, $79.50

Reference textbook covering the entire spectrum of neurologic disease in depth. Organization of topics is variable.

# HIGH-YIELD TOPICS

## ROTATION OBJECTIVES

Probably the most important things to learn are both the screening and complete neuro exams as well as the workup and management of common neurologic problems such as headache, seizure, low back pain, and stroke. You should focus on the history, physical, and studies; on the development of differentials; and on the recognition of emergency conditions. It's also a good time to learn about the indications for and interpretation of investigational studies, especially CT, MRI, and LP, and perhaps EMG and EEG as well.

The following is a list of topics that you may want to review during this rotation. Topics in italics are discussed in greater detail in this chapter.

*The complete neurologic examination*

### Movement disorders

- *Parkinsonism*
- Other major movement disorders

### Headache

- *Subarachnoid hemorrhage*
- *Temporal arteritis*
- *Intracranial tumor*
- *Subdural hematoma*
- *Migraine*
- *Cluster headache*

### Seizures

- *Focal seizures*
- *Absence (petit mal) seizures*
- *Tonic-clonic (grand mal) seizures*
- *Status epilepticus*

### Stroke

- Recognize the clinical features of the major types of stroke.
- Learn risk factors and preventive therapies.
- Study the approach to workup, treatment, and management.

### Altered mental status/coma

- Distinguish acute confusional states from dementia.
- Identify common and treatable causes of dementia.
- Understand Wernicke's encephalopathy and its treatment.
- Differential diagnoses of coma (mass lesion, metabolic encephalopathy).

### Dysequilibrium

- Differentiate central from peripheral dysequilibrium.
- Recognize common etiologies.
- Understand the basis of nystagmus.

### Weakness

- Develop an approach toward a patient with weakness.
- Recognize common patterns of weakness and learn to localize by exam.

## CNS infections

- Bacterial meningitis.
- HIV infection (both primary and opportunistic).
- TB and HSV infection.
- CSF profiles of types of meningitis.

## Low back pain, spinal cord injuries

- Cord lesions, cord compression, and common myelopathies (such as $B_{12}$ deficiency)
- Differential diagnosis and workup of back pain and a protocol for workup.
- Cervical spine injury.

## Mass lesions and hydrocephalus

- Epidural and subdural hematomas.
- Common types of brain tumors.
- Management of elevated intracranial pressure.

## THE COMPLETE NEUROLOGIC EXAMINATION

Learning to do a complete neuro exam is one of the most important objectives of your rotation. Don't expect to master it in a few weeks; rather, spend time learning to feel comfortable with the components and creating a systematic order to the exam that makes sense to you. Perhaps the best advice is to carefully observe the exams of your residents and attendings, taking note of how (and why) they choose to abbreviate or focus their exam and what tricks help them find subtle deficits. Tables 1–4 provide information for a complete exam. Below is the abbreviated version. Good luck!

### Screening exam for mental status

1. Assess level of consciousness and orientation.

2. Pay attention to patients' use of language and comprehension of your requests during the exam. Ask if they know what's going on with their care/condition. Consider a quick check of repetition and naming (a sensitive test of aphasia).

3. Again, use information from interaction: can the patient attend to commands? Can he or she concentrate on giving a history? If not, check a digit span or similar test.

4. To check memory, you can use information from the history: how did the patient get to hospital? How long has he or she been there? What tests were done today?

### Screening exam for cranial nerves

1. Focus on the eyes: check acuity, visual fields (confrontation), pupillary size/shape/constriction to light and accommodation, and extraocular movements. Ask about diplopia. Don't leave out the funduscopic exam.

2. Check light touch/temperature to face; check corneals if the patient has a depressed level of consciousness.

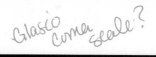
Glasco Coma Scale?

| What You're Testing | What You're Looking For | What You're Doing |
|---|---|---|
| **TABLE 1.** Mental status exam | | |
| Level of consciousness | Alertness<br>Orientation | Observe (eyes open? drowsy looking?).<br>Can patient answer: What's your name? What is the day of week, date, month, year? Where are you? What floor? |
| | Response to voice<br>Response to pain | Call patient's name; ask to open eyes.<br>Try sternal rub, pinching extremities, and watch response for purposefulness. |
| Language | Comprehension of spoken word | Ask patient to close eyes, show three fingers, and touch right ear with left thumb. |
| | Comprehension of written word<br>Repetition of phrases | Hold up card reading "Close your eyes."<br>Have patient repeat, "No ifs, ands, or buts" or "Around the rugged rock the ragged rascal ran," and write "Today is a sunny day." |
| | Fluency of speech | Is it intelligible, fluent, grammatical? Can patient write a complete sentence? |
| | Naming | Try pointing to watch and parts to elicit "watch, band, buckle," or use a pen: "Pen, cap, tip/point." |
| Attention | Ability to focus on a task | Ask patient to repeat digit spans, eg, "02139." |
| Concentration | Ability to maintain focus | Have patient serially subtract 7 from 100 (or 3 from 20) or spell "world" backwards. |
| Mood, insight, thought process and content | Look for signs of depression, other psychiatric disturbance, denial | Ask patient, "How are your spirits?" "Do you know why you are here in the hospital?" |
| Memory | Registration | List three words, eg, "Apple, England, and John Lennon," and ask patient to repeat. |
| | Short term | Three minutes later, ask patient to recall three items. Offer prompts if patient is unable to do so (such as "a kind of fruit," "a country in Europe," "the best Beatle"); can also try current events. |
| | Long term | Ask for birthdate, SSN, history. |
| Higher cognitive function | Fund of knowledge<br>Calculations | Ask for names of current/past presidents.<br>Try simple addition and division (how many quarters in $2.50), subtraction (making change from $5.00 for $1.39). |
| | Abstractions | Ask patient to interpret a proverb such as "A rolling stone gathers no moss." Be aware of cultural differences. |
| | Constructions | Ask patient to copy sketches (square, cube) and to draw a clock (analog). |

3. Observe the face for asymmetries; check the facial muscles.

4. Listen to the voice for hoarseness, dysarthria.

### Screening exam for motor coordination

1. Observe! Does the patient have atrophy, abnormal movements or postures, or a tendency to favor one side of the body? Other localizing findings?

## TABLE 2. Cranial nerve exam

| What You're Testing | What You're Looking For | What You're Doing |
|---|---|---|
| I Olfactory nerve | Ability to discern smells | Usually omitted—can check with coffee, ammonia, orange or lemon extract. |
| II Optic nerve | Visual acuity<br>Visual fields<br><br>Ocular fundi (funduscopic exam) | Use Snellen eye chart.<br>Test by confrontation if patient cooperates, or estimate by visual threat otherwise.<br>Look for papilledema, retinal/subhyaloid hemorrhages, retinopathy, and/or optic atrophy. |
| III Oculomotor nerve | Pupillary function<br><br><br>Function of levator palpebrae<br>Function of superior rectus<br>Function of inferior rectus<br>Function of inferior oblique | Check baseline size, shape, and symmetry; direct and consensual constriction (using penlight); and accommodation.<br>Check for elevation of eyelid and ptosis.<br>EOM (elevate gaze).<br>EOM (depress gaze).<br>EOM (elevate adducted eye). |
| IV Trochlear nerve | Function of superior oblique | EOM (depress adducted eye). |
| VI Abducens nerve | Function of lateral rectus<br>Assessment of EOMs | EOM (abduction).<br>Ask patient to follow target in H shape, looking for full movement and coordination. |
| V Trigeminal nerve | Motor: temporal, masseter muscles<br>Sensory: V1, V2, V3<br>Reflex: corneal blink | Palpate muscles as patient clenches teeth.<br>Check sensation to forehead, cheek, and jaw.<br>Touch cornea with cotton thread or tissue. |
| VII Facial nerve | Motor to facial muscles (also checked in motor response to the corneal reflex) | Check raised eyebrows, tightly squinted eyes, smile, and puffed-out cheeks, looking for asymmetries. |
| VIII Vestibulocochlear nerve | Auditory function<br><br>Vestibular function | Grossly test hearing by rubbing fingers together by each ear or scratching pillow.<br>Check for nystagmus, h/o vertigo. |
| IX Glossopharyngeal nerve | Sensory: palate, pharynx | Check gag reflex (stroke back of throat). |
| X Vagus nerve | Motor: palate, pharynx, vocal cords | Check voice for hoarseness, articulation; check palatal elevation, uvular position, gag reflex. |
| XI Spinal accessory nerve | Motor: trapezius<br>Motor: sternocleidomastoid | Have patient shrug shoulders with resistance.<br>Have patient check SCM strength. |
| XII Hypoglossal nerve | Motor: tongue | Look at tongue in mouth for position, atrophy, and fasciculations; have patient protrude tongue and move side to side (again, check for asymmetry and movement). |

2. Check pronator drift by asking the patient to raise both arms to a 90° angle (palms up) with eyes closed. Weakness shows as pronation or downward drift.

3. Raise arms overhead and maintain against resistance (proximal muscles).

4. Check strength of finger extension, index finger abduction, and big toe dorsiflexion.

5. Rapid hand movements such as quickly tapping index finger on thumb show weakness or loss of coordination. Also check rapid foot tapping.

## TABLE 3. Motor and coordination exam

| What You're Testing | What You're Looking For | What You're Doing |
|---|---|---|
| Appearance | Bulk (atrophy, hypertrophy), fasciculations, spasms, spontaneous motion. | Observing. |
| Tone | Resistance to passive motion. | Check wrists, elbows, ankles, knees; remind patient to relax, shake gently, move evenly through range of motion, then move abruptly (note pattern of resistance). |
| Descriptions of tone | Rigidity: Increased in full range of motion, not dependent on rate or location; may be constant (lead-pipe rigidity) or ratchety (cogwheel rigidity). Spasticity: Tone increased most in arm flexors and leg extensors, increases as rate of motion increases, more noted at initiation of motion than continuation. Flaccidity: Decreased tone, joints tend to flop and hyperextend like a rag doll. Paratonia: Changes in tone over time/position caused by an inability to relax. | |
| Power | Discover pattern of weakness (or absence of weakness). Explore extent of weakness and elucidate possible etiologies. | History (weakness, clumsiness). Screening exam (see below). Focused motor exam based on information given in history and screen. Also use functional testing (see *gait* below). Examination tips: give patient mechanical advantage (start with joint in midposition) and apply force to overcome patient's strength, not to match it. Palpate muscle belly during exam. |
| Reflexes | Deep tendon reflexes (jaw, biceps, brachioradialis, triceps, finger flexors, patellar, thigh adductors, ankle jerk). Superficial reflexes (abdominal, cremasteric). Pathological reflexes (Babinski, frontal release). | Ask patient to relax, position limbs, alternate from side to side for comparison. Watch for clonus, and record briskness (0–4+). Pay attention to symmetry! For Babinski (plantar response), stroke the lateral plantar surface of the foot with a key; look for direction of big toe motion (dorsiflexion = Babinski sign). |
| Coordination | Point-to-point testing. Rapid movements (strength and coordination). | Upper: have patient touch his nose, then your finger, repeat. Lower: have patient run heel up and down opposite shin from knee to foot. Index finger tapping on thumb, foot tapping on the ground or on your palm. |
| Gait | Normal gait. Important for testing power of the lower extremities; functional testing is more sensitive than manual testing. Test for ataxia (tandem gait). Test for distal weakness. Test for proximal weakness. | Is gait balanced and coordinated with feet no wider than shoulders and arms swinging? Can patient walk in a line heel-to-toe? Have patient walk on toes (plantar flexion) and on heels (dorsiflexion of ankles). Have patient hop on one foot or try a knee bend (standing on one foot). Can patient get out of chair w/o using arms? |

| TABLE 4. Sensory exam | | |
|---|---|---|
| **What You're Testing** | **What You're Looking For** | **What You're Doing** |
| **Sensory modalities**—Seeking to identify a pattern of sensory loss/disruption. | | |
| Pain | Ability/inability to identify "sharp." | Pricking with a safety pin or a Q-tip stick broken in half. |
| Temperature | Ability/inability to identify "cold." | Touching with cool tuning fork. |
| Vibration | Ability/inability to identify "buzz." | Buzzing tuning fork touched to bone and joint. |
| Joint position sense | Ability to sense direction of motion. | Moving patient's finger or toe up or down. Romberg test: Stand with feet together and eyes closed for 10 seconds. If patient is OK with eyes open but not closed, test is positive. |
| Light touch | Ability/inability to identify touch. | Lightly touch patient with finger or cotton. |
| **Higher sensory function**—Deficits in the discriminative sensations, testing cortical/peripheral. | | |
| Graphesthesia | Ability to recognize object by feeling. | Ask patient to identify object in hand without seeing it, such as a paper clip, or to identify heads/tails of a coin. |
| Point localization | Ability to localize sensory input. | Quickly touch patient, then ask to identify location. |
| Extinction | Ability to recognize dual, bilateral stimuli. | Touch same areas bilaterally and ask patient to identify location of stimulus. |

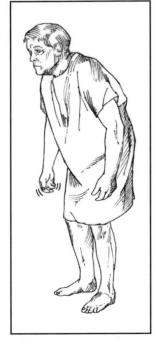

**FIGURE 1.** Patient with parkinsonism in typical flexed posture. Note the masklike facies and resting hand tremor. Aminoff, *Clinical Neurology,* Third Edition, Stamford, CT: Appleton & Lange, 1996, page 220.

6. Check gait as described in Table 3 (great assessment of leg power and coordination).

7. Check tone, DTRs (biceps, triceps, patellar), and plantar responses.

**Screening exam for sensation**

1. Check pain (or cold) sensation in the hands and feet.

2. Check vibration (or joint position sense) in the hands and feet.

3. Check light touch on arms and legs, looking for asymmetry.

## PARKINSONISM

Parkinsonism describes a movement disorder characterized by tremor, rigidity, bradykinesia, and abnormal gait and posture (see Figure 1). Most cases of parkinsonism result from idiopathic degeneration of the dopaminergic nigrostriatal tract, with a resulting imbalance between dopamine and acetylcholine; these cases are termed Parkinson's disease. Other insults that decrease dopaminergic activity can lead to parkinsonism, including postencephalitic, toxic (such as carbon disulfide, manganese, "designer drugs"), ischemic, and iatrogenic (especially neuroleptics) insults.

## Signs and Symptoms

"The Parkinson's tetrad":

1. Resting tremor (especially "pill-rolling" tremor of hands, but may affect all extremities, head, and trunk).
2. Rigidity (in particular, cogwheeling).
3. Bradykinesia, with difficult initiation and with typical shuffling, festinating gait without arm swing.
4. Postural instability.

Mild dementia is common as well but typically is not profound. Other telltale signs include masked facies and decreased amplitude of movements (seen in micrographia and hypophonia).

## Differential

It is important to consider treatable causes of tremors, psychomotor slowness, and instability, such as depression, essential tremor, normal pressure hydrocephalus, and Wilson's disease. Other conditions in the differential include Creutzfeldt-Jakob disease, Shy-Drager's syndrome, and Huntington's disease.

## Treatment

Treatment for parkinsonism seeks to improve the balance between dopamine and acetylcholine by increasing dopaminergic tone with agonists such as levodopa and bromocriptine, decreasing dopamine-antagonizing neuroleptics, or decreasing acetylcholine with anticholinergic medications. Amantadine can be useful as well (mechanism unknown). Some studies have shown that selegiline, an MAO-B inhibitor, can be used as an adjunct to levodopa to slow disease progression. Surgical management may be helpful in intractable cases; pallidotomy has recently reemerged as a potentially important treatment.

# HEADACHE

Headache is a common reason to seek medical attention. Headache is also among the first presenting symptoms of serious neurologic disease—so it is essential to remember that headache is a complaint that should be taken seriously. It is your job to differentiate between benign and life-threatening conditions.

## Workup

There are four important questions that you should ask with regard to headache:

1. **"Is this a new or an old headache?"**

   You should ask if the patient has ever had a headache like this one before. Is it qualitatively different from headaches they've had in the past? Is it the "worst headache of their life"? Any new, severe headache warrants an emergent workup.

2. **"What are the characteristics of the pain?"**

   You should obtain a temporal profile of the headache and ask what makes it better or worse. Be on the lookout for clues to differentiate between the different headache syndromes.

   Also ask about present and past medical conditions. A new headache in a patient with a history of cancer or with AIDS is even more likely to be serious; this information is crucial to your differential.

3. **"Are there other signs or symptoms of systemic (or neurologic) disease?"**

   Look for fever, nausea and vomiting, weight loss, jaw claudication. Ask about associated sensory symptoms (eg, flashing lights, funny smell).

4. **"Are there associated neurologic findings?"**

   The neuro exam is crucial here to determine if the patient has either positive (paresthesias, visual stigmata) or negative (weakness, numbness, ataxia) symptoms. Always remember to check the neck for stiffness/meningeal signs. A focal exam needs immediate workup.

## Differential

Headaches are classified as acute, subacute, or chronic.

"Worst headache of my life" gets a CT and an LP.

- **Acute:** *Subarachnoid hemorrhage*, hemorrhagic stroke, TIA, meningitis, seizure, acute elevated intracranial pressure, hypertensive encephalopathy, postcoital, post-lumbar puncture, ocular (glaucoma, iritis).
- **Subacute:** *Temporal arteritis*, *intracranial tumor*, *subdural hematoma*, pseudotumor cerebri, trigeminal/glossopharyngeal neuralgia, postherpetic neuralgia, hypertension.
- **Chronic:** *Migraine*, *cluster headache*, tension headache, subacute sinusitis, dental disease, neck pain, intracranial mass.

Items in italics are discussed in more detail below.

## SUBARACHNOID HEMORRHAGE

Subarachnoid hemorrhage (SAH) is commonly caused by a ruptured aneurysm (berry, hypertensive), stroke, AVM, or trauma (see Figure 2).

### Signs and Symptoms

SAH is characterized by a sudden-onset, intensely painful headache, often with neck stiffness, fever, nausea and vomiting, and changing level of consciousness.

### Differential

The differential diagnosis of SAH includes hemorrhagic stroke, trauma, meningitis, and first presentation of migraine.

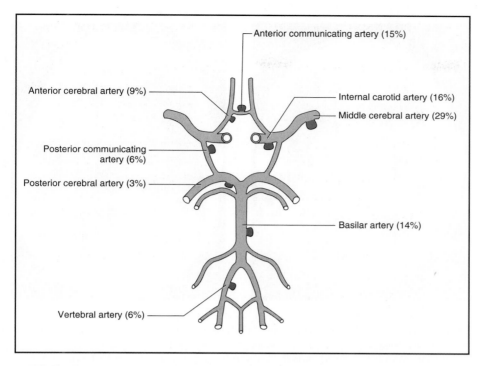

**FIGURE 2.** Frequency distribution of intracranial aneurysms. Aminoff, *Clinical Neurology*, Third Edition, Stamford, CT: Appleton & Lange, 1996, page 77.

## Workup

- Stat head CT (Figure 3) (looking for blood in the subarachnoid space—don't use contrast!).
- Immediate LP if CT is negative (looking for elevated red cells, a xanthochromia, and/or elevated ICP).
- Four-vessel angiography once SAH is confirmed (if patient is a surgical candidate).

## Treatment

Medical treatment focuses on preventing the elevation of ICP by raising the head of the bed, limiting IV fluids, and avoiding hypertension (while ensuring adequate cerebral perfusion) together with the use of calcium-channel blockers (nimodipine) and seizure prophylaxis (phenytoin). Surgical treatment may involve open or interventional radiologic clipping or coiling of an aneurysm or AVM.

## Complications

- Rebleeding (more common in aneurysm than in AVM).
- Extension into the brain parenchyma (more common with AVM).
- Arterial vasospasm (occurs in one-third of SAHs from aneurysmal rupture).

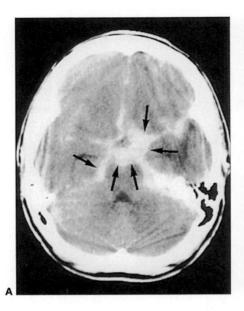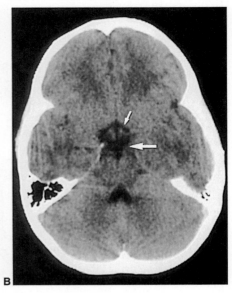

**FIGURE 3.** Head CT scans. (A) Acute SAH. Areas of high density (arrows) represent blood in the subarachnoid space. (B) A normal scan; note the interpeduncular cistern (large arrow) and suprasellar cistern (small arrow). Aminoff, *Clinical Neurology,* Third Edition, Stamford, CT: Appleton & Lange, 1996, page 78.

## TEMPORAL ARTERITIS

Generally not seen before age 50, this condition affects twice as many women as men. Causes include subacute granulomatous inflammatory process involving the external carotid (especially the temporal branch) and vertebral arteries. Thrombosis of the affected arteries leads to complications. The most serious complication is thrombosis of the ophthalmic artery (branch of the ICA), which can cause ipsilateral blindness.

### Signs and Symptoms

Signs and symptoms may include a new headache that is unilateral or bilateral associated with scalp pain and temporal tenderness, as well as transient or permanent monocular blindness. Associated with weight loss, jaw claudication, myalgia/arthralgia, and fever.

### Workup

- ESR (> 50, usually >100).
- Temporal artery biopsy.

### Treatment

Treatment should consist of prednisone, 40–60 mg PO qd, for 3 months, followed by q.o.d. dosing over 1–2 years. Treatment should be started on an empiric basis (ie, before confirmation with temporal artery biopsy) to prevent serious complications such as blindness.

## INTRACRANIAL TUMOR

May be primary or metastatic (most commonly from lung, melanoma, breast, colon, or kidney).

### Signs and Symptoms

Only 30% of patients present with headache. Headache is typically dull and steady, worse in the morning, exacerbated by coughing/changing position/exertion, and associated with nausea and vomiting. May be associated with focal findings on neuro exam, seizures, lethargy.

### Workup

Workup should include CT with contrast and MRI.

### Treatment

Management depends upon tumor type. Some types (eg, meningioma) can be cured with resection, radiation therapy, and/or chemotherapy. Other types (eg, glioblastoma multiforme) may be poorly responsive and require conservative and supportive care.

## SUBDURAL HEMATOMA

Subdural hematoma is typically a result of trauma (especially in the elderly or alcoholics, secondary to rupture of bridging veins).

### Signs and Symptoms

Signs and symptoms include headache, change in mental status, contralateral hemiparesis, or other focal changes. Changes can be either subacute or chronic and may present as a new-onset dementia.

### Workup

Workup should include CT (see Figure 4) or MRI.

### Treatment

Surgical evacuation if symptomatic; otherwise, observe.

## MIGRAINE

Migraine is more commonly seen in women under the age of 30 and runs in families. The etiology is not fully understood; vascular abnormalities (such as intracranial vasoconstriction and extracranial vasodilation) are perhaps secondary to a disorder of serotonergic neurotransmission or other primary disturbances of neurologic function.

**Many migraines do not present "classically."**

A                                    B

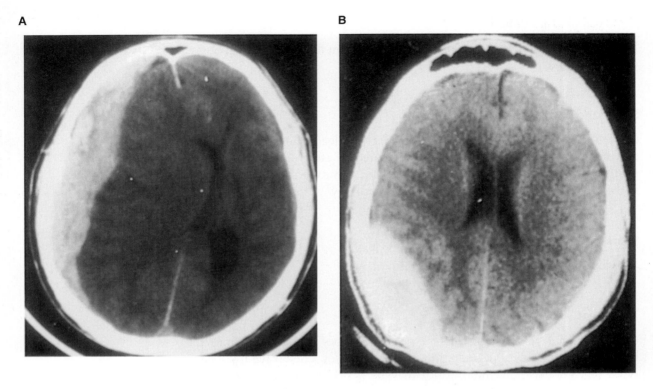

**FIGURE 4.** Head CT scans. (A) Subdural hematoma. Note the crescent shape and the mass effect with midline shift. (B) Epidural hematoma with classic biconvex lens shape. Aminoff, *Clinical Neurology,* Third Edition, Stamford, CT: Appleton & Lange, 1996, page 296.

### Signs and Symptoms

Headache is either throbbing or dull, often unilateral (but can be bilateral or occipital), and associated with nausea and vomiting, photophobia, and noise sensitivity (Figure 5). "Classic migraines" are usually unilateral and defined by visual symptoms such as scintillating lights, scotomas, and field cuts; "common migraines" are not. Migraines typically last between 2 and 20 hours and occur less frequently than once a week.

### Workup

CT or MRI is warranted on first presentation, especially if there are focal findings on examination (migraine itself can be associated with transient focal neurologic deficits).

### Treatment

Abortive therapy seeks to end the headache once it has started and may be sufficient for the patient with a reliable prodrome or a tolerable occasional breakthrough. Abortive therapy includes aspirin/NSAIDs, sumatriptan (a 5HT agonist), ergots (partial 5HT agonists), Midrin, Fiorinal, and opiates. Prophylaxis includes NSAIDs, beta blockers, ergots, tricyclic antidepressants, calcium-channel blockers, and valproic acid. Narcotics should not be used prophylactically.

Pain

**FIGURE 5.** Pain in migraine headache is most commonly hemicranial. Pain can also be holocephalic, bifrontal, or unilateral frontal. Aminoff, *Clinical Neurology,* Third Edition, Stamford, CT: Appleton & Lange, 1996, page 91.

## CLUSTER HEADACHE

Cluster headaches affect men more often than women, with onset usually in the 20s.

### Signs and Symptoms

Cluster headache is a brief, severe, unilateral headache usually occurring around the eye (Figure 6). Attacks tend to occur in clusters, affecting the same part of the head and taking place at the same time of day (usually at night). Associated symptoms include ipsilateral tearing of the eye and conjunctival injection, Horner's syndrome, and nasal stuffiness. Cluster headache may be precipitated by intake of alcohol or vasodilators.

### Workup

No workup is necessary if presentation is classic.

### Treatment

Cluster headaches are relieved acutely by 100% oxygen, ergots, or sumatriptan. Therapy for the prevention of recurrence during an acute attack includes ergots, calcium-channel blockers, prednisone, and lithium.

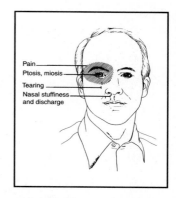

**FIGURE 6.** Distribution of pain in cluster headache. Pain is commonly associated with ipsilateral conjunctival injection, tearing, nasal stuffiness, and Horner's syndrome. Aminoff, *Clinical Neurology*, Third Edition, Stamford, CT: Appleton & Lange, 1996, page 92.

## SEIZURES

Seizures are cortical events characterized by excessive or hypersynchronous discharge by cortical neurons; they are caused by a primary nervous system disorder or are secondary to a systemic disturbance. Epilepsy describes the predisposition to recurrent, unprovoked seizures (not everyone with seizures has epilepsy!). Most seizures are self-limited and last less than 2 minutes; prolonged or repetitive seizures are called "status epilepticus" and constitute a medical emergency.

The evaluation and treatment of a patient with a recent history of seizure should seek to answer the following questions:

1. **Did the patient actually have a seizure?**

   A syncopal event can easily be confused with a seizure. In taking a history from the patient and observers, ask about the onset, course, and postspell period (see Table 5).

2. **Was the seizure caused by a systemic process?**

   It is important to consider the systemic causes of seizure in the workup. If there is a clear, treatable, nonneurologic cause, further neurologic investigation may be unnecessary. Such disorders include hypoglycemia, hyponatremia, hypocalcemia, hyperosmolar states, hepatic encephalopathy, uremia, porphyria, drug overdose (especially cocaine, antidepressants, neuroleptics, methylxanthines, and lidocaine), drug withdrawal (especially alcohol and other sedatives), eclampsia, hyperthermia, hypertensive encephalopathy, and cerebral hypoperfusion. Therefore, workup should focus on reversible causes first.

| TABLE 5. Seizure versus syncope | | |
|---|---|---|
| | **Seizure** | **Syncope** |
| Onset | Sudden onset without prodrome. Focal sensory or motor phenomena. Sensation of fear, smell, memory. | Progressive lightheadedness. Dimming of vision, faintness. |
| Course | Sudden LOC with tonic-clonic activity. May last 1–2 minutes. May see tongue laceration, head trauma, and bowel/urinary incontinence. | Gradual LOC, limp or with jerking. Rarely lasts longer than 15 seconds. Less commonly injured. |
| Postspell | Postictal confusion and disorientation. | Typically immediate return to lucidity. |

**Tonic-clonic movements do not exclude syncope.**

3. **Was the seizure caused by an underlying neurologic disorder?**

Patients without a known cause for their seizures should undergo neurologic evaluation, particularly in search of treatable causes (Table 6). Seizures with focal onset (or focal postictal deficit) suggest focal CNS pathology. Seizures may be the presenting sign of a tumor, stroke, AVM, infection, or hemorrhage, or they may represent the delayed presentation of a developmental abnormality. The history should include past seizures, birth/childhood or recent trauma, and developmental delays. For both treatment and prognosis, it is important to try to determine the etiology. In a patient with a known seizure disorder, you must ask the question, "Why did this seizure occur?" and consider subtherapeutic levels of meds or a new provoking factor, such as infection or trauma (see Table 6).

4. **Is anticonvulsant therapy indicated?**

Patients with a first seizure are often not treated when the underlying cause is unknown. However, 40–60% of idiopathic seizures will recur. Recurrence is higher in patients with abnormal EEGs or MRIs, with focal exams, and with irreversible predisposing factors (Figure 7).

## FOCAL SEIZURES

Focal seizures arise from a discrete region in one cerebral hemisphere.

| TABLE 6. Common etiologies of seizures by age | | | | |
|---|---|---|---|---|
| **Infant** | **Child (2–10)** | **Adolescent** | **Adult (18–35)** | **Adult (35+)** |
| Perinatal injury/ ischemia | Idiopathic | Idiopathic | Trauma | Trauma |
| Infection | Infection | Trauma | Alcoholism | Stroke |
| Metabolic disturbance | Trauma | Drug withdrawal | Brain tumor | Metabolic disorders |
| Congenital/ genetic disorders | Febrile seizure | AVM | Drug withdrawal | Alcoholism |

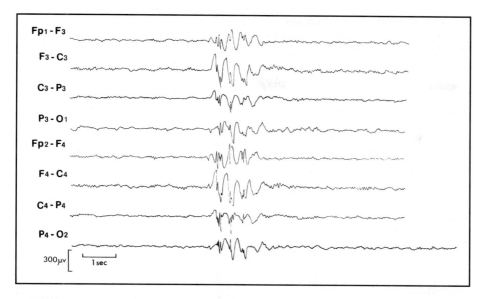

**FIGURE 7.** EEG in idiopathic seizures. Note the burst of generalized epileptiform activity on a relatively normal background. Aminoff, *Clinical Neurology,* Third Edition, Stamford, CT: Appleton & Lange, 1996, Page 241.

## Signs and Symptoms

The clinical effects of focal seizure activity depend on the region of the cortex that is affected. Seizure foci in the motor or sensory areas (frontal or parietal lobes) might lead to phenomena such as twitching of the face or tingling of the hand. Involvement of the insular cortex can result in autonomic phenomena. If the patient's level of consciousness is unaffected during these seizures, they are called "simple partial seizures." Postictally, there may be a focal neurologic deficit known as Todd's paralysis that resolves over one to two days and often indicates a focal brain lesion.

Involvement of the temporal lobe or medial frontal lobe leads to more complex manifestations, such as memories (déjà vu), feelings of fear, or complex actions such as lip smacking or walking. The patient's contact with the outside world is often affected during these seizures, which are called "complex partial seizures." Both simple and complex partial seizures can generalize; that is, the electrical activity can spread to involve both hemispheres.

## Workup

The standard seizure workup includes CBC, electrolytes, calcium, glucose, ABG, LFTs, renal panel, FTA, ESR, and tox screen to rule out systemic causes and diagnostic tests such as the EEG (to look for epileptiform waveforms) and CT or MRI (preferable).

## Treatment

Treatment should consist of management of the underlying cause if feasible. Otherwise, phenytoin (Dilantin), carbamazepine (Tegretol), valproate (Depakote), lamotrigine (Lamictal), or gabapentin (Neurontin) can be administered.

## ABSENCE (PETIT MAL) SEIZURES

Absence seizures begin in childhood, are often familial, and typically subside before adulthood.

### Signs and Symptoms

Absence seizures are characterized by brief, often unnoticeable episodes of impaired consciousness lasting only seconds and occurring up to hundreds of times per day.

### Workup

The EEG shows a classic 3-per-second spike-and-wave tracing (see Figure 8).

### Treatment

Valproate or ethosuximide.

## TONIC-CLONIC (GRAND MAL) SEIZURES

### Signs and Symptoms

Tonic-clonic seizures begin suddenly with loss of consciousness and tonic extension of the back and extremities, continuing with 1–2 minutes of repetitive, symmetric clonic movements. Consciousness is slowly regained in the postictal period.

### Treatment

Treatment consists of management of the underlying cause. Otherwise, valproate, phenytoin, or carbamazepine is administered.

## STATUS EPILEPTICUS

Status epilepticus is characterized by prolonged or repetitive seizures without a return to baseline consciousness in between. Common causes include anticonvulsant withdrawal/noncompliance, EtOH/sedative withdrawal or other drug intoxication, metabolic disturbances, trauma, and infection.

### Signs and Symptoms

Continuous seizure activity or multiple episodes of seizure activity occur without return of consciousness.

### Workup

Check CBC, electrolytes, calcium, glucose, ABG, LFTs, renal panel, FTA, ESR, tox screen. EEG and brain imaging is deferred until patient is stabilized.

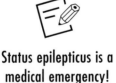

Status epilepticus is a medical emergency!

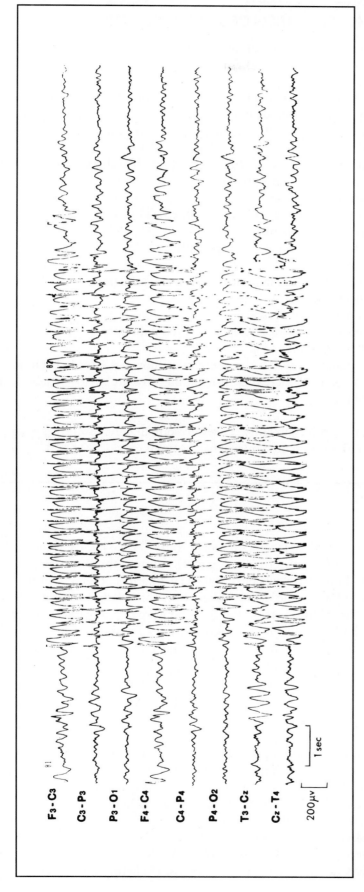

F3 - C3

C3 - P3

P3 - O1

F4 - C4

C4 - P4

P4 - O2

T3 - Cz

Cz - T4

200μV

1 sec

**FIGURE 8.** EEG of absence seizures with the classical 3-spikes-per-second pattern. Aminoff, *Clinical Neurology*, Third Edition, Stamford, CT: Appleton & Lange, 1996, page 240.

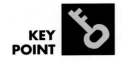

**EMERGENCY EVALUATION OF STATUS EPILEPTICUS**

Treatment with anticonvulsants should be instituted immediately (Table 7) while the following measures are taken:
- Vital signs:
  - **Blood pressure:** Exclude hypertensive encephalopathy and shock.
  - **Temperature:** Exclude hyperthermia.
  - **Pulse:** Exclude life-threatening cardiac arrhythmia.
- Draw venous blood for serum glucose, calcium, electrolytes, hepatic and renal function blood studies, complete blood count, erythrocyte sedimentation rate, and toxicology.
- Insert intravenous line.
- Administer glucose (50 mL of 50% dextrose) intravenously.
- Obtain any available history.
- Rapid physical examination, especially for:
  - Signs of trauma.
  - Signs of meningeal irritation or systemic infection.
  - Papilledema.
  - Focal neurologic signs.
  - Evidence of metastatic, hepatic, or renal disease.
- Arterial blood gases.
- Lumbar puncture, unless the cause of seizures has already been determined or signs of increased intracranial pressure or focal neurologic signs are present.
- EKG.
- Calculate serum osmolality: 2 (serum sodium concentration) + serum glucose/20 + serum urea nitrogen/3 (normal range: 270–290).

### Treatment

On admission, attend to cardiopulmonary status (ABCs). Give thiamine (100 mg) and glucose (50 mL of 50% dextrose). Correct the underlying disorder when found. Immediately begin sequential pharmacotherapy with Ativan (lorazepam) and a loading dose of phenytoin (or fos-phenytoin if available) (Table 7). If the seizures persist after first 18 mg/kg of phenytoin is given (rate not to exceed 50 mg/min), infuse another 7 mg/kg at the same rate. If seizures continue, intubate and add IV phenobarbital (at the same dose and rate as phenytoin—first 18 mg/kg, then 7 mg/kg). If the patient fails therapy, admit to the ICU and treat with an IV anesthetic such as midazolam.

### STROKE

Stroke is a clinical syndrome defined by the acute onset of a focal neurologic deficits as a result of a disturbance in blood flow (either ischemia or hemorrhage). If the deficit reverses within 24 hours, the event is renamed a transient ischemic attack (TIA). A reversible ischemic neurologic deficit (RIND) reverses within the first week.

The risk of stroke increases with age, is higher for men than for women, and is higher for African-Americans than for Caucasians. Intracranial vascular disease is particularly common in Asians. Diabetes and hypertension are

## TABLE 7. Drug treatment of status epilepticus

| Drug | Dosage/Route | Advantages/Disadvantages/Complications |
|------|--------------|----------------------------------------|
| Lorazepam[1] or diazepam | 10 mg IV over 2 minutes.<br>0.1 mg/kg IV rate not greater than 2 mg/min. | Fast-acting. Effective half-life 15 minutes for diazepam and 4 hours for lorazepam. Abrupt respiratory depression or hypotension in 5%, especially when given in combination with other sedatives. Seizure recurrence in 50% of patients; therefore must add maintenance drug (phenytoin or phenobarbital). |
| **IMMEDIATELY PROCEED TO PHENYTOIN** | | |
| Phenytoin or fos-phenytoin | 1000–1500 mg (18 mg/kg) IV rate not greater than 50 mg/min (cannot be given in dextrose solution). Fos-phenytoin at 100–150 mg/min. | Little or no respiratory depression. Drug levels in the brain are therapeutic at completion of infusion. Effective as maintenance drug. Hypotension and cardiac arrhythmias can occur, probably more often with phenytoin than with fos-phenytoin. |
| **IF SEIZURES CONTINUE FOLLOWING TOTAL DOSE, PROCEED IMMEDIATELY TO PHENOBARBITAL** | | |
| Phenobarbital | 1000–1500 mg (18 mg/kg) IV slowly (50 mg/min). | Peak brain levels within 30 minutes. Effective as maintenance drug. Respiratory depression and hypotension common at higher doses. (Intubation and ventilatory support should be immediately available.) |
| **IF ABOVE IS INEFFECTIVE, PROCEED IMMEDIATELY TO GENERAL ANESTHESIA** | | |
| Pentobarbital or midazolam[1] | 15 mg/kg IV slowly, followed by 0.5–4 mg/kg/h.<br>0.2 mg/kg IV slowly, followed by 0.75–10 mg/kg/min. | Intubation and ventilatory support required. Hypotension is limiting factor. Pressors may be required to maintain blood pressure. |

[1]Investigational in the United States.

important risk factors, as are smoking and atrial fibrillation. Cocaine use and IV drug use are also risk factors, particularly in young people. Hyperlipidemia and heavy alcohol intake are less significantly associated with stroke.

The most common vascular cause of stroke is atherosclerosis of the large extracranial vessels (internal and common carotids, basilar and vertebral arteries). The main risk factors for atherosclerosis are hypertension and diabetes. Lacunar infarcts occur in regions supplied by small perforating vessels and result from either atherosclerotic or hypertensive occlusion. Other causes include fibromuscular dysplasia, inflammatory diseases, arterial dissection, migraine, and venous thrombosis.

Cardiac causes of stroke include atrial fibrillation (the most common cause of cardioembolic stroke) as well as embolism of mural thrombi, thrombi from diseased or prosthetic valves, other arrhythmias, endocarditis (septic, fungal, or marantic emboli), and paradoxic (venous) emboli in patients with right-to-left shunt in the heart (from atrial septal defect or patent foramen ovale).

Hematologic disorders implicated in stroke include sickle-cell disease, polycythemia, thrombocytosis, leukocytosis, and other hypercoagulable states (such as those seen in malignancy, hereditary coagulopathies, or collagen vascular diseases).

Intraparenchymal hemorrhage tends to result from hypertensive rupture of small vessels, AVMs, hemorrhage conversion of ischemic strokes, amyloid angiopathy, cocaine use, and bleeding diatheses.

## Signs and Symptoms

On physical exam, listen carefully to the heart and the carotid and subclavian arteries. The deficits on neurologic examination correlate with the region of the brain affected (see Table 8). Classically, thrombotic strokes evolve over minutes to hours and may be preceded by TIAs; embolic strokes may present with full deficit acutely and do not evolve; and hemorrhagic strokes may be preceded by headache and altered mental status and may have deficits that do not comply with strict vascular territories (although these rules are much too general to be definitive).

## Workup

The workup of a stroke patient seeks to localize the lesion, distinguish between ischemic and hemorrhagic stroke, rule out other lesions, and determine the etiology of the stroke. Studies include:

- CT without contrast to differentiate ischemic from hemorrhagic stroke (see Figure 9).
- MRI to identify early ischemic changes, to identify neoplasms, and to adequately image the brain stem/posterior fossa.

**TABLE 8.** Stroke sites and resulting neurologic deficits

| Vessel | Region Supplied | Neurologic Deficit |
|---|---|---|
| **Anterior circulation** | | |
| Middle cerebral (MCA) | Lateral cerebral hemisphere; deep subcortical structures | See deficits of superior/inferior divisions combined; may see coma/symptoms of increased ICP. |
| Superior division | Motor/sensory cortex of face, arm, hand; Broca's area | CL hemiparesis of face, arm, and hand; expressive aphasia if dominant hemisphere. |
| Inferior division | Parietal lobe (visual radiations, Wernicke's area), macular visual cortex | Homonymous hemianopsia, receptive aphasia (dominant), impaired cortical sensory functions, gaze preference, apraxias and neglect. |
| Anterior cerebral (ACA) | Parasagittal cerebral cortex | CL leg paresis and sensory loss. |
| Ophthalmic artery | Retina | Monocular blindness. |
| **Posterior circulation** | | |
| Posterior cerebral (PCA) | Occipital lobe, thalamus, rostral midbrain, medial temporal lobes | CL homonymous hemianopsia, memory or sensory disturbances. |
| Basilar | Ventral midbrain, brain stem, postlimb internal capsule, cerebellum, PCA distribution | Coma, cranial nerve palsies, apnea, cardiovascular instability. |
| **Deep circulation** | | |
| Lenticulostriate, paramedian, thalamoperforate, circumferential arteries | Basal ganglia, pons, thalamus, internal capsule, cerebellum | "Lacunes." Pure motor or sensory deficits, ataxic hemiparesis, "dysarthria–clumsy hand" syndrome. |

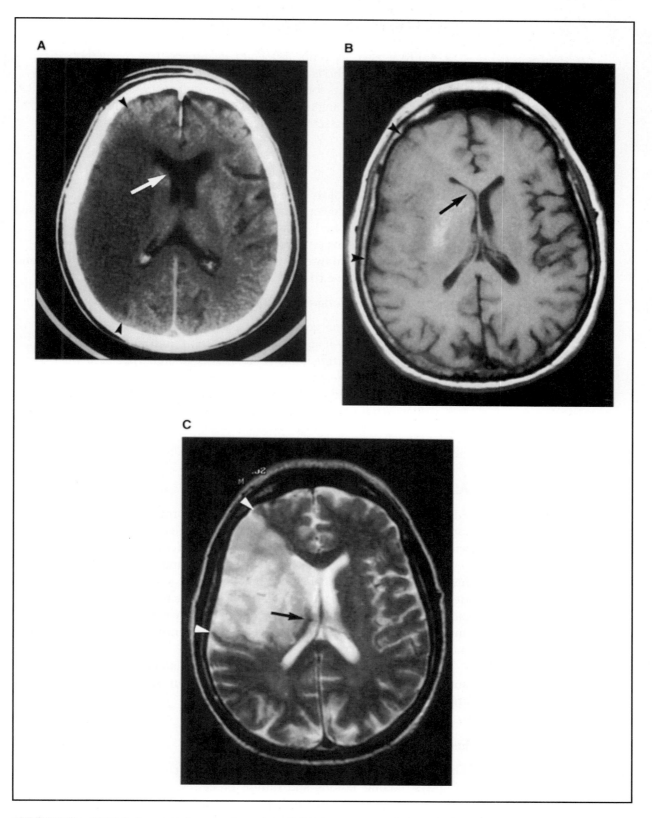

**FIGURE 9.** CT-MRI findings in ischemic stroke in the right MCA territory. (A) CT shows low density and effacement of cortical sulci (between arrowheads) and compression of the anterior horn of the lateral ventricle (arrow). (B) T1-weighted MRI shows loss of sulcal markings (between arrowheads) and compression of the anterior horn of the lateral ventricle (arrow). (C) T2-weighted MRI scan shows increased signal intensity (between arrowheads) and ventricular compression (arrow). Aminoff, *Clinical Neurology,* Third Edition, Stamford, CT: Appleton & Lange, 1996, page 275.

- CBC and glucose; consider lipid workup, ESR, and a treponemal assay.
- EKG; also an echocardiogram if suspected to be embolic (trans-esophageal echo is most sensitive for thrombi).
- Vascular studies for extracranial disease by carotid ultrasound; MRA or traditional angiography looking for intracranial disease.
- Blood cultures; screen for hypercoagulable states (if indicated).

### Treatment

- Heparin if etiology is suspected to be embolic or hypercoagulable.
- Vigilance in detecting symptoms or signs of brain swelling, increased ICP, herniation.
- Avoid hypotension, hypoxemia, hypoglycemia.
- Investigational interventions include revascularization with tPA and neuroprotective trials.

Preventive and long-term treatments include:

- Aspirin 325 mg qd if stroke is secondary to small vessel disease or thrombosis, or if anticoagulation is contraindicated.
- Carotid endarterectomy if stenosis is greater than 70% with corresponding clinical deficits.
- Anticoagulation (heparin initially, then warfarin) if cardiac emboli, new atrial fibrillation, or a hypercoagulable state is present (possibly for intracranial vascular disease as well).
- Manage hypertension.

## ALTERED MENTAL STATUS/COMA

Altered mental status (AMS) describes an abnormal level of consciousness ranging from agitated or somnolent and disoriented to unarousable and without meaningful response to external stimuli (comatose). There are many terms that describe mental status, such as alert and oriented, delirious, confused, somnolent, and comatose, but it is more useful to describe the patient's response to a stimulus, such as "opens eyes to voice" or "withdraws to pain." Acute changes in mentation may be easily explained as the effects of anesthesia or sedation but may also be the presenting sign of serious illness, such as an infection or intracranial hemorrhage.

Change in mental status localizes to the bilateral cerebral hemispheres and to the reticular activating system in the brain stem above the midpons and has a long list of potential etiologies.

### Etiology

The causes of altered mental status and coma can be divided into two groups: structural lesions and diffuse processes. Structural lesions include those that involve the hemispheres (supratentorial) and those that involve the brain stem (infratentorial). It is important to detect supratentorial processes in order to try to prevent potential advancement toward herniation and subsequent compression of the midbrain and brain stem. Supratentorial processes include hemorrhage (epidural, subdural, or intraparenchymal), infarction, abscesses, and tumors. Infratentorial lesions include hemorrhages of the pons, cerebellum, or posterior fossa, vertebrobasilar strokes, and tumors of the brain stem or cerebellum.

Diffuse processes include those that depress consciousness with endogenous disturbances in electrolytes, endocrine, or metabolic function; exogenous toxins such as medications, ethanol, and other drugs; infectious or inflammatory disease; subarachnoid blood; or generalized seizure activity (or postictal state).

## Differential

Patients with an apparent decreased level of conciousness may actually be awake, as may be the case with abulic, catatonic, hysterical, or "locked-in" patients.

## Workup

Discussed with treatment below.

## Treatment

1. Stabilize the patient. Attend to Airway, Breathing, and Circulation.

2. Reverse the reversible. Administer thiamine, glucose, naloxone, and supplemental oxygen.

3. Localize the lesion. This requires differentiation between structural and diffuse processes.

   a. Labs should be sent to check glucose, electrolytes, LFTs, BUN/Cr, PT/PTT, CBC, and ABG.

   b. History should focus on onset of altered mental status and course as well as on past medical history. In the history, the progression from awake to comatose gives valuable information. Onset may be sudden, as is seen in brain stem infarctions or subarachnoid hemorrhage, or initially focal but rapidly progressive, as in intracerebral hemorrhage. Subacute presentations include cases such as tumor, abscess, or subdural hematoma. Structural lesions may initially present with focal neurologic deficits. Diffuse processes, such as metabolic or drug intoxication, are more likely to present without signs of focality.

   c. Physical exam should check for vital signs, trauma, nuchal rigidity, and funduscopic changes.

   d. Neurologic exam should focus on pupillary response, ocular motor reflexes, motor response to pain, and pattern of respiration. Signs of focal localization point to a structural lesion. Reactive pupils in a patient with absent oculocephalic reflexes cannot be truly localized and point to a toxic/metabolic insult.

   e. CT scan is indicated, particularly if a structural lesion, trauma, or SAH is suspected.

4. Prevent further damage. This requires recognition of the progressive and/or treatable etiologies of coma. A few things to look for include the following:

   a. Signs of herniation can be managed by decreasing intracerebral pressure and/or surgical decompression. It is important to detect supratentorial processes early on and to follow neurologic changes vigilantly.

b. Signs of meningitis include fever and nuchal rigidity; patients with possible meningitis should receive IV antibiotics immediately and an LP within 4 hours.

c. Signs of subarachnoid hemorrhage warrant a CT and an LP emergently.

d. Seizure activity should be considered and treated if verified by clinical findings or EEG.

e. Signs of trauma may suggest possible cervical spine injury and warrant cervical x-rays and/or a CT.

After the above emergent conditions have been attended to or excluded, management can shift to the treatment of metabolic disturbances and further investigation, if indicated, by EKG, CXR, tox screens, and EEG.

## DYSEQUILIBRIUM

It is not uncommon for a patient to present to the ER with complaints of feeling "dizzy." "Dizziness" is a vague, nonlocalizing term that may mean presyncope, lightheadedness, or vertigo. Through the history, determine if the patient has vertigo (an errant sense of motion of body or surroundings) or other manifestations of dysequilibrium (defined as the inability to maintain orientation of the body in relation to its surroundings).

**Vertical nystagmus is pathognomonic for a central lesion.**

Equilibrium is maintained through the input of visual, vestibular, and proprioceptive sensory systems and through processing by the cerebellum and brain stem. Dysequilibrium manifests clinically as vertigo or ataxia (incoordination without weakness of voluntary movement of eyes, speech, gait, trunk, or extremities) and can be localized along this axis. The first step is to determine if the process is peripheral (dysfunction of the labyrinthine structure or the vestibular nerve) or central (brain-stem or cerebellar processes, such as stroke, tumor, or multiple sclerosis).

### Signs and Symptoms

Peripheral lesions more commonly present with severe, intermittent vertigo, often associated with nausea and vomiting; nystagmus that is usually unidirectional and not vertical; and hearing loss or tinnitus without signs of ataxia or pyramidal involvement (see Tables 9 and 10). Central lesions are often associated with constant vertigo that is less severe. Nystagmus, if present, may be in one or more directions and may be vertical. Only rarely are there signs of hearing loss or tinnitus. Cerebellar and brain-stem signs such as ataxia, dysarthria, cranial nerve abnormalities, and motor system dysfunction are often present.

### Workup

Workup seeks to determine the location of the lesion and its etiology, which will in turn govern treatment.

In the neuro exam, be sure to focus on the patient's stance and gait, checking his or her ability to stand still with eyes closed (Romberg's sign)

| **TABLE 9.** Etiologies of peripheral and central dysequilibrium | | |
|---|---|---|
| **Peripheral Vestibular Disorders** | **Acute Central Ataxias** | **Chronic Central Ataxias** |
| Benign positional vertigo | Drug intoxication | Multiple sclerosis |
| Ménière's disease | Wernicke's encephalopathy | Cerebellar degeneration |
| Acute peripheral vestibulopathy | Vertebrobasilar ischemia | Hypothyroidism |
| Otosclerosis | Vertebrobasilar infarction | Wilson's disease, CJD |
| Cerebellopontine-angle tumor | Inflammatory disorders | Posterior fossa masses |
| Vestibulopathy/acoustic neuropathy | Cerebellar hemorrhage | Ataxia–telangiectasia |

and to march in place. A patient with a cerebellar lesion will be unable to stand still; if the lesion is vestibular, the patient will often turn or fall in the ipsilateral direction. Check for nystagmus, paying attention to direction and character, and check hearing (grossly). Test for dysmetria, checking finger-to-nose and heel-to-shin coordination; this should be unimpaired in peripheral processes. Don't ignore the rest of the neuro exam, especially the cranial nerves and motor exams.

Specific testing includes positional testing (Nylen-Barany maneuver, in which vertigo is elicited with change in position of the patient's head) and caloric testing (injecting cold or warm water into the ear to assess the vestibulo-ocular reflex, which may be impaired in peripheral disease). An MRI should be done if the patient has signs of central involvement or evidence that a peripheral disturbance cannot be explained by a benign etiology.

Other tests might include assessment of thyroid, $B_{12}$ level, CSF cells and oligoclonal bands, and electrophysiologic studies.

## Treatment

Reducing the symptoms of vertigo may be achieved medicinally with antihistamines (especially meclizine), anticholinergics such as scopolamine, benzodiazepines, and sympathomimetics; these are appropriate in the treatment of benign conditions such as benign positional vertigo and Ménière's disease. Vestibulotoxic drugs such as quinidine, alcohol, and aspirin should be dis-

| **TABLE 10.** Central vs. peripheral dysequilibrium | | |
|---|---|---|
| | **Peripheral** | **Central** |
| Vertigo | Often intermittent; severe. | Often constant; usually less severe. |
| Nystagmus | Always present; unidirectional, never vertical. | May be absent, uni- or bidirectional; may be vertical. |
| Associated findings | | |
| Hearing loss or tinnitus | Often present. | Rarely present. |
| Intrinsic brainstem signs | Absent. | Often present. |

continued. When possible, the underlying disorder, such as thiamine deficiency or hypothyroidism, should be dealt with promptly.

## WEAKNESS

The key to working up a patient with complaints of weakness is to think anatomically. True weakness describes a loss of motor power or strength and is exclusively a disorder of the motor system, localizing somewhere between the motor cortex and the muscles themselves. It is your job to find a pattern in the patient's weakness and to make an anatomic diagnosis; from there, you can go on to create a differential by etiology. You should seek to differentiate upper motor neuron (UMN) from lower motor neuron (LMN) disease and then try to pinpoint location using your exam, thinking about what the affected muscles have in common (eg, all are proximal, all are innervated by one nerve). As always, the history, the physical, and the remainder of the neurologic examination are crucial in this process.

### Etiology

#### Supraspinal lesions

- Stroke
- Other structural lesions

#### Spinal cord lesions

- **Infective:** Poliomyelitis, coxsackievirus infection
- **Inflammatory:** Transverse myelitis, multiple sclerosis
- **Compressive:** Tumor, disk protrusion, abscess
- **Vascular:** Infarction, hematomyelia

#### Peripheral neuropathy

- Guillain-Barré syndrome
- Diphtheria
- Shellfish poisoning
- Porphyria
- Arsenic poisoning
- Organophosphate toxicity

#### Disorders of neuromuscular transmission

- Myasthenia gravis
- Botulism
- Aminoglycoside toxicity

#### Muscle disorders

- Necrotizing myopathies
- Acute hypo- or hyperkalemia
- Periodic paralyses

Tables 11–14 may be helpful in finding patterns and etiologies.

## TABLE 11. Lesions in the motor pathways

| Location of Lesion | Disease Term | Weakness Pattern | Etiologies |
|---|---|---|---|
| Intracranial | | UMN, as described below | Stroke, neoplasm, MS, hemorrhage, trauma, infection |
| Spinal cord | Myelopathy | UMN at spinal level | Compression, trauma, MS |
| Anterior horn cell | Motor neuron disease | UMN/LMN: variable | ALS, spinal muscular atrophy, poliomyelitis |
| Nerve root | Radiculopathy | LMN at root level | Compression, infection, meningeal mets, trauma |
| Plexus | Plexopathy | LMN, mixed roots | Trauma, neoplastic infiltration, idiopathic |
| Peripheral nerve | Neuropathy | LMN, by nerve | Metabolic, toxic, inflammatory, neoplastic |
| Neuromuscular junction | | Diffuse weakness | Myasthenia gravis, Lambert-Eaton syndrome |
| Muscle | Myopathy | Proximal weakness | Muscular dystrophy, polymyositis, EtOH |

## TABLE 12. Anatomic localization: upper versus lower motor neuron disease

| Clinical Features | UMN | LMN |
|---|---|---|
| Pattern of weakness | Pyramidal (arm extensors, leg flexors) | Variable |
| Function | Slowed FFM | Impaired secondary to weakness |
| Tone | Spastic (increased: initially flaccid) | Flaccid (decreased) |
| DTRs | Increased (initially decreased) | Normal, decreased, absent |
| Miscellaneous signs | Babinski's, other CNS signs | Atrophy, fasciculations |

## TABLE 13. Clinical localization of UMN weakness

| Specific Location | Clinical Features |
|---|---|
| Parasagittal cerebrum | Bilateral legs more than arms |
| Discrete cortical lesion | Monoparesis with or without sensory involvement |
| Extensive cortical/ subcortical lesion | Hemiparesis: Contralateral face, arm, leg weakness with associated signs (aphasia, sensory deficits, visual field cuts) |
| Internal capsule | Contralateral face, arm, leg; can be motor without sensory |
| Brain stem lesion | Bilateral paresis, or contralateral limbs with ipsilateral face |
| Spinal cord | Spastic paraparesis or quadriparesis; LMN symptoms or signs at level of lesion with sensory level |

| Test | Spinal Cord | Anterior Horn Cell Disorders | Peripheral Nerve or Plexus | Neuromuscular Junction | Myopathy |
|---|---|---|---|---|---|
| Serum enzymes | Normal. | Normal. | Normal. | Normal. | Normal or increased. |
| Electromyography | Reduced number of motor units under voluntary control. With lesions causing axonal degeneration, may be abnormal spontaneous activity (eg, fasciculations, fibrillations) if sufficient time has elapsed after onset; with reinnervation, motor units may be large, long, and polyphasic. | | | Often normal, but individual motor units may show abnormal variability in size. | Small, short, abundant polyphasic motor unit potentials. Abnormal spontaneous activity may be conspicuous in myositis. |
| Nerve conduction velocity | Normal. | Normal. | Slowed, especially in demyelinative neuropathies. May be normal in axonal neuropathies. | Normal. | Normal. |
| Muscle response to repetitive motor nerve stimulation | Normal. | Normal, except in active stage of disease. | Normal. | Abnormal decrement or increment depending on stimulus frequency and disease. | Normal. |
| Muscle biopsy | May be normal in acute stage but subsequently suggestive of denervation. | | | Normal. | Changes suggestive of myopathy. |
| Myelography or spinal MRI | May be helpful. | Helpful in excluding other disorders. | Not helpful. | Not helpful. | Not helpful. |

**TABLE 14.** Investigation of patient with weakness

Aminoff, *Clinical Neurology,* Third Edition, Stamford, CT: Appleton & Lange, 1996, page 156.

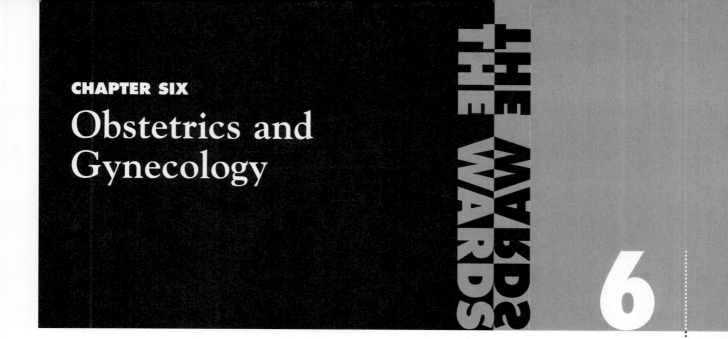

**CHAPTER SIX**

# Obstetrics and Gynecology

**6**

# Ward Tips

Welcome to obstetrics and gynecology! This rotation is dedicated to acquainting future MDs with the basic principles and skills of delivering babies and managing basic gynecologic issues ranging from surgical to medical to social. Keep in mind that this rotation does not simply start with a pregnant patient and end with the delivery of a baby. You will be involved in prenatal care and counseling, antepartum checkups, and numerous surgical procedures from C-sections to complicated oncology cases. Obstetricians/gynecologists are surgeons by nature who keep extremely demanding schedules and thus spend minimal time rounding and discussing differentials on a regular basis. For the next few weeks, you will enjoy a whirlwind of activities covering a wide range of issues. In whatever field you enter, more than half your patients will be women with potential gynecologic problems, so take advantage of this learning opportunity.

## WHAT IS THE ROTATION LIKE?

OB/GYN rotations last approximately 6–8 weeks and differ vastly from school to school and from site to site. The basic setup consists of inpatient obstetrics, inpatient gynecology, and the outpatient clinic, where both obstetrics and gynecology are covered. Obstetrics can be one of the most rewarding and pleasant experiences in medical school. It is not, however, an easy-going discipline. It will provide you with the opportunity to handle an acute situation primarily on your own (with resident backup), thereby representing perhaps the most responsibility you have had thus far in your medical training.

You will spend much of your time in the labor and delivery (L&D) suite. Responsibilities include prerounding on postpartum patients and presenting those patients on ward rounds. Other responsibilities include admission history and physical, working closely with residents and nurses in monitoring the progress of laboring patients, delivering babies, writing progress and delivery notes, and checking labs.

You should get to know the nursing staff very well; in many instances much of the labor and delivery is taken care of by nurses or midwives. You

**Obstetricians/ gynecologists are surgeons by nature.**

**Try to follow a patient from admission to the delivery.**

should also try to follow the patient from the beginning of her L&D admission to the delivery of her baby. Such longitudinal care allows for a better relationship with the patient while simultaneously enabling you to see the complete picture of labor management. Prior to the rotation, you should also read about the basics of labor and delivery (steps of labor, signs and symptoms of true labor, steps of delivery, fetal heart tracing) and learn about common complications that can arise and their management (failure to progress, hypertension, fetal distress). Always keep in mind that competence is only half the story; knowing your patient well by periodically checking in on her to see if she needs anything or just to comfort her will impress not only your patient but your attendings and residents as well.

As a surgically oriented specialty, inpatient gynecology is very similar to general surgery with the exception that all of your patients are female. Your responsibilities consist of note writing (preop, operative, postop) on the patients whose surgeries you are involved with, prerounding on postoperative patients, and presenting patients on ward rounds. Rounding is early and fast; all the notes, rounding, and daily management planning for the patients must be done prior to surgeries planned for the day, which can start at 7:30 AM. Prior to leaving the day before, you should try to plan out which surgery you want to participate in, read up on the surgery and on relevant anatomy, and learn something about the patient's history. Surgeries will differ depending on which type of hospital you are working at; they can range from a half-hour laparoscopy for tubal ligation to a 6-hour gynecologic oncology case.

You or your resident should always introduce yourself to the attending surgeon, especially if the surgeon is from a private practice. You should practice some basic suturing and knotting skills in case you are presented with a rare opportunity to help close up an incision. You should also learn some of the medical jargon common to surgeries and be willing to ask questions pertaining to technique or to the prognosis of the surgery being performed.

Outpatient clinics are a great place to see both common and uncommon nonacute cases. Common gynecologic clinic issues are requests for birth control, routine health maintenance (breast and pelvic exams and Pap smears), abnormal vaginal bleeding, vaginal discharge, and lower abdominal pain. In clinics, obstetrics patients are seen to assess the adequacy of pregnancy progression, to screen for potential maternal–fetal complications, to help mothers adjust to their pregnancies, and to prepare mothers for childbirth. In addition, postpartum patients are seen for their regular 6-week checkup or for any postpartum complications that may arise. The clinic experience is extremely helpful because the skills and knowledge acquired there are potentially applicable to most fields you may want to pursue, such as internal medicine, family practice, or surgery.

## WHO ARE THE PLAYERS?

Team OB/GYN consists of a senior resident (R3 or R4), at least one junior resident (R2), and an intern (from OB/GYN, family practice, psychiatry, or medicine). There may also be a fourth-year medical student doing his or her senior elective as well as one or two third-year medical students. Usually there is one ward attending, although there may be several private attendings, subspecialty attendings (maternal–fetal, gynecologic oncology), and fellows. Other very important players include the nursing staff and midwives (especially in L&D), who can teach you invaluable obstetrics skills, and the anesthesiologists, who are needed for pain control both during labor and postoperatively.

## HOW IS THE DAY SET UP?

A typical day on an OB/GYN service may look like this:

| | |
|---|---|
| 5:30–6:30 AM | Prerounds |
| 6:30–7:30 AM | Work rounds |
| 7:30 AM–4:00 PM | L&D or OR |
| 12:00 NOON–1:00 PM | Lunch conference |
| 1:00–4:00 PM | L&D, OR, or student conferences |
| 4:00–6:00 PM | Wrap up work, do postop checks if possible |

Call days are usually busy and are always in-house. After you are done with your regular work day, you start call in the L&D and follow any laboring patient. You and your resident will also admit any potential patients from the ER for obstetric or gynecologic acute care. You are usually up all night or, if you are lucky, get 1–2 hours of sleep. This is because there will often be someone delivering in the early hours of the morning or an emergency to keep you busy.

## WHAT DO I DO DURING PREROUNDS?

Depending on the size of your inpatient gynecologic service, prerounds should begin 30 minutes to an hour before work rounds. Like surgery, most of your patients will be postop. You are expected to check the vital signs overnight, check labs, do a quick physical exam, check the surgical wound, review the chart for new notes, and write a concise progress note—all before work rounds. On the obstetrics service, you will probably preround on your postpartum patients. In addition to the usual preround chores, you will also want to check fundus size, extent of vaginal bleeding, and any wounds, such as sewn episiotomies.

## HOW DO I DO WELL IN THIS ROTATION?

**Be assertive.** This is key to furthering your education and to scoring points with the people who evaluate you. Ask good questions (you should know a bit about the subject matter before asking the questions), take initiative to ask for demonstrations of procedures, know other patients on the service (for your own learning and in case you are asked to fill in), volunteer for drawing blood (you need to practice anyway), do pelvic exams, and dig up interesting/informative articles for the team.

**Be the intern for your patients.** You will have patients assigned to you by your residents. Among other things, you are responsible for the patient's H&P, writing progress notes, following up on diagnostic studies, and presenting your patients to the team. In order to fulfill your responsibilities dili-

Don't go to bed if you're missing too many night deliveries.

Don't get shut out of learning the pelvic exam.

gently, you need to know and do everything you can for your patient. This means reading up on the patient's case, carefully reviewing the patient's history, and talking to your patient. This will allow you to actively participate in your patient's care as her strongest advocate.

**Be knowledgeable in the general sense.** Realize that once residents become involved in a specialty, they tend to forget everything else they learned in medical school. You can be a great asset by providing information about the patient's medical problem (diabetes, hepatitis, hypertension), reminding residents of nongynecologic surgical differentials (appendicitis, bowel obstruction, hernia), and recognizing psychiatric issues (postpartum depression, drug dependence).

**Work quickly, independently, and efficiently.** Residents appreciate any student who can effectively contribute to the team. Order lab tests, make necessary phone calls, and write notes for patients. Be focused and brief when presenting the patient. In many ways, this rotation is similar to surgery. Gynecologic oncology, for example, is really just a surgical subspecialty.

**Know the expectations.** At the beginning of the rotation, be straightforward and ask the residents what exactly is expected of you. You should ask your attending his or her preferred format of patient presentation. Midway through the rotation, it is very important to get feedback both from residents and from attendings you have worked with. Try to be assertive and ask for constructive feedback on what you should continue to do and what you can improve on. Be tactful, and communicate with the goal of maximizing your performance, education, and contribution to the team while on the OB/GYN clerkship.

You may fall in love with OB/GYN and want to pursue it as a career. If this is the case, you should take additional steps. Let your team know of your sincere interest; they will be more than happy to lead you down the right track. Ask the interns and residents for advice on the politics of residency (eg, which programs are good, who are the key people to get to know better, whom to ask for letters of recommendation, which senior electives to take). If possible, try to work with one of the key faculty members, who can write an influential letter of recommendation or be your adviser in your quest to match into the residency of your choice.

## Survival Tips

Do not be discouraged if a patient does not want a medical student to deliver her baby or even to be involved in her care. Many mothers want as little intrusion as possible into a sacred, personal moment of their lives, while others may be concerned about the inexperienced hands of a student touching their newborn infant. Occasionally, male students may find some gynecology patients who are uncomfortable with the notion of a man in the examining room, much less a male student. On a rotation such as this, in which you are working very hard with long hours, it can be very easy to feel frustrated and rejected when something like this occurs. But it is important to respect a patient's wishes and to keep in mind that there may be very specific, personal reasons for such a request. Do not take it personally if a patient does not want you in the examination room. If this continues to happen frequently, however, you should discuss it with your resident. Being with an affable yet

**Don't be discouraged if the patient initially does not want you in the exam room or delivering her baby.**

assertive female resident who cares about your educational experience is of great help in getting your foot in the door as a male medical student.

A few tips are as follows:

- Talk to OB patients early in labor and throughout the delivery. Establishing a rapport early on will increase the likelihood that you will be able to help with the delivery.
- Learn how to "count" and coach a patient through labor. A calm yet clear and assertive voice is usually appreciated.

## KEY NOTES

**Admission note.** The obstetrical H&P is similar to a standard H&P with the following additions:

- **HPI:** Include gravida, para, TAB (therapeutic abortion), SAB (spontaneous abortion), menstrual frequency.
- Gestational age, LMP (last menstrual period), EDD (estimated date of delivery—same as due date), full term vs. preterm.
- **Contractions:** Time of onset, frequency, intensity; rupture of membranes (time, color).
- **Vaginal bleeding:** Duration, consistency, number of pads; fetal movement.

**Prenatal care.** Date of first exam, total number of visits, infections, diabetes, HTN, appropriate weight gain, approximate size based on dates.

- **Prenatal labs:** VDRL/RPR, rubella, Rh, blood type, antibody screen, glucose testing, hepatitis panels, urine C&S.
- **Diagnostic tests:** Ultrasound, amniocentesis, CVS (chorionic villi sampling).
- **Obstetric history:** Dates of pregnancies with gestational age, route (vaginal, C-section), complications (including preeclampsia, abruption, previa, preterm labor, unusually long labor).
- **Gynecologic history:** Menstrual history, STDs, OCPs.
- **Family history:** Congenital abnormalities, twins, bleeding disorders.
- **Social history:** Any tobacco, EtOH, or drug use during pregnancy, occupational exposures (eg, nurse preparing chemotherapy agents).

**L&D (labor and delivery) note.** Some hospitals have preprinted L&D forms that allow you to simply fill in the blanks and check off appropriate boxes. If this is not the case, here is a summary of the information that should be in an L&D note:

- Age, gravida, para, TAB, SAB, gestational age.
- Onset of labor, ROM (rupture of membranes with or without meconium), ? induction (indications).
- Anesthesia/pain control.
- Time of birth, type of birth (normal spontaneous vaginal delivery [NSVD], forceps assist, vacuum suction, C-section), presentation (eg, left occiput anterior).
- Bulb suction, sex, weight, APGAR scores, ? nuchal cord (×1, ×2) reduced, number of cord vessels.
- Time of placenta delivery, ? expressed spontaneously, ? intact.
- Episiotomy (degree) repaired, ? lacerations.

- Estimated blood loss (EBL).
- Disposition: Mother to recovery room in stable condition; infant to newborn nursery in stable condition.

## KEY PROCEDURES

Delivering babies, cervical checks, Pap smears, cervical/vaginal cultures, external fetal monitoring, IV lines, basic suturing and knotting, and bladder retraction are the principal procedures on this rotation. Descriptions of most of these procedures can be found in major textbooks. However, the best way to learn is by observing and practicing. So let your residents know you are interested in these procedures.

## WHAT DO I CARRY IN MY POCKETS?

**Checklist**

- ❏ Pregnancy wheel
- ❏ OB/GYN handbook of choice
- ❏ Penlight
- ❏ Stethoscope
- ❏ Index cards to keep track of your patients. Create cards with high-yield information, including:
  - ❏ Steps of a vaginal delivery
  - ❏ Normal labor patterns (duration, cervical dilation, etc)
  - ❏ Indications for cesarean section
  - ❏ Outlines of frequently written notes (preop, op, postop, delivery notes)
  - ❏ The diagnosis and management of preeclampsia/eclampsia

Most of the equipment needed for obstetric or gynecologic exams is provided in the examination room.

# Top-Rated Books

## HANDBOOK/POCKETBOOK

**Current Clinical Strategy: Gynecology & Obstetrics**
Chan
Current Clinical Strategies, 1995, 106 pages, ISBN 1881528278, $12.75

Quick, readable pocketbook containing the essentials necessary immediately prior to the patient encounter. Includes signs/symptoms, risk factors, treatment, and complications. Inexpensive and remarkably compact.

**Handbook of Gynecology & Obstetrics**
Brown
Appleton & Lange, 1993, 626 pages, ISBN 0838536085, $27.95

A concise, easily read pocketbook which lacks detail in therapeutics. Provides good conceptual information with tables, illustrations, and a free pregnancy wheel. Some may find this book too simplistic.

**Benson and Pernolls's Handbook of Obstetrics and Gynecology**
Benson
McGraw-Hill, 1994, 817 pages, ISBN 0071054057, $32.00

Thorough but somewhat bulky pocketbook with excellent tables and graphics. Dry writing style in some sections, and small print makes for difficult reading.

**Obstetrical Pearls: A Practical Guide for the Efficient Resident**
Benson
F. A. Davis, 1994, 214 pages, ISBN 0803607024, $18.95

A practical, easily read, clinically oriented pocketbook that is most useful as prerotation orientation material. Includes useful information on clinical procedures. Expensive when combined with its gynecology companion.

**Obstetrics and Gynecology (House Officer Series)**
Rayburn
Williams & Wilkins, 1996, 423 pages, ISBN 0683071815, $24.95

Paragraph-format pocketbook geared toward house officers. Particularly complete with respect to obstetric topics; however, does not include discussion of normal H&P. Best used by students with some grounding in OB/GYN issues.

**Obstetrics & Gynecology On Call**
Horowitz
Appleton & Lange, 1993, 640 pages, ISBN 0838571743, $24.95

Organized by clinical problems with focus on differential diagnosis. Assumes good knowledge base in OB/GYN. Minimal discussion in some areas. Excellent section on pharmacology. Bonus chapters on diagnostic studies, procedures, and management.

**B+**

**Obstetrics and Gynecology: Resident Survival Guide and Handbook**
Gordon
Stanford University Bookstore, 1995, 232 pages, ISBN 0964546728, $12.95

Fast, practical pocketbook to common OB/GYN problems designed as a resident survival guide. Many excellent figures and charts, but requires background knowledge for optimal utility. Contains no discussion of pathophysiology.

**B**

**Danforth's Handbook of Obstetrics & Gynecology**
Scott
Lippincott, 1996, 554 pages, ISBN 0397512813, $29.95

Pocketbook listing key facts relevant to a wide range of OB/GYN issues. Contains many useful tables and figures. Useful to get a quick bullet, but weak with respect to the differential diagnosis, approach to, and treatment of common problems. Geared toward residents.

**B**

**Manual of Obstetrics**
Niswander
Little, Brown, 1996, 538 pages, ISBN 0316611727, $32.95

Same format as the *Washington Manual*. Skimps on signs, symptoms, and differential diagnoses in favor of therapeutics. Otherwise, well organized and practical. Good labor and delivery chapter. No discussion of maternal/fetal physiology during pregnancy. More appropriate for interns or subinterns.

**B**

**Practical Gynecology**
Jacobs
Appleton & Lange, 1994, 528 pages, ISBN 0838513360, $28.95

A large pocketbook written in an expanded outline format with good coverage of signs and symptoms as well as therapeutics. Provides a quick read on a broad range of topics. Features a handy appendix of differential diagnoses for common presenting complaints.

**B-**

**Gynecologic Pearls: A Practical Guide for the Efficient Resident**
Benson
F. A. Davis, 1995, 268 pages, ISBN 0803600054, $18.95

Good prerotation introductory material, but not sufficient for the wards. Useful as easy, quick supplementary reading. Requires separate purchase of another book for obstetrics. Some pearls have been found to be incorrect.

**B-**

**Practical Guide to the Care of the Gynecologic-Obstetric Patient**
Danakas
Mosby, 1996, 800 pages, ISBN 0815123167, $39.95

Same format as the popular Ferri handbook for medicine, but not as "practical." Bulky handbook with unnecessary epidemiology and background material, but misses some key topics such as third-trimester bleeding and care of the surgical patient. Placement of sections on lab tests and differential diagnoses of common complaints in middle of book makes it harder to use.

OBSTETRICS AND GYNECOLOGY

216

# REVIEW/MINI-REFERENCE

### Basic Gynecology & Obstetrics
Gant
Appleton & Lange, 1993, 472 pages, ISBN 0838596339, $38.95

Excellent short reference for the core rotation. Thorough and well written with just enough information for a junior student on the wards. Excellent use of graphics to highlight the text.

### Current Obstetric and Gynecologic Diagnosis & Treatment
DeCherney
Appleton & Lange, 1994, 1227 pages, ISBN 0838514472, $45.00

Great reference book overall. Good use of graphics. Minimal emphasis on differential diagnosis, however. Good value. New edition expected in early '98.

### Essentials of Obstetrics & Gynecology
Hacker
Saunders, 1992, 674 pages, ISBN 0721636683, $36.95

Well organized. Has excellent discussions on patient workups and good background material on women's health. Overall very readable, but lacks the depth of a true reference book.

### NMS Obstetrics & Gynecology
Beck
Williams & Wilkins, 1993, 510 pages, ISBN 0683062417, $28.00

Concise overview of fundamental concepts on OB/GYN pathophysiology presented in outline form. Includes practice questions at end of each chapter for reinforcement. An easy read for a student who likes the outline format, but may be boring reading for others. Good sections on ultrasound and fetal heart monitoring/tocometry. Geared more toward USMLE Step 2.

### Obstetric & Gynecologic Secrets
Frederickson
Mosby, 1991, 308 pages, ISBN 0932883958, $34.95

Presented in question-and-answer format, with a highly variable level of detail. Some find that this book lacks a cohesive, organized approach, while others welcome the information presented in small, discrete chunks.

### Obstetrics and Gynecology
Willson
Mosby, 1991, 658 pages, ISBN 080165542, $53.95

An introductory hardcover text geared toward medical students. Features concise, readable chapters with multiple figures and tables. Covers the basics.

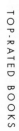

**B** **Obstetrics and Gynecology for Medical Students**
Beckmann
Williams & Wilkins, 1995, 682 pages, ISBN 0683005030, $36.00

Short textbook featuring case-based approach with brief coverage of topics. An easy read with some helpful tables, figures, and diagrams. Sometimes overly simplistic. Enough to get by, but lacks the depth of other texts.

**B** **Oklahoma Notes Obstetrics and Gynecology**
Miles
Springer-Verlag, 1996, 219 pages, ISBN 0387946322, $17.95

Rapid review of common topics in obstetrics and gynecology presented in outline format. Some good charts and illustrations. Variable coverage of topics.

## TEXTBOOK/REFERENCE

**A** **Danforth's Obstetrics & Gynecology**
Scott
Lippincott, 1994, 1121 pages, ISBN 0397513534, $135.00

Very readable, organized, and comprehensive reference book of obstetrics and gynecology with numerous illustrations. Excellent for the serious OB/GYN student, but too detailed and expensive for other students.

**A-** **Gynecology & Obstetrics: A Longitudinal Approach**
Moore
Churchill Livingstone, 1993, 966 pages, ISBN 044308811X, $115.00

Concise yet highly informative. Excellent diagrams with good differential diagnosis and charts. A good reference book, but perhaps a little less comprehensive than others.

**A-** **Williams Obstetrics**
Cunningham
Appleton & Lange, 1993, 1448 pages, ISBN 0838596347, $90.00

Excellent reference book on obstetrics for the serious student. Divided by organ system and includes good use of graphics to highlight the material. Includes maternal–fetal medicine. Lacks gynecology.

# HIGH-YIELD TOPICS

## ROTATION OBJECTIVES

In OB/GYN you should be able to generate a differential diagnosis for common problems, perfect a systematic way of working up a patient, gain experience in performing a thorough pelvic examination with a Pap smear, and, hopefully, find an appreciation of the process of birth. You can also learn about commonly used studies such as ultrasonography (the imaging tool of OB/GYN), cervical biopsies, and fetal monitoring. The following list outlines common disease entities, conditions, and topics that you are likely to confront during your OB/GYN rotation. Topics that are further discussed in this chapter are listed in italics.

### Obstetrics

- *Normal physiology of pregnancy*
- *Prenatal care*
- *Normal labor*
- Abnormal labor
- *First-trimester bleeding*
- *Ectopic pregnancy*
- *Third-trimester bleeding*
- *Gestational diabetes*
- *Pregnancy-induced hypertension*
- *Preterm labor*
- *Abnormal labor patterns*
- *Postpartum hemorrhage*
- Fetal heart rate monitoring
- Postpartum fever

### Gynecology

- *Pelvic inflammatory disease*
- *Sexually transmitted diseases*
  - *Genital herpes*
  - *Chlamydia trachomatis*
  - *Gonorrhea*
  - *Condylomata acuminata (venereal warts)*
  - *Syphilis*
- *Common vaginal infections (vaginitis)*
- *Endometriosis*
- *Amenorrhea*
- *Abnormal uterine bleeding*
- *Menopause*
- *Gynecologic oncology*
- Pelvic relaxation
- Contraceptives
- Premenstrual syndrome
- Infertility

## NORMAL PHYSIOLOGY OF PREGNANCY

In pregnancy, multiple adaptations occur in each of the mother's organ systems to support the maternal–fetal unit (see Table 1).

## PRENATAL CARE

Prenatal care is extremely critical to the outcome of an uneventful delivery of a healthy baby. Once the pregnancy is confirmed, the patient's prenatal visits should be scheduled as follows:

| TABLE 1. Maternal changes during pregnancy | | |
|---|---|---|
| System | Changes | Effects |
| Metabolic | Increased proteins, lipids<br>Increased need for iron, folate<br>Increased insulin sensitivity early in pregnancy, decreased glucose tolerance later in pregnancy | Increased maternal fat deposition<br>Maternal anemia<br>Narrow euglycemic range (normal 84 ±10) |
| Blood | Hyperplasia of hematopoietic system<br>50% increase in plasma volume with corresponding increase of 20–40% in red blood cell mass | Increased white blood cells, fibrinogen, coagulation factors 7, 8, 9, 10<br>Physiologic anemia of pregnancy |
| Endocrine | Increased estrogen, progesterone, prolactin, aldosterone | Water retention<br>Breast engorgement, preparation for milk production<br>Mood changes |
| Skin, hair | Increased estrogen, progesterone | Increased skin pigmentation (areola, axilla, vulva)<br>Hirsutism |
| Respiratory | Increase in minute tidal volume, slight increase in respiratory rate<br>Upward displacement of diaphragm late in pregnancy | Dyspnea<br>Mild respiratory alkalosis |
| Cardiovascular | Cardiac output increases up to 45% (mostly due to increase in stroke volume)<br>Decreased arterial blood pressure and peripheral vascular resistance | Dependent edema<br>Physiologic flow murmur<br>Decreased blood pressure, supine hypotensive syndrome |
| Renal | Dilation of collecting system, decreased peristalsis<br>Increased renal blood flow, glomerular filtration rate by 30–50%<br>Decreased renal glucose absorption<br>Increased aldosterone, renin, ADH | Increased urinary tract infection, hydroureters<br>Urinary frequency, nocturia<br>Glucosuria<br>Salt and water retention |
| Gastrointestinal | Decreased muscle tone leading to hypomotility<br>Decreased lower esophageal sphincter tone<br>Bile stasis | Constipation, hemorrhoids<br>Gastric reflux, hiatal hernia<br>Gallstones |

- **0–28 weeks' gestation:** Once every 4 weeks
- **28–36 weeks' gestation:** Once every 2 weeks
- **36 weeks' gestation until delivery:** Once every week

At each visit, the following questions and documentation should be addressed:

### Questions

- Fetal movement
- Vaginal discharge, bleeding
- Abdominal cramps/uterine contractions
- Blurred vision, headache, rapid weight gain, edema

### Documentation

- Weight
- Blood pressure
- Dipstick urine protein and glucose
- Fetal heart tones (FHTs)
- Fundal height
- Edema
- Deep tendon reflexes
- Confirmation of estimated date of delivery

**Accurate determination of estimated due date is key.**

Fundal height is measured from the top of the symphysis pubis. At 12 weeks' gestation, the fundal height should be palpable at the pubic symphysis. At 16 weeks, it should be midway between the pubis and the umbilicus (see Figure 1); at 20 weeks, at the umbilicus; at 20–32 weeks, the fundal height in centimeters above the symphysis should equal the gestational age in weeks (ie, "size equals dates").

Nutrition is a crucial factor in ensuring the health of the mother and the fetus. Iron and folate supplementation is recommended. The normal weight gain is about 20–30 pounds for the entire pregnancy. In the first trimester, the patient should gain an average of 2.5 pounds. From 8 to 20

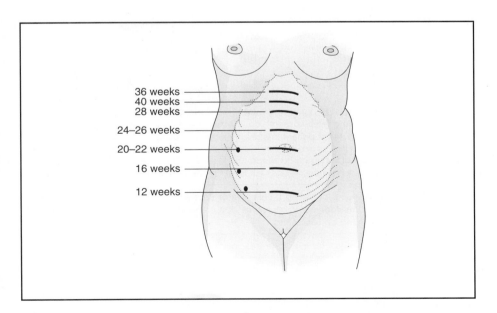

**FIGURE 1.** Height of fundus at various times during pregnancy. DeCherney, *Current Obstetric & Gynecological Diagnosis & Treatment*, Eighth Edition, Stamford, CT: Appleton & Lange, 1994, page 187.

weeks, the patient should gain about 0.7 pound a week. From 20 weeks to delivery, the patient should usually gain about 1 pound a week. Weight gain is excessive when it is greater than 4 pounds a month and inadequate when it is less than one-half pound a week or less than 2 pounds a month.

Basic labs should be obtained during the prenatal visits and carefully charted (see Table 2).

## NORMAL LABOR

Labor has two components:

1. Uterine contractions of sufficient frequency, duration, and intensity resulting in . . .
2. Cervical changes, such as effacement (thinning) and dilation.

Labor is divided into three stages, as shown in Table 3 and Figure 2.

Babies undergo seven stereotypical cardinal movements for successful delivery; the movements constitute the second stage of labor. As the baby descends, he or she moves from station −5 to +5 cm or from −3 to +3 station units:

1. Engagement
2. Descent
3. Flexion
4. Internal rotation
5. Extension
6. Restitution
7. External rotation

| TABLE 2. Standard prenatal labs and studies | |
| --- | --- |
| Gestation | Labs to Be Obtained |
| Initial visit | CBC<br>Type, Rh, and antibody screen<br>Rubella antibody titer<br>Cervical gonorrhea and chlamydia cultures<br>VDRL for syphilis screening<br>Hepatitis B surface antigen test<br>Pap smear<br>Urinalysis<br>PPD<br>Sickle prep in high-risk groups<br>HIV testing (with consent), counseling in high-risk groups<br>Glucose test if patient has risk factors for diabetes |
| 15–20 weeks | Maternal serum alpha-fetoprotein level should be measured to screen for any neural tube defect (very high level) or risk of trisomy 21 (low level). |
| 18–20 weeks | Ultrasound for dating if unknown or uncertain. This is the best time during fetal development to assess the age of the fetus if there is only one chance of obtaining an ultrasound. |
| 24–28 weeks | Glucose test for everyone (risk factors or not). |
| 28–30 weeks | RhoGAM administered to patients initially determined to be Rh antibody negative. |
| 34–38 weeks | CBC |
| 36–40 weeks | Cervical chlamydia and gonorrhea cultures in high-risk patients. |

**TABLE 3.** The three stages of labor

| Stage | Starts/End | Events | Average Duration (hours) Nulli* | Multi** |
|---|---|---|---|---|
| First Latent | Regular uterine contractions/cervix dilated to 4 cm | Highly variable duration, cervix effaces and slowly dilates | 6–11 | 4–8 |
| Active | 4-cm cervical dilation/ complete cervical dilation (10 cm) | Regular and intense uterine contractions, cervix effaces and dilates more quickly, fetal head progressively descends into pelvis | 4–6 | 2–3 |
| Second | Complete cervical dilation/delivery of the baby | Baby undergoes all stages of cardinal movements | 1–2 | 0.5–1 |
| Third | Delivery of baby/ delivery of placenta | Placenta separates and uterus contracts to establish hemostasis | 0–0.5 | 0–0.5 |

*Nulli = nulliparous (first-time mother)

**Multi = multiparous (pregnant and delivered before)

The orientation of the baby is described in relation to the maternal pelvis:

- **Fetal lie:** Long axis of baby in relation to long axis of mother (longitudinal, transverse, oblique).
- **Fetal presentation:** Part of the fetus that enters the pelvis first (vertex [head first], breech [buttocks or leg first], face, brow).

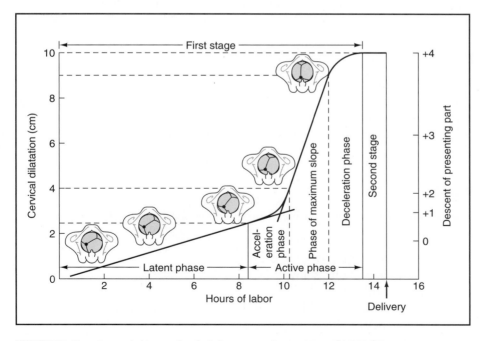

**FIGURE 2.** Cervical dilation, level of descent, and orientation of occipitoanterior presentation during various stages of labor. DeCherney, *Current Obstetric & Gynecological Diagnosis & Treatment*, Eighth Edition, Stamford, CT: Appleton & Lange, 1994, page 211.

- **Fetal position:** Reference point of the fetal presenting part (for vertex presentation, the presenting part is the occiput; for breech presentation, the presenting part is the sacrum) to the maternal pelvis (right, left, anterior, posterior).

Note that the most common fetal orientation is longitudinal, vertex, occiput anterior (ie, baby's face emerges facing mom's rectum).

### FIRST-TRIMESTER BLEEDING

First-trimester bleeding occurs anytime from 0 to 12 weeks' gestational age and complicates some 20–30% of all pregnancies; 50% of these cases will end up in a miscarriage. However, only 5% of cases with the presence of a fetal heart rate on ultrasound end in miscarriage. The etiologies include abortion, ectopic pregnancies, molar pregnancies, and local causes (cervicitis, genital tract trauma or infection). It is best to place abortion and ectopic pregnancy on the top of your list and rule out one or both of these two most common causes of first-trimester bleeding.

Abortion is a termination of pregnancy at less than 20 weeks' gestational age or estimated fetal weight of less than 500 g. The different types of abortion are listed in Table 4.

### Signs and Symptoms

Besides vaginal bleeding (which can be significant), abortion is associated with tissue passage, opened/partially opened cervical os, and hemodynamic instability. Ectopic pregnancy is associated with adnexal mass, cervical motion tenderness, and bleeding between 6 and 12 weeks' gestational age. A ruptured ectopic pregnancy may present with shock and peritoneal signs.

### Differential

The differential diagnosis of first-trimester bleeding includes ectopic pregnancy, complete abortion, incomplete abortion, missed abortion, threatened abortion, septic abortion, intrauterine fetal death, molar pregnancies, and local causes (cervicitis, genital tract trauma or infection).

### Workup

The workup of first-trimester bleeding involves obtaining/performing the following:

- Qualitative/quantitative β-HCG
- Transvaginal ultrasound
- Culdocentesis
- Consideration of dilation and curettage (if patient does not want pregnancy)
- Serum progesterone

**The presence of fetal cardiac activity on ultrasound is reassuring.**

## TABLE 4. Types of spontaneous abortion

| Abortion | Definition | Treatment |
|---|---|---|
| Complete abortion | Less than 20 weeks' gestation<br>All products of conception expelled<br>Internal cervical os is closed<br>Uterine bleeding present | RhoGAM if appropriate |
| Incomplete abortion | Less than 20 weeks' gestation<br>Some products of conception expelled<br>Internal cervical os is open<br>Uterine bleeding present | Dilation and curettage (D&C)<br>RhoGAM if appropriate |
| Threatened abortion | Less than 20 weeks' gestation<br>No products of conception expelled<br>Membranes remain intact<br>Internal cervical os is closed<br>Uterine bleeding is present<br>Abdominal pain may be present<br>Fetus still viable | Avoid heavy activity<br>Pelvic rest<br>Bed rest<br>RhoGAM if appropriate |
| Inevitable abortion | Less than 20 weeks' gestation<br>No products of conception expelled<br>Membranes have ruptured<br>Internal cervical os is open<br>Uterine bleeding and cramps | Emergent D&C<br>RhoGAM if appropriate |
| Missed abortion | No cardiac activity<br>No products of conception expelled<br>Retained fetal tissue<br>Uterus not growing<br>Internal cervical os is closed<br>No uterine bleeding<br>Nonviable tissue not expelled in 4 weeks | Evacuate uterus<br>D&C<br>RhoGAM if appropriate |
| Septic abortion | Infection associated with abortion<br>Endometritis leading to septicemia<br>Maternal mortality 10–50% | Complete uterine evacuation<br>D&C<br>Intravenous antibiotics<br>RhoGAM if appropriate |
| Intrauterine fetal death | No cardiac activity (fetal heart tones)<br>Greater than 8 weeks' gestation, with 15 mm or larger crown–rump length | Evacuate uterus<br>D&C<br>RhoGAM if appropriate |

In an **abortion**, β-HCG is not appropriate for gestational age unless the abortion occurred in the distant past. The progesterone level is usually less than 15 ng/mL unless the abortion occurred a long time ago; intrauterine pregnancy is visualized (gestational sac) on ultrasound, no blood is obtained from culdocentesis (aspiration of fluid from the cul de sac), and villi are evident on uterine dilation and curettage.

In an **ectopic pregnancy**, β-HCG is abnormally low for gestational age, no intrauterine pregnancy with or without adnexal mass is visualized on ultrasound, at least 5 mL of nonclotting blood is obtained with culdocentesis, and no villi are evident on dilation and curettage.

If there is a diagnostic dilemma and ectopic pregnancy cannot be ruled out, laparoscopy should be performed as a diagnostic and potentially therapeutic procedure.

### Treatment

As in any case of hemorrhage, the patient needs to be hemodynamically stabilized if there has been significant bleeding. RhoGAM should be given to all antibody-negative patients experiencing abortions or ectopic pregnancy (see Figure 3). The treatment for abortions, described above, essentially consists of uterine evacuation and prevention of infection. The treatment for ectopic pregnancy is described below.

## ECTOPIC PREGNANCY

Any pregnancy occurring outside the uterine cavity is considered ectopic. Ectopic pregnancies commonly occur in the fallopian tubes (98%) in the ampulla region (90%). The incidence is 17/1000 pregnancies. Etiologies include anything that causes abnormal tubal motility. The number-one risk factor for ectopic pregnancy is a history of PID. Other risk factors include prior ectopic pregnancy, tubal/pelvic surgery, DES exposure in utero, and IUD use.

### Signs and Symptoms

The signs and symptoms of an ectopic pregnancy include:

- Symptoms of pregnancy (nausea, vomiting).
- Abdominal/pelvic pain and tenderness, usually on the side of the ectopic pregnancy.
- Abnormal bleeding, including amenorrhea.
- Pelvic mass on examination.
- Ruptured ectopics can also present with orthostatic hypotension, tachycardia, local and then generalized abdominal tenderness, shoulder pain, and shock.

### Differential

The differential diagnosis of an ectopic pregnancy includes intrauterine pregnancy, threatened abortion, PID, ruptured ovarian cyst, endometriosis, appendicitis, ovarian torsion, renal stones, and diverticulitis.

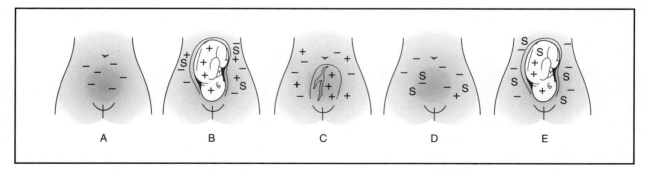

**FIGURE 3.** Why it is important to identify Rh-negative mothers and give RhoGAM. (A) Rh-negative woman before pregnancy. (B) Pregnancy occurs. The fetus is Rh-positive. (C) Separation of the placenta. (D) Following delivery, Rh-isoimmunization occurs in the mother, and she develops antibodies (S = antibodies). (E) The next pregnancy with an Rh-positive fetus. Maternal antibodies cross the placenta, enter the bloodstream, and attach to Rh-positive red cells, causing hemolysis. RhoGAM (Rh IgG) is given to the Rh-negative mother to prevent sensitization. DeCherney, *Current Obstetric & Gynecological Diagnosis & Treatment,* Eighth Edition, Stamford, CT: Appleton & Lange, 1994, page 339.

## Workup

Quantitative β-HCG is used to confirm pregnancy and to check for subnormal doubling time and low levels (80% of ectopics have β-HCG < 6500). Also consider serum progesterone (ectopics usually have < 15 ng/mL). Transvaginal ultrasound should be performed to identify the possibility of intrauterine gestation. The following possibilities exist:

1. The gestational sac is visualized, indicating an intrauterine pregnancy; or

2. No gestational sac is visualized, in which case the possible scenarios include very early intrauterine pregnancy, ectopic pregnancy, recent abortion, or a false-positive pregnancy test (very rare).

The next step is to correlate the β-HCG level with ultrasound findings and/or with time elapsed since the last menstrual period (see Table 5).

On ultrasound, also look for evidence of an ectopic pregnancy (eg, noncystic adnexal mass, fluid in the cul de sac). Other diagnostic tests include culdocentesis (at least 5 mL of nonclotting blood), dilation and curettage (only if the patient does not wish to be pregnant) to look for the absence of chorionic villi, and diagnostic laparoscopy.

Maintain a high level of suspicion for ectopic pregnancy.

## Treatment

For clinically stable patients in whom the diagnosis of ectopic pregnancy is uncertain and for patients in the "β-HCG discriminatory zone," expectant management of serial β-HCG and ultrasound should be performed.

For patients with confirmed ectopic pregnancy, medical and surgical options are available. For unruptured ectopic pregnancies of less than 3 cm with a β-HCG level of less than 1000 in a clinically stable patient, methotrexate can be administered. Surgical options depend on the reproductive plans of the patient, the age of the patient, and clinical status and consist of salpingostomy (the tube is incised and only the product of conception is removed), salpingectomy (the entire tube is removed), and salpingo-oophorectomy (the tube and the ovary are removed).

## THIRD-TRIMESTER BLEEDING

Third-trimester bleeding is any bleeding that occurs after 20 weeks of gestation. It complicates approximately 5% of all pregnancies.

**TABLE 5.** Correlation of ultrasound findings, β-HCG levels, and time since last menstrual period

| Transvaginal Ultrasound Findings | β-HCG Level | Time Elapsed Since Last Menstrual Period (days) |
|---|---|---|
| Gestational sac* | 1500 | 35 |
| Fetal pole | 5000 | 40 |
| Fetal heart motion | 17,000 | 45 |

\* For transabdominal ultrasound, the gestational sac should be visualized at a β-HCG level of 6000–6500 and/or 42 days since the last menstrual period.

## Signs and Symptoms

Table 6 describes the characteristics, diagnosis, and management of abruptio placentae and placenta previa (see Figure 4), the two causes of third-trimester bleeding associated with the most significant maternal and fetal morbidity and mortality.

## Differential

**Never do a vaginal exam prior to an ultrasound in third-trimester bleeding.**

The differential diagnosis of third-trimester bleeding includes abruptio placentae (30%), placenta previa (20%), early labor, marginal separation, and genital tract lesions. Other causes of third-trimester bleeding include bloody show (dilation of the cervix and loss of mucous plug associated with cervical dilation during the first stage of labor), ruptured vasa previa, ruptured uterus, and cervical carcinoma.

## Workup

The general principles in approaching a patient with third-trimester bleeding are as follows:

- Stat ultrasound to rule out placenta previa before vaginal or speculum exam.
- Cautious sterile speculum exam to evaluate the source of bleeding or ruptured membranes.
- Prepare cervical cultures.
- Perform abdominal exam.
- Check for fetal heart tones.
- Perform non–stress test to check fetal status.
- Consider amniocentesis for phosphatidylglycerol, lecithin-sphingomyelin ratio.

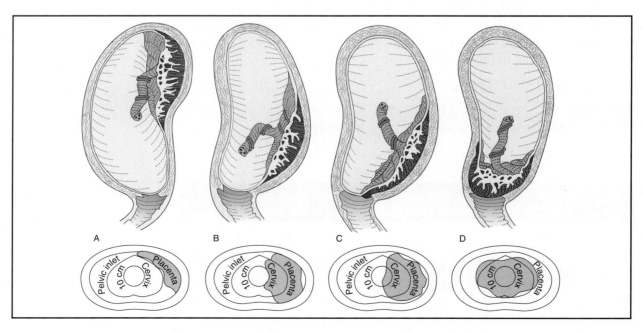

**FIGURE 4.** (A) Normal placenta. (B) Low implantation. (C) Partial placenta previa. (D) Complete placenta previa. DeCherney, *Current Obstetric & Gynecological Diagnosis & Treatment,* Eighth Edition, Stamford, CT: Appleton & Lange, 1994, page 404.

OBSTETRICS AND GYNECOLOGY

Other tests include type and cross for at least two units of packed RBCs, CBC, PT/PTT, Betke-Kleihauer test (a slide test that looks for fetal RBCs among those of the mother), urinalysis, and drug screen.

## Treatment

Treatment generally includes bed rest and tocolytics (drugs used to arrest uterine contractions) for the stable patient. In a mature fetus or with severe placental abruption, close fetal monitoring, amniotomy, and cesarean section are indicated as listed in Table 6.

**TABLE 6.** Abruptio placentae versus placenta previa

| | Placenta Abruptio | Placenta Previa |
|---|---|---|
| Pathophysiology | Premature (before the onset of labor) separation of normally implanted placenta. | Abnormal implantation of placenta near or at the cervical os, classified as:<br>• Total: placenta covers cervical os<br>• Partial: placenta partially covers os<br>• Marginal: edge of placenta extends to margin of os<br>• Low-lying: placenta within reach of the examining finger reached through the cervix |
| Incidence | 1/100 | 1/200 |
| Risk factors | Hypertension, abdominal/pelvic trauma, tobacco or cocaine use. | Prior cesarean sections, grand multiparous. |
| Symptoms | **Painful** vaginal bleeding (although 10% of the cases are concealed and there will be no bleeding); bleeding usually does not spontaneously cease. Abdominal pain, uterine hypertonicity, tenderness. Fetal distress present. | **Painless,** bright red bleeding (bleeding source is purely mom's), with the first bleeding episode averaging 29–30 weeks' gestation. Bleeding often ceases in 1–2 hours with or without uterine contractions. Usually no fetal distress present. |
| Diagnosis | Transabdominal/transvaginal ultrasound: look for retroplacental clot; can only rule in diagnosis but cannot rule out! | Transabdominal/transvaginal ultrasound: look for abnormally positioned placenta; this test is very sensitive to rule out this diagnosis. |
| Management | Stable patient with premature fetus: expectant management with continuous or frequent monitoring. Moderate to severe abruption: immediate delivery (vaginal delivery with amniotomy if fetal heart rate is stable; cesarean section if mom or fetus is in distress). Close fetal monitoring at all times. | NO vaginal exam! Stable patient with premature fetus: bed rest. Tocolytics (magnesium sulfate). Serial ultrasound to check fetal growth, resolution of partial previa. Amniocentesis to check fetal lung maturity; administer betamethasone to augment fetal lung maturity. Delivery by cesarean section or vaginal route depending on the lie of the placenta. Delivery if persistent labor, blood loss of more than 500 mL, unstable bleeding requiring multiple transfusion, coagulation defects, documented fetal lung maturity, 36 weeks' gestational age. |
| Complications | Hemorrhagic shock. Coagulopathy: DIC complicates 10% of all abruptions. Ischemic necrosis of distal organs. Recurrence risk is 5–16%; this risk increases to 25% after two previous abruptions. Fetal anemia. | Placenta accreta (up to 25% with one previous cesarean section). Vasa previa. Twofold increase in congenital abnormalities. Increased risk of postpartum hemorrhage. Fetal anemia. |

## GESTATIONAL DIABETES

Gestational diabetes occurs in 3–5% of all pregnancies. Physiologically, early in pregnancy there is increased insulin release, although as the pregnancy progresses there is a tendency toward insulin resistance. A pregnant patient has a narrow euglycemic range of 84 ± 10 mg/dL, beyond which pathology must be considered.

Risk factors for gestational diabetes include a past history of gestational diabetes, glycosuria or polyuria, obesity, a previous history of a macrosomic baby, habitual abortions/stillbirths, recurrent UTIs, a family history of diabetes, and a fetus that is large for gestational age on ultrasound or by fundal height.

### Signs and Symptoms

Gestational diabetes is largely asymptomatic in the mother and is usually noted only clinically through the evidence of glycosuria, hyperglycemia, and/or an abnormal glucose-tolerance test on routine prenatal screening at 24–28 weeks' gestation. Findings include a fetus large for gestational age on ultrasound or by fundal height.

### Differential

The differential diagnosis of gestational diabetes includes diabetes mellitus type I or II, volume overload, simple sugar overload, and urinary tract abnormalities.

### Workup

An abnormal 3-hour glucose test (see below in labs) in a patient with no history of diabetes prior to pregnancy is diagnostic.

In patients with risk factors for gestational diabetes (> 30 years old, family/personal history of diabetes, macrosomic child, obesity, hypertension), a 50-g oral glucose test should be administered at the initial visit to check for nonfasting blood glucose levels 1 hour following administration. If the glucose level is less than 140 mg/dL, retest at 24–28 weeks' gestation; if greater than 140 mg/dL, proceed to the 3-hour glucose tolerance test. The 50-g oral glucose test is administered to all pregnant patients at 24–28 weeks, and if found to be greater than 140 mg/dL, the 3-hour glucose tolerance test is administered.

In the 3-hour glucose tolerance test, 100 g of glucose is administered orally and the blood glucose level is checked at fasting (initial reading) and at 1-, 2-, and 3-hour time invervals:

- **Fasting:** > 105 mg/dL is considered abnormally high serum glucose.
- **1 hour:** > 195 mg/dL is considered abnormally high serum glucose.
- **2 hour:** > 165 mg/dL is considered abnormally high serum glucose.
- **3 hour:** > 145 mg/dL is considered abnormally high serum glucose.

The diagnosis of gestational diabetes is established if the patient has abnormally high blood glucose levels at any two of those four time points.

## Treatment

For uncomplicated cases, start with the American Diabetic Association (ADA) diet and monitor fasting blood glucose and 2-hour postprandial glucose levels. If a persistent (1- to 2-week) fasting blood glucose level greater than 105 mg/dL or 2-hour postprandial glucose level greater than 120 mg/dL is found despite dietary compliance, then start insulin. Patient education and diabetic clinic/dietitian consults are important in the management of the patient.

## Complications

Complications from gestational diabetes can be divided into maternal and fetal complications (see Table 7).

## PREGNANCY-INDUCED HYPERTENSION

Hypertension in pregnancy is diagnosed when there are two blood pressure measurements of 140/90 mmHg measured two times at least 6 hours apart. Pregnancy-induced hypertension (PIH) is hypertension that is present after 20 weeks of gestation. The two most common causes of PIH are preeclampsia and eclampsia.

Preeclampsia is defined as PIH, proteinuria (300 mg/24 hours), and/or edema. Severe proteinuria of greater than 5 g/day defines severe preeclampsia. A variant of preeclampsia with a poor prognosis is known as HELLP syndrome (Hemolysis, Elevated Liver enzymes, Low Platelets). Eclampsia manifests as seizures (not due to neurologic disease) in a patient with preeclampsia.

Preeclampsia is thought to result from systemic endothelial damage that causes vascular spasm, capillary hyperpermeability, and an imbalance in which the thromboxane level (vasoconstrictor) is much higher than the prostacyclin level (vasodilator). The pathology is linked to the placenta; the only cure is to remove the placenta (ie, delivery). Eclampsia results from CNS damage secondary to endothelial damage.

Risk factors for preeclampsia include nulliparity, extremes of age when pregnant (< 15, > 35), multiple gestations, vascular disease (secondary to lupus or diabetes), and chronic hypertension.

> **HELLP syndrome**
> **H**emolysis
> **E**levated **L**FTs
> **L**ow **P**latelets
> (thrombocytopenia)

---

| TABLE 7. Complications of gestational diabetes | |
| --- | --- |
| **Maternal Complications** | **Fetal Complications** |
| Preterm labor | Macrosomia |
| Pregnancy-induced hypertension | Shoulder dystocia |
| Polyhydramnios | Perinatal mortality 2–5% |
| Cesarean section for macrosomia | Congenital defects |
| Preeclampsia/eclampsia | |
| Glucose intolerance or diabetes mellitus type I later on (50% of gestational diabetes patients have impaired glucose tolerance later in life) | |

### Signs and Symptoms

Mild preeclampsia and severe preeclampsia share the same spectrum of signs and symptoms (see Table 8). Eclampsia is present if seizures occur in a preeclamptic patient.

### Differential

As cited above, the two most common causes of pregnancy-induced hypertension are preeclampsia and eclampsia. A common cause of pregnancy-induced hypertension occurring in the first or second trimester is a molar pregnancy. Other diseases in the differential for preeclampsia include renal disease, renovascular hypertension, primary aldosteronism, Cushing's disease, pheochromocytoma, and lupus erythematosus. Consider primary seizure disease and thrombotic thrombocytopenic purpura in the workup of eclampsia.

### Workup

As discussed in Table 8, the diagnostic criteria for preeclampsia include two blood pressure readings of 140/90 mmHg or greater measured at least 6 hours apart, a median arterial pressure increase of 15 mmHg over baseline (or 105 mmHg), proteinuria (300 mg/24 hours or 1 mg/L), and/or edema. The diagnosis of eclampsia is made when seizures (not due to neurologic disease) are present in a patient with preeclampsia.

Labs and diagnostic tests to obtain in the workup of preeclampsia include:

- CBC and platelet count
- BUN/creatinine
- Fibrinogen, fibrinogen split products (where indicated)
- Urinalysis, serial urine protein
- Amniocentesis (to check for fetal lung maturity)
- Liver function tests
- PT/PTT
- Urine toxicology screen
- Ultrasound
- Non–stress test and biophysical profiles as indicated

**Preeclamptic and eclamptic patients are at risk for seizures up to 24 hours postpartum.**

| **TABLE 8.** Signs and symptoms of preeclampsia and eclampsia | | |
| --- | --- | --- |
| **Mild Preeclampsia** | **Severe Preeclampsia** | **Eclampsia** |
| Blood pressure greater than 140/90 measured two times 6 hours apart | Signs and symptoms of mild preeclampsia plus . . . | The three most common symptoms preceding an eclamptic attack include headache, visual changes, and right upper quadrant/epigastric pain |
| Cerebral changes (headaches, somnolence) | Blood pressure greater than 160/110 measured two times 6 hours apart | |
| Visual changes (blurred vision, scotomata) | Proteinuria (> 5 g over 24 hours, or over 3 on urine dipstick) | Seizures; severe if not controlled with anticonvulsant therapy |
| GI symptoms (epigastric pain) | Oliguria | |
| Rapid weight gain, edema | Right upper quadrant/epigastric pain | |
| Jugular venous distention | Pulmonary edema/cyanosis | |
| Hyperactive reflexes, clonus | Increased liver function tests, decreased platelets | |
| | Oligohydramnios | |
| | IUGR | |

## Treatment

The only cure for preeclampsia is delivery of the fetus and placenta (see Table 9).

## PRETERM LABOR

Preterm labor complicates 5–10% of all pregnancies. Risk factors (think MAPPS) for preterm labor include multiple gestations, abdominal surgery during pregnancy, previous preterm labor, previous preterm delivery, and surgery of the cervix. Half of all cases of preterm labor, however, occur in patients without any risk factors.

> **Risk factors for preterm labor—MAPPS**
>
> **M**ultiple gestations
>
> **A**bdominal surgery during pregnancy
>
> Previous **P**reterm labor
>
> Previous **P**reterm delivery
>
> **S**urgery of the cervix

## Signs and Symptoms

The signs and symptoms of preterm labor include abdominal/pelvic pain, cramps, back pain, vaginal discharge, bloody show, uterine contractions, cervical dilation and/or effacement, and rupture of membranes.

## Differential

The differential diagnosis of preterm labor includes false labor, appendicitis, local causes (cervicitis, trauma, physiologic discharge), and genital tract infections.

## Workup

Diagnostic criteria are based on the presence of preterm (< 37 weeks' gestation) and true labor (uterine contractions of sufficient duration and intensity to result in cervical dilation of > 2 cm or effacement of > 80%).

| **TABLE 9.** Management of preeclampsia and eclampsia | |
| --- | --- |
| **Preeclampsia** | **Eclampsia** |
| If term or fetal lung maturity, deliver.<br>If severe, expedite delivery regardless of maturity.<br>Modified bed rest, check blood pressure, reflexes, daily weight and urine protein output, labs, fetal surveillance, patient education.<br>Control blood pressure with antihypertensives (hydralazine, labetalol, diazoxide) if diastolic blood pressure is higher than 110 mmHg. The goal is to maintain a blood pressure lower than 160/110, preferably with a diastolic blood pressure of 90–100 mmHg.<br>If severe, immediately hospitalize, check urine output, check for pulmonary edema, keep diastolic blood pressure 90–105 with antihypertensive, give magnesium sulfate for seizure prophylaxis, deliver as soon as possible by labor induction and/or cesarean section.<br>Postpartum: continue magnesium sulfate for at least the first 24 hours; check blood pressure, pulmonary status, and fluid retention. Follow heme, renal, and liver labs.<br>General course of disease: 30% of preeclampsia cases occurs before 30 weeks' gestational age, with the maximum number of cases occurring at 34 weeks' gestational age. | Insert padded tongue blade.<br>Supplemental oxygen. Place in lateral decubitus position.<br>Prevent maternal trauma.<br>Control seizure with magnesium sulfate and consider diazepam if seizures are poorly controlled.<br>Control blood pressure if severe hypertension (blood pressure > 160/110, or diastolic blood pressure > 110).<br>General measures: limit fluid intake, Foley catheter, monitor inputs and outputs, monitor magnesium blood level, carefully monitor fetal status, initiate steps to delivery!<br>Postpartum: same as preeclampsia.<br>General course of disease: 50% of seizures occur antepartum, 25% occur intrapartum, 25% occur within 24 hours postpartum. |

Labs to obtain include CBC with differential, DIC panel, urine tox screen, urine culture, vaginal and cervical culture for group B strep/chlamydia/gonorrhea, sterile speculum exam if there is suspicion of premature rupture of membranes, and ultrasound to assess estimated fetal weight and presentation.

### Treatment

Outpatient management is as follows:

- Bed rest, pelvic rest
- Education
- Self-monitoring at home
- Weekly cervical exams (from week 20 to week 37 gestational age)

For inpatients, the above labs should be obtained and pediatrics should be notified. Serial exams—if possible performed by the same examiner—should be performed more often than weekly, and the patient should be observed for possible signs of infection, especially if there is premature rupture of the membranes. For mom, consider the use of tocolytics (terbutaline, magnesium sulfate, nifedipine, ritodrine) if there are no contraindications (see the mnemonic labeled "CHAMPS"). There is, however, no uncontested evidence that the use of tocolytics prolongs premature delivery; tocolytics are ineffective if the patient is in active labor (cervical dilation at 4 cm).

In monitoring the fetus, a daily non–stress test and interval ultrasound should be performed to monitor fetal growth and presentation. Consider betamethasone if the following conditions exist: an estimated gestational age of 24–34 weeks, absence of chorioamnionitis, absence of uncontrolled maternal diabetes, and no need for immediate delivery. Note that betamethasone has been proven most effective with a singleton pregnancy between 28 and 34 weeks' gestational age. Amniocentesis may be considered, especially at 35–36 weeks' gestational age, to check for fetal lung maturity (lecithin: sphingomyelin ratio > 2:1).

## ABNORMAL LABOR PATTERNS

A diagnosis of abnormal labor is considered in any case where there is a variation in the normal pattern of cervical dilation or descent of the fetal presenting part. It occurs in 8–11% of all cephalic deliveries.

### Signs and Symptoms

Labor is abnormal when the duration of an event is too long or too short. Table 10 describes patterns of abnormal labor.

Also beware of false labor, which has the following distinguishing characteristics:

- Irregular intervals and duration of uterine contractions.
- Contraction intensity unchanged.
- No cervical dilation.
- Lower back and abdominal discomfort.
- Relief with sedation.

> **Contraindications for tocolytics— CHAMPS**
>
> **C**horioamnionitis
>
> **H**emorrhage
>
> **A**bruption of placenta
>
> Fetal **M**aturity
>
> **P**reeclampsia/ eclampsia
>
> **S**evere intrauterine growth retardation

**TABLE 10.** Abnormal labor patterns

| Abnormal Pattern | Threshold Duration of Labor Nulliparous | Multiparous | Possible Causes |
|---|---|---|---|
| Precipitous | Completion of stages 1 and 2 in less than 3 h | | Unknown |
| Prolonged latent phase | More than 20 h | More than 14 h | Ineffective uterine contractions<br>Unripe cervix<br>Excess sedation<br>Abnormal fetal position<br>False labor |
| Protracted active phase | More than 12 h<br><br>Less than 1.2 cm/h<br><br>Less than 1 cm/h | More than 6 h or cervical dilation<br>Less than 1.5 cm/h or fetal descent<br>Less than 2 cm/h | Abnormal fetal position<br>Fetopelvic disproportion<br>Excess sedation<br>Ineffective uterine contrations |
| Arrest of dilation in active phase* | Cervical dilation stops for more than 2 h | | Ineffective uterine contractions<br>Fetopelvic disproportion<br>Abnormal fetal lie, presentation, or position |
| Arrest of fetal descent (late in active phase and throughout second stage) | Fetal descent stops for more than 1 h | | Ineffective uterine contractions<br>Fetopelvic disproportion |

\* Indicates immediate attention; potential complications can emerge quickly.

## Differential

The differential diagnosis of abnormal labor includes normal labor, false labor, ineffective uterine contractions, incompetent cervix, fetal malposition, and fetopelvic disproportion.

## Workup

Workup consists of the following:

1. Accurately assessing the specific abnormal pattern the patient is experiencing:

   a. Graphic demonstration of cervical dilation and effacement.

   b. Documenting on each vaginal exam the dilation of the cervix, the station of the fetal presenting part, the presence of the caput or molding of the fetal head, and the position of the fetal presenting part. The results of each examination should be assessed dynamically.

2. Systematically assessing the "3 P's of labor":

   a. **Powers (uterine forces):** Frequency and duration can be evaluated by manual palpation of the gravid abdomen during a con-

> **Causes of abnormal labor— the "3 P's"**
>
> **P**owers (uterine contractions)
>
> **P**assenger (fetus)
>
> **P**assage (pelvic)

traction; by a tocodynamometer; and by an internal pressure catheter (this also provides information about the pressure generated by each uterine contraction).

b. **Passenger:** Estimation of fetal weight and clinical evaluation of fetal lie, presentation, and position.

c. **Passage:** Measurement of the bony pelvis is often a poor predictor of abnormal labor unless the pelvis is extremely contracted; also assess for other physical obstacles (distended bladder or colon, uterine myoma, cervical mass, size of the baby).

### Treatment

Precipitous labor:

- Tocolytics may be administered to slow down uterine activity.
- Complications include uterine atony leading to postpartum hemorrhage and genital tract trauma.

Prolonged latent phase:

- Rest or augmentation of labor with oxytocin if powers are the problem.
- Amniotomy.

Protracted/arrested active phase:

- Artificial rupture of membranes.
- Rest and then augmentation with oxytocin if powers are the problem.
- Cesarean section if fetopelvic disproportion or maternal/fetal distress.

Arrest in second stage:

- Attempt vaginal delivery if mom and baby are doing well.
- Oxytocin augmentation and lots of support for mom.
- Operative vaginal delivery (forceps, vacuum) if vertex is low in pelvis.
- Cesarean section if maternal/fetal distress, breech, or fetopelvic disproportion.

Prolonged labor predisposes the mother to increased risk of infection, exhaustion, laceration, uterine atony, and operative delivery. The fetus experiences an increased risk of asphyxia, infection, trauma, and possible cerebral damage.

## POSTPARTUM HEMORRHAGE

The clinical diagnosis of postpartum hemorrhage is established when there is more than a 500-mL blood loss within the first 24 hours of delivery. Hemorrhage can be sudden and profuse, or blood loss can occur more slowly but persistently. Either way, excessive bleeding is a serious and potentially fatal complication. The following discussion outlines the three most common causes of postpartum hemorrhage together with their diagnosis and management.

**Don't forget serial HCTs in postpartum hemorrhage.**

| | Uterine Atony | Genital Tract Trauma | Retained Placental Tissue |
|---|---|---|---|
| **TABLE 11.** Common causes of postpartum hemorrhage | | | |
| Risk factors | Overdistention of the uterus (multiple gestations, macrosomia)<br>Abnormal labor (prolonged labor, precipitous labor)<br>Conditions interfering with uterine contractions (uterine myomas, magnesium sulfate, general anesthesia)<br>Uterine infection | Precipitous labor<br>Operative vaginal delivery (forceps, vacuum extraction)<br>Large infant<br>Inadequate episiotomy repair | Placenta accreta/increta/pecreta<br>Preterm delivery<br>Placenta previa<br>Previous cesarean section/curettage<br>Uterine leiomyomas |
| Diagnosis | Palpation of a softer, flaccid, "boggy" uterus without a firm fundus | Careful visualization of the lower genital tract looking for any laceration greater than 2 cm in length | Careful inspection of the placenta for missing cotyledons. Ultrasound may also be used to examine the uterus. |
| Treatment | Most common cause of postpartum hemorrhage (90%)<br>Bimanual uterine massage, which is usually successful<br>Oxytocin infusion<br>Methylergonovine maleate (Methergine) if not hypertensive and/or prostaglandin F2-alpha if patient is not asthmatic or hypertensive | Surgical repair of the physical defect | Manual removal of the remaining placental tissue.<br>Curettage with suctioning may also be used with care taken to avoid perforating the uterine fundus.<br>In cases of true placenta accreta/increta/pecreta where the placental villi invade into the uterine tissue, hysterectomy is often required as a life-preserving therapy. |

## Differential

The three most common causes of postpartum hemorrhage are uterine atony (most common cause), genital tract trauma, and retained placental tissue; all are discussed in Table 11. Other causes of postpartum hemorrhage include uterine inversion, uterine rupture, and cervical carcinoma.

## Workup/Treatment

The diagnosis and treatment of the three major causes of postpartum hemorrhage are discussed in Table 11.

# GYNECOLOGY

## PELVIC INFLAMMATORY DISEASE (PID)

PID is an upper genital tract infection usually resulting from an ascending infection from the cervix. Approximately one-third of all cases are caused by *N. gonorrhoeae* alone, another third by *N. gonorrhoeae* and anaerobes/aerobes (including *C. trachomatis*), and the remaining third by anaerobes/aerobes alone. The lifetime risk is 1–3%. Risk factors for PID include multiple sex partners, a new partner within 30 days before becoming symptomatic, a high frequency of intercourse, a young age at first intercourse, and possibly IUD use.

### Signs and Symptoms

Patients usually present with a 1- to 3-day history of lower abdominal pain with or without fever, vaginal discharge, recent menses, a history of sexual exposure, and a past history of PID. On physical exam, there is lower abdominal tenderness with cervical motion tenderness together with adnexal mass and/or tenderness.

### Differential

The differential diagnosis of PID includes ectopic pregnancy, endometriosis, ovarian torsion, hemorrhagic ovarian cyst, appendicitis, UTI, and diverticulitis.

### Workup

Specific criteria are required to establish the diagnosis of PID. The following three criteria should be present:

1. History of abdominal pain and finding of abdominal tenderness with or without rebound
2. Cervical motion tenderness (CMT)
3. Adnexal tenderness

One of the following criteria is also required to establish the diagnosis:

1. Temperature higher than 38°C
2. WBC greater than 10K
3. Presence of an inflammatory mass (tubo-ovarian abscess) on exam, sonography, or culdocentesis yielding peritoneal fluid with bacteria and white blood cells; or the presence of *N. gonorrhoeae* and/or *C. trachomatis* on the endocervix (mucopurulent cervicitis, evidence of gram-negative diplococci, positive chlamydia antigen test, > 10 WBC/hpf).

Laboratory tests that should be obtained in the workup of pelvic inflammatory disease include CBC (WBC > 10K), ESR (> 15 mm/hr), β-HCG (check for pregnancy status), Gram stain of cervical discharge (gram-negative intracellular diplococci), RPR/VDRL (to rule out syphilis), HIV, hepatitis screen, ultrasound (inflammatory mass), culdocentesis (peritoneal fluid with bacteria and white blood cells), and laparoscopy (for definitive diagnosis of edema and erythema of fallopian tubes and purulent exudate). Note that laparoscopy has established the definitive diagnosis and has been shown to confirm the clinical diagnosis in approximately 60% of cases.

### Treatment

Surgery is needed only if there is a complication, such as a tubo-ovarian abscess (TOA). The inpatient regimen includes cefotetan and doxycycline. Outpatients are usually managed with ceftriaxone and doxycycline.

Sequelae of PID include a tenfold increase in the risk of an ectopic pregnancy and a fourfold increase in the risk of chronic pelvic pain, infertil-

"Chandelier sign": severe CMT on exam that makes the patient "jump for the chandelier."

ity, and recurrent PID. An often-pimped complication of PID is Fitz-Hugh-Curtis syndrome, a perihepatitis characterized by inflammation of the liver capsule and the undersurface of the diaphragm. Patients often present with pleuritic right upper quadrant pain limiting chest expansion. The Fitz-Hugh-Curtis syndrome complicates 15–30% of PID cases.

## SEXUALLY TRANSMITTED DISEASES

Taken together, STDs are one of the most common gynecologic problems encountered in the outpatient setting. All sexually active patients must thus be examined with an awareness of a possible STD. Often patients have had a past history of STDs, which can be elicited through careful and tactful history taking.

On physical examination, the following should be noted:

- **Inguinal area:** rashes, lesions, adenopathy.
- **Vulva:** lesions, ulcerations, abnormal discharge, abnormal swelling/thickening.
- **Vagina/cervix:** lesions, discharge.

Also check out the glands (Bartholin's, Skene's), the urethra, and the perineum and perianal area.

Cultures of the urethra and cervix for chlamydia, gonorrhea, or other infectious agents should be obtained for any suspicious case. It is important to note that 20–50% of patients with STD have coexisting infections, creating a low threshold for detecting other infectious diseases. All contacts of the patient must be treated.

## GENITAL HERPES

Herpes simplex is the most common STD and is highly infectious (75% rate).

### Etiology

Herpes simplex virus type II (90%); type I (10%).

### Signs and Symptoms

The prodromal phase (mild paresthesia, burning) progresses to painful vesicular lesions 3–7 days after exposure; in primary infections, patients may often have malaise, low-grade fever, and adenopathy. Physical findings often reveal clear vesicles that may have lysed, progressing to painful ulcers with red borders that coalesce and become secondarily infected. These lesions can be found on the vulva, vagina, cervix, perineum, and perianal area.

### Workup

Workup consists of obtaining a history and physical findings, a Tzank smear of lesions, and viral cultures.

Pregnant patients with active herpes at the time of labor often necessitate C-section.

### Treatment

Expectant (keep lesions dry and clean, antimicrobial cream to prevent secondary bacterial infections), acyclovir (ointment for duration of flare-up, oral for decreasing frequency and severity of recurrence, intravenous for hospitalized cases of severe outbreaks).

## CHLAMYDIA TRACHOMATIS

*Chlamydia trachomatis* is the second most common STD, is 10 times more common than *Neisseria gonorrhoeae*, and has an infection rate 5 times higher in women with 3 partners and 4 times higher in women using no barrier methods. It can manifest as cervicitis, PID, or lymphogranuloma venereum (rare) and often coexists with gonorrhea.

### Etiology

*Chlamydia trachomatis* is an obligate intracellular parasite.

### Signs and Symptoms

Mild cases can be asymptomatic or patients may present with dysuria, abnormal vaginal discharge, ectopic pregnancy, or infertility. Physical findings are subtle and nonspecific; mucopurulent cervical discharge is often a clue. Findings may be masked by coexisting gonorrheal infection.

### Diagnosis

A diagnosis of *Chlamydia trachomatis* is usually suspected on clinical grounds; cultures are performed to confirm the diagnosis. Two screening tests are now available: a monoclonal antibody test (faster) and an enzyme immunoassay of the cervical secretion (95% specificity). Always check for concomitant gonorrheal infection (cultures, smear).

### Treatment

Treatment consists of tetracycline or doxycycline; erythromycin may be substituted in allergic or pregnant patients. Treatment has about a 95% cure rate. The main sequelae from chlamydia infection arise from insidious tubal damage leading to infertility.

## GONORRHEA

Gonorrhea is still a very common infection; an increased frequency has also been observed with penicillin-resistant strains in asymptomatic infections.

### Etiology

*Neisseria gonorrhoeae* is a gram-negative intracellular diplococcus.

### Signs and Symptoms

*Neisseria gonorrhoeae* lower genital tract infection is characterized by a malodorous, purulent, yellow-green discharge from the cervix, vagina, Skene's ducts, urethra, or anus. In heterosexual women, 10–20% also have gonorrhea infection in the pharynx. Acute upper genital tract infection occurs in approximately 15% of women infected with gonorrhea (see PID section).

## Workup

Workup consists of obtaining a Gram stain of discharge for intracellular gram-negative diplococci, cultures from the discharge on Thayer-Martin medium (80–95% sensitivity), and enzyme immunoassay for gonorrhea antigen.

## Treatment

Have a low threshold for treating patients for gonorrhea; it is valid to treat on clinical grounds alone. Antibiotics used are dependent on the site of infection. For urethral/cervical/rectal infection, use ceftriaxone, cefixime, ciprofloxacin, ampicillin, or amoxicillin with probenecid; for pharyngeal infection, use ceftriaxone, ciprofloxacin, aqueous penicillin with probenecid, or tetracycline.

## Complications

Infertility occurs in 15% of patients after a single episode and in 75% of patients after 3 episodes of PID. The risk of ectopic pregnancy is increased by seven- to tenfold.

Other complications include recurrent infection and chronic pelvic pain.

## CONDYLOMATA ACUMINATA (VENEREAL WARTS)

Condylomata acuminata are almost as common as gonorrhea infection; unlike other STDs, however, the sequelae may take years to manifest.

## Etiology

Human papillomavirus (HPV). Three subtypes of HPV have a very high association with cervical neoplasia: 16, 18, and 31 (see Pap-smear section).

## Signs and Symptoms

Patients may present with painless bumps, discharge, and pruritus. Physical findings include soft, fleshy, exophytic, papular, verrucous, flat, or macular growths on the cervix, vagina, vulva, urethral meatus, perineum, or perianal area. Lesions are often symmetrical; coinfection with *Trichomonas* or *Gardnerella* is common.

## Diagnosis

Presumptive diagnosis is made with physical findings. Diagnosis is confirmed with biopsy of warts following 5% acetic acid staining. Note that Pap smear of the cervix diagnoses only about 5% of patients infected with HPV.

## Treatment

External and vaginal lesions are treated with Condylox, cryotherapy, $CO_2$ laser, colposcopy, and biopsy of the cervix to rule out cervical cancer.

Cervical lesions are treated with colposcopy and biopsy of the cervix, cryotherapy, laser, or loop electrosurgical excision procedure (LEEP).

Lesions are often more resistant to therapy during pregnancy, in diabetic patients, or in immunosuppressed patients. Any patient infected with HPV must have at least once-yearly Pap-smear evaluation of the cervix.

## SYPHILIS

The incidence of syphilis has been rising over the past few years owing to penicillin-resistant gonorrhea strains. In the past, gonorrhea treatment with penicillin would also treat syphilis.

### Etiology

*Treponema pallidum*, a motile spirochete.

### Signs and Symptoms

The signs and symptoms of syphilis according to the stage of the infection are as follows:

- **Primary (10–60 days after infection):** Painless ulcer (chancre) found in or near vulva, vagina, cervix, anus, rectum, pharynx, lips, and fingers; often missed the first time around; heals spontaneously in 3–9 weeks.
- **Secondary (4–8 weeks after appearance of chancre):** Low-grade fever, headache, malaise, anorexia, generalized lymphadenopathy; diffuse, symmetric, asymptomatic maculopapular rash in soles and palms; highly infective secondary eruptions (mucous patches) can coalesce, forming condylomata lata; lesions heal spontaneously in 2–6 weeks.
- **Tertiary (1–20 years after the initial infection):** Destructive, granulomatous gummas cause systemic damage to the CNS, heart, or great vessels.

### Workup

Workup consists of dark-field microscopy (motile spirochetes) of primary or secondary lesions, VDRL/RPR (rapid, nonspecific screening test), and FTA-ABS/MHA-TP (specific, diagnostic).

### Treatment

Penicillin is the treatment of choice for primary/secondary/tertiary syphilis. Alternatively, tetracycline or penicillin desensitization can be used for allergic patients and erythromycin for pregnant patients. Of note is the fact that transplacental spread can occur at any stage of syphilis, leading to congenital syphilis.

# COMMON VAGINAL INFECTIONS (VAGINITIS)

The normal vaginal flora consists of approximately 25 bacterial species. The vaginal environment is normally acidic (pH 3.3–4.2) secondary to colonizing lactobacilli producing lactic acid. This acidic environment inhibits the growth of organisms. A less acidic environment can lead to bacterial proliferation and hence to possible clinical infection.

## Signs and Symptoms

The signs and symptoms of vaginitis include vulvovaginal itch with or without burning sensation, abnormal odor, and increased vaginal discharge. Occasionally vaginal discharge is physiologic, although this type of discharge is usually white and odorless, and the patient is asymptomatic. In examining the patient, always check for the quantity, odor, and color of vaginal discharge. See Table 12 for helpful hints in differentiating the etiologies of vaginitis.

## Differential

The differential diagnosis for increased vaginal discharge includes STDs and UTIs.

## Workup

Laboratory tests required to establish the diagnosis of vaginitis include slide smears with saline and KOH. In addition, a Gram stain of the vaginal discharge and a chlamydia antigen test should be performed to rule out STDs. A urinalysis of a clean-catch urine specimen rules out UTIs.

Table 12 describes the three most common causes of vaginitis.

| **TABLE 12.** Causes of vaginitis | | | |
|---|---|---|---|
| | Bacterial Vaginosis (usually *Gardnerella*) | *Trichomonas* | Yeast (usually *Candida*) |
| Relative frequency | 50% | 25% | 25% |
| Discharge | Homogenous, grayish-white, watery, fishy and stale odor | Profuse malodorous, grayish, frothy, "strawberry spots" on cervix, vaginal wall | Thick, white, cottage-cheese texture |
| Vaginal pH | Higher than 4.5 | Higher than 4.5 | Normal vaginal pH |
| Saline smear** | Clue cells (epithelial cells coated with bacteria) | Motile trichomonads | Nothing |
| KOH smear | Fishy odor | Nothing | Pseudohyphae |
| Treatment | Metronidazole* | Metronidazole* Treat partner; this is considered an STD | Nystatin |

*Patients taking metronidazole should not drink alcohol, which would lead to an Antabuse-like effect.

** Saline smear: if you see lots of WBCs and no organism, suspect chlamydia.

## Treatment

Treatments for the specific types of vaginitis are discussed in Table 12.

## ENDOMETRIOSIS

Endometriosis is characterized by the presence of endometrial glands and stroma outside the uterine cavity. In descending frequency, most endometriosis lesions are found in the ovaries (usually bilateral), broad ligament, and cul de sac (see Figure 5). It afflicts 5–15% of premenopausal women and accounts for 40–50% of all surgeries for infertility. Evidence exists, however, for a genetic disposition in first-degree relatives. Classically, endometriosis lesions have been described as having the appearance of "mulberry," "raspberry," "powder burns," and "chocolate cysts" found in the ovaries.

Although the exact mechanisms are unknown, the following hypotheses for the pathogenesis of endometriosis have been proposed:

- Direct implantation of endometrial cells by retrograde menstruation.
- Vascular and lymphatic dissemination of endometrial cells.
- Celomic metaplasia of multipotential cells in the peritoneal cavity.

## Signs and Symptoms

Classic and often-quoted symptoms of endometriosis are dysmenorrhea (beginning a few days prior to and lasting throughout the entire menstrual cycle), deep dyspareunia, chronic pelvic pain, abnormal bleeding, and infertility. The nature and severity of the symptoms depend on both the extent and the location of the disease. On pelvic examination, findings indicative of more established disease include nodular thickening along the uterosacral ligament; a fixed, retroverted uterus; and tender, fixed adnexal masses (endometriomas). Physical findings in early-stage endometriosis are often subtle and even nonexistent despite the patient's complaints.

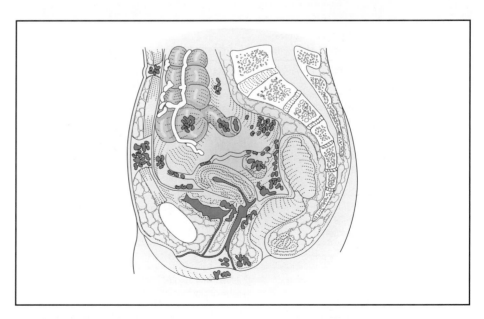

**FIGURE 5.** Common sites of endometriosis (dark ovals). DeCherney, *Current Obstetric & Gynecological Diagnosis & Treatment*, Eighth Edition, Stamford, CT: Appleton & Lange, 1994, page 802.

## Differential

Patients with endometriosis can present with a wide range of symptoms, and the differential list depends on the patient's specific complaints. For chronic abdominal pain, chronic pelvic inflammatory disease and pelvic adhesions should be entertained. In patients presenting with amenorrhea, causes of primary and/or secondary amenorrhea should be on the differential. If sudden-onset lower abdominal pain is the chief complaint, ectopic pregnancy, appendicitis, PID, adnexal torsion, rupture of the corpus luteum, or endometrioma must be considered.

## Workup

The definitive diagnosis of endometriosis is established by laparoscopic examination and biopsy of "endometriosis-appearing lesions" revealing functional endometrial glands and stroma together with hemosiderin-laden macrophages. Laboratory tests to be obtained should include a pregnancy test, a urinalysis, CA-125, and ultrasound to rule out differential diagnoses.

## Treatment

Treatment should be individualized according to age, reproductive plans, and extent of disease.

Medical treatment is aimed at inducing inactivity/atrophy of endometrial tissue. These options include hormonal manipulation, including OCP, progestin, danazol, and GnRH agonist. All medical treatments are for symptomatic relief, not for cure; they have no effect on the adhesions and fibrosis caused by endometriosis.

Conservative surgical options include laparoscopic removal of implants (excision, electrocauterization, laser ablation) that allows for future pregnancy. Definitive surgeries are appropriate for severe disease uncontrolled by medical and conservative surgical treatment or for patients who are willing to forgo future pregnancy. Surgery includes total abdominal hysterectomy, bilateral salpingo-oophorectomy, lysis of adhesions, and removal of all implants. In younger patients, some ovarian tissue may be left intact to prevent early menopause, although there may be a recurrence of endometriosis. In patients without endogenous estrogen production (ie, who have no ovaries), hormonal replacement therapy must be instituted.

Note that endometriosis is a chronic disorder requiring long-term therapy. Treatment often improves the chances of successful conception. This disease is hormone-dependent and usually improves after menopause. The risk of malignant transformation is very low.

## AMENORRHEA

Amenorrhea is defined as the complete absence of menstruation and is divided into primary and secondary amenorrhea.

## Signs and Symptoms

By definition, primary amenorrhea is the absence of menses and the lack of secondary sexual characteristics by age 14, whereas secondary amenorrhea is the absence of menses for 3 cycles or for 6 months with normal prior menses.

## Differential

The causes of primary amenorrhea include gonadal failure/agenesis, Müllerian abnormality, androgen insensitivity syndrome, hypopituitary failure, and constitutional delay. Common causes of secondary amenorrhea include pregnancy, hypothyroidism, polycystic ovarian syndrome, premature menopause, pituitary failure, galactorrhea, hyperprolactinemia, and eating disorders.

## Workup/Treatment

The workup of amenorrhea should follow a logical order:

1. Does the patient have primary (see Figure 6) or secondary (see Figures 7 and 8) amenorrhea? Making this distinction will help you narrow down your differential workup.

2. The causes of amenorrhea can be systemically broken down into pregnancy, genital tract outflow obstruction, ovarian dysfunction, and hypopituitary axis abnormalities.

   a. **Pregnancy:** It is essential to rule out pregnancy given that it is the most common cause of amenorrhea. A history of breast fullness, weight gain, and morning sickness are supportive evidence. The diagnosis can be easily and economically confirmed or ruled out with a pregnancy test.

Pregnancy is a common cause of amenorrhea (always check a pregnancy test).

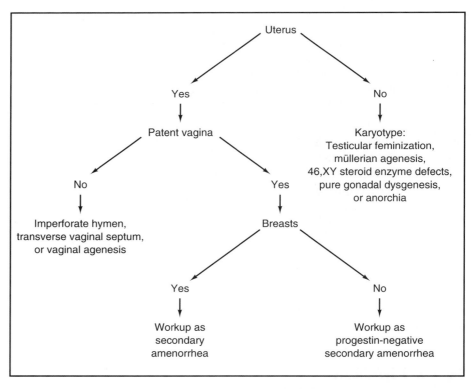

**FIGURE 6.** Workup for primary amenorrhea. DeCherney, *Current Obstetric and Gynecological Diagnosis and Treatment,* Eighth Edition, Stamford, CT: Appleton & Lange, 1994, page 1010.

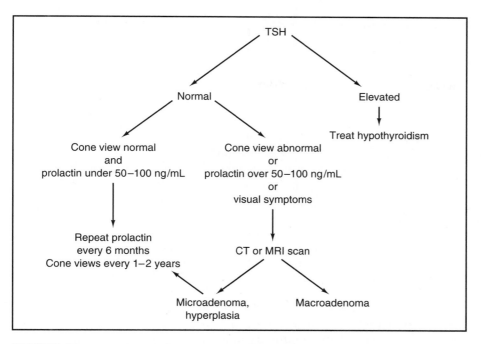

**FIGURE 7.** Workup for patients with secondary amenorrhea and galactorrhea–hyperprolactinemia. DeCherney, *Current Obstetric and Gynecological Diagnosis and Treatment,* Eighth Edition, Stamford, CT: Appleton & Lange, 1994, page 1010.

b. **Genital tract outflow obstruction:** Obstruction is a physical cause of amenorrhea and is more common in cases of primary amenorrhea. It commonly results from congenital anomalies in the development and canalization of the müllerian ducts. Physical examination may readily reveal an imperforate hymen or absence of a uterus and/or a vagina. Occasionally, scarring of the uterus (also known as Asherman's syndrome) may result from uterine dilation and curettage or from infection and may subse-

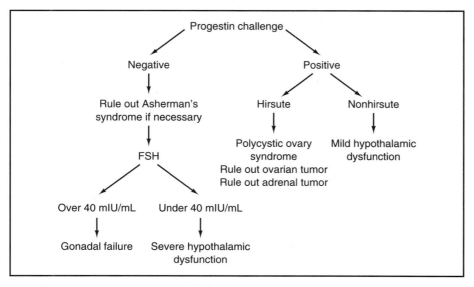

**FIGURE 8.** Workup for patients with secondary amenorrhea without galactorrhea–hyperprolactinemia. DeCherney, *Current Obstetric and Gynecological Diagnosis and Treatment,* Eighth Edition, Stamford, CT: Appleton & Lange, 1994, page 1010.

quently lead to secondary amenorrhea. This information may be elicited from the patient's history. In mild cases of scarring, surgical lysis of the adhesions by dilation and curettage or hysteroscopy may be curative; more severe cases may be refractory.

c. **Ovarian–pituitary–hypothalamic axis:** History information should focus on more common problems that can occur in any of these three areas. For primary amenorrhea, look for any incongruence in sexual characteristics and amenorrhea, systemic symptoms suggesting lack of pituitary-regulated hormones, and age. In patients with secondary amenorrhea, check for stress (nutritional, physical, emotional) and for signs and symptoms of hypothyroidism (goiter) or hyperprolactinemia (milky nipple discharge), hirsutism, obesity, and hot flashes/mood changes.

A systematic approach to working up the endocrine axis is much more efficient than a shotgun approach. The following is recommended:

1. If the pregnancy test is negative, check blood TSH (if high, evaluate hypothyroidism) and/or prolactin (if high, evaluate pituitary tumor, drugs affecting pituitary function).

2. If blood TSH/prolactin, are normal, do progesterone challenge (if there is withdrawal bleeding, there is adequate estrogen production and the diagnosis is anovulation).

3. If there is no withdrawal bleeding (there is inadequate estrogen production secondary to LH/FSH abnormalities), check LH and FSH levels.

Low to normal levels of LH/FSH indicate that the main problem lies in the hypothalamus–pituitary axis (stress, nutritional imbalance, tumors) or constitutional delay in a patient with primary amenorrhea. High levels of LH/FSH indicate that the problem lies in the ovaries (failure of or resistance to stimulation by gonadotropins). Check the patient's age; if the patient is more than 40 years old, she is going through the climacteric period toward menopause; if the patient is less than 40 years old, she is suffering from premature ovarian failure and needs to have endocrine disorders ruled out.

## ABNORMAL UTERINE BLEEDING

Uterine bleeding is considered abnormal in any postmenopausal woman; in premenopausal women, uterine bleeding is abnormal if any of the following exist: a menstrual cycle lasting more than 8 days, a menstrual interval of less than 21 days, and/or a total blood loss/menstrual cycle greater than 80 mL (see Table 13).

### Etiology

Causes of abnormal bleeding during the reproductive years are as follows:

• Pregnancy is the most common cause. Keep in mind abnormal pregnancies such as ectopic pregnancy, threatened abortion (internal cervical os closed), and incomplete abortion (internal cervical os opened).

| TABLE 13. Abnormal uterine bleeding patterns | |
|---|---|
| Term | Definition |
| Menorrhagia | Prolonged cycle (> 8 days) or increased total blood loss (> 80 mL) with regular intervals |
| Metrorrhagia | Irregular bleeding between menses with frequent intervals |
| Menometrorrhagia | Irregular, prolonged, and heavy menstrual bleeding with frequent intervals |
| Polymenorrhea | Regular intervals of less than every 21 days |
| Oligomenorrhea | Regular intervals of greater than 35 days to 6 months |

- Organic causes such as blood dyscrasias, hypersplenism, hypothyroidism, sepsis, ITP, and leukemia.
- Anatomic causes include malignancies, infections, endometriosis, ruptured corpus luteum cyst, and trauma.
- Dysfunctional uterine bleeding (DUB).

The most common cause of postmenopausal vaginal bleeding is atrophic vaginitis.

Other causes of postmenopausal bleeding include endometrial cancer and atrophic endometrium (due to D&C), as well as estrogen and medroxyprogesterone acetate (Provera).

## Workup

On physical examination, assess rate of bleeding, hemodynamic status, orthostatic vitals, skin and hair changes, thyroid enlargement, galactorrhea, obesity, hirsutism, cervical motion tenderness, uterine size, cervical lesions, and adnexal tenderness.

Laboratory tests should include CBC, pregnancy test, coagulation studies if coagulopathy is suspected, endocrine tests (TSH, prolactin, LH, FSH), endometrial biopsy for women greater than 35 years old, and transvaginal ultrasound to check for masses/endometrial thickening (normally < 5 mm in postmenopausal women).

To work up abnormal uterine bleeding:

1. Obtain CBC to check hematocrit; do a pregnancy test.
2. Determine whether the patient is having ovulatory or anovulatory cycles. The patient is ovulating if she has menstrual cycles at regular intervals.
3. If the patient is not ovulating, she has dysfunctional (irregular, excessive bleeding with no organic cause) uterine bleeding, most likely secondary to hormonal irregularities.
4. If the patient is ovulating, she is having abnormal uterine bleeding and further workup is required to rule out pathology. Obtain platelet count, bleeding time, prothrombin time, and partial thromboplastin time. Check for cervical masses/polyps, do dilation and curettage or hysteroscopy, and obtain a biopsy if necessary.

**Pregnancy is the most common cause of abnormal uterine bleeding (always check a pregnancy test).**

### Treatment

**Anovulatory bleeding.** After ruling out pathologies (uterine polyps, endometrial cancer), patients are placed on medroxyprogesterone acetate (Provera). Also consider hormone replacement therapy, especially if the patient is perimenopausal (see Table 14).

### Dysfunctional uterine bleeding:

- For mild cases (hemoglobin > 11), treat patient with iron supplement, Colace, ibuprofen to reduce menorrhagia, and oral contraceptives. Alternately, medroxyprogesterone acetate can be used to normalize menses. In more severe cases (hemoglobin < 8), the patient needs to be hemodynamically stabilized (blood transfusion, saline) and placed on oral hormone therapy (conjugated estrogen, Provera) or OCPs.
- For recurrent, severe, dysfunctional uterine bleeding, suppression can be achieved by placing the patient on OCPs, Provera, or Depo-Provera with or without an estrogen supplement.
- Surgical options for dysfunctional uterine bleeding include hysteroscopy with dilation and curettage, endometrial ablation with laser or electrocautery, and hysterectomy.

## MENOPAUSE

Menopause is the permanent cessation of natural menses and marks the end of a woman's reproductive life. The average age ranges from 45 to 55 years, with the median age 51 years. The climacteric period is the extended period of decreased ovarian function beginning several years before and lasting years after menopause itself.

## Signs and Symptoms

Perimenopausal symptoms include irregular and infrequent menses accompanied by hot flashes, sleep disturbances, vaginal dryness, volatility of affect, sexual dysfunction, and hair and nail brittleness. All of these changes progress over a few months to a few years. Some may continue into the postmenopausal period. Postmenopausal symptoms include genital tract atrophy (eg, urinary incontinence), osteoporosis, and cardiovascular diseases.

**TABLE 14.** General management of abnormal uterine bleeding

| Acute Uterine Bleeding | Chronic Uterine Bleeding |
|---|---|
| High-dose estrogen | GnRH agonists (Lupron) |
| Oral contraceptives | Danazol |
| D&C | |
| Endometrial ablation | |
| Total abdominal hysterectomy | |

## Differential

The differential diagnosis of menopause includes premature ovarian failure (menopause occurring prior to 42 years) due to alkylating chemotherapy, smoking, autoimmune diseases, and hysterectomy.

## Workup

Menopause is definitively diagnosed when serum FSH is higher than 40 mIU/mL × 2 or when LH/FSH is higher than 2.

Baseline laboratory tests for the workup of menopause include FSH, mammography, Pap smear, LFTs, cholesterol panel, CBC, urinalysis, and possibly a bone density study (if necessary).

## Treatment

All of the signs and symptoms of the climacteric period result from declining estrogen production by the ovarian follicles. Exogenous estrogen administration to perimenopausal and postmenopausal women will obviate most of these changes. Because unopposed estrogen can lead to endometrial hyperplasia and adenocarcinoma, it is routine practice to supplement it with progestin in women who still have an intact uterus. Daily administration of estrogen combined with progestin is the most popular regimen to alleviate peri- and postmenopausal changes without subjecting the patient to menstrual cycles. Patients should also be advised to take calcium supplements, stop smoking, and exercise to prevent/reduce osteoporotic changes. An annual pelvic exam, Pap smear, and mammogram should be performed.

Common side effects of hormone replacement therapy (HRT) include irregular bleeding, especially in the first 6 months. With continuous HRT, the patient may see weight gain, fluid retention, and endometrial hyperplasia (rare if the patient is also taking progesterone).

## GYNECOLOGIC ONCOLOGY

Table 15 summarizes the essentials of the three important gynecologic cancers.

Most common cancers in women:
1. Breast
2. Lung
3. Colorectal
4. Uterine

## TABLE 15. Common gynecologic cancers

| | Cervical Cancer | Endometrial Cancer | Ovarian Cancer |
|---|---|---|---|
| Symptoms | Postcoital bleeding<br>Foul discharge<br>May be asymptomatic | Postmenopausal uterine bleeding | Increased abdominal girth (ascites)<br>Palpable abdominal and pelvic masses<br>GI and GU complaints<br>Thrombophlebitis<br>Lower abdominal pain/pressure |
| Risk factors | Anything that increases the risk of or indication of HPV infection:<br>• Venereal warts<br>• Early sexual activity<br>• Multiple sexual partners<br>• Smoking<br>• Family history | Chronic, unopposed estrogen stimulation (eg, PCO)<br>Obesity<br>Nulliparity<br>Postmenopausal<br>Diabetes mellitus<br>Hypertension<br>Early menarche<br>Late menopause<br>Anovulation<br>Family history<br>Endometrial hyperplasia | Nulliparity<br>Breast cancer<br>Family history<br>(Oral contraceptives may have a protective role in decreasing the risk of ovarian cancer) |
| Screening tests | Pap smear (performed at least once a year for sexually active women) | None (Pap smear is only 50% effective in detecting uterine cancer) | None (routine ultrasound, CA-125 are not cost-efficient) |
| Diagnostic tests | Punch and/or cone biopsy | Endometrial biopsy<br>D&C | U/S, abdominal CT, CA-125 for epithelial cancers, AFP and β-HCG for germ cell cancers, surgical biopsy |
| Treatment | Early stage: radiotherapy, radical hysterectomy, and lymphaden-ectomy<br>Advanced stage: irradiation/chemotherapy only (surgery would harm bladder and rectum without being effective) | Total abdominal hysterectomy/bilateral salpingo-oophorectomy (TAH-BSO) and peritoneal washing for cytology ± pelvic and aortic node sampling<br>Radiotherapy<br>Chemotherapy<br>Progesterone | TAH-BSO and peritoneal washing for cytology with or without pelvic and aortic node sampling<br>Tumor debulking<br>Chemotherapy |
| Prevention | Safe sex (condoms) to decrease risk of HPV infection<br>Smoking cessation<br>Routine Pap smears | Progesterone to oppose estrogen<br>Low-fat diet<br>Weight control | Oral contraceptives<br>Oophorectomy in patients with a strong family history of ovarian cancer |
| Notes | 85% are squamous-cell carcinoma, 15% adenocarcinoma<br>Uremia is the most common cause of death in patients with end-stage cervical cancer | Most common gynecologic cancer<br>Fourth most common cancer in women (after breast, colorectal, lung)<br>Most are adenocarcinoma<br>Endometrial hyperplasia is the precursor lesion and is treated with progesterone | Most lethal gynecologic cancer<br>Complications of ovarian cancer include ovarian rupture, torsion, hemorrhage, infection, and infarction<br>Most common cause of death in end-stage ovarian cancer is bowel obstruction |

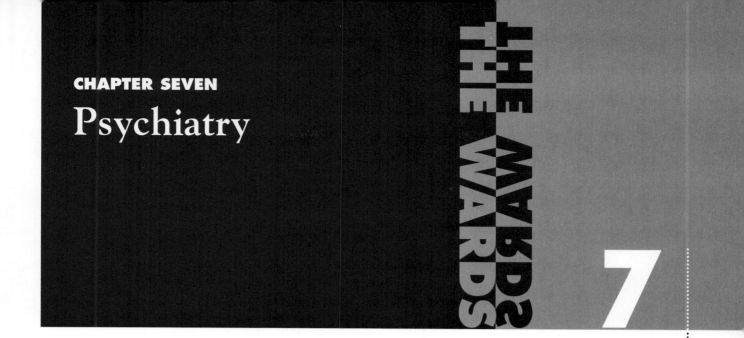

## CHAPTER SEVEN
# Psychiatry

# WARD TIPS

Welcome to psychiatry. Psychiatry is the study and management of behavioral disorders. Given recent advances in the neurobiological understanding of major psychiatric disorders as well as continuing additions to the psychiatrist's pharmacologic arsenal, many find psychiatry to be an increasingly exciting field in which to practice and conduct research. Even if you do not intend to enter psychiatry, the rotation will offer you valuable exposure to common psychiatric disorders (eg, depression, schizophrenia, bipolar disorder, anxiety disorders, dementia, and delirium) that you will see for the rest of your career regardless of your specialty.

## WHAT IS THE ROTATION LIKE?

In general, the psychiatry core rotation is one of the more relaxed and laid-back rotations that you will experience as a medical student. Thus, if you have the option of choosing the order in which to take your third-year medical-student core rotations, psychiatry would be a good rotation to take after surgery or OB/GYN to "catch your breath." On the other hand, expectations and the mechanics of this rotation are much different from those of the more conventional rotations. For example, medical students' exposure to the outpatient setting is often limited owing to the private nature of the activity. Consultation and liaison as well as emergency crisis services also play an important role for most psychiatric departments. Medical schools that are associated with a VA or children's hospital will allow students to focus on a unique psychiatric population, and students may rotate through any one or combination of these services.

Outpatient psychiatry encompasses a spectrum of activities, from one-time consultations to brief crisis intervention to long-term psychotherapy. Patients requiring psychiatric hospitalization are admitted to an inpatient psychiatric service. Patients on other hospital services, as well as those in the emergency room, may develop or have a psychiatric illness; these services may consult psychiatry for advice.

**Psychiatry is more relaxed but can be emotionally intense.**

## WHO ARE THE PLAYERS?

### Attending

As in every other specialty, the psychiatry attending bears ultimate responsibility for the patient. Unlike most other specialties, however, the attending will not necessarily see all inpatients each day but will usually lead rounds. Many outpatients may never be seen by an attending at all.

### Chief Resident

Each inpatient service usually has its own chief—a PGY-4 or PGY-5 who acts as a quasi-attending and who holds responsibility for the day-to-day organization of the ward as well as for decision making, supervising residents, and often leading rounds. Even more than is the case in other specialties, your residents, especially the chief, will make or break your psychiatry rotation. A good chief will be your principal guide, teacher, judge, and jury during the rotation, so try to sit down with him or her on your first day (or even set up a meeting beforehand, if you are really interested in psychiatry) to discuss your goals for the rotation, the structure and rules of the ward/team, and your role on the team.

### Resident

As a core member of the team, the resident may be the "primary clinician" (ie, may bear full responsibility for all aspects of patient care), or he or she may act as "med backup" to non-MD primary clinicians, doing physicals and mental status exams, prescribing medications, and dealing with concurrent medical issues. PGY-1's, also known as "interns" in other specialties, are often called residents in psychiatry.

### "Primary Clinician"

Some psychiatry services utilize psychologists, social workers, or nurse clinicians to take care of admission interviews, paperwork, phone calls, discharge dictations, etc, with residents acting as "med backup." Although they may be skilled professionals and are often highly knowledgeable about community services, disposition, and other issues critical to managing psychiatric patients, these clinicians tend to have more limited knowledge of the mental status exam, diagnostic categories, and pharmacologic treatments.

### Clinical Psychologist ("PhD" or "PsyD")

Psychologists perform assessments, conduct psychological testing, and perform psychotherapy (eg, IQ tests, Rorschachs). Some psychometric tests are dull, but try to see a Rorschach (or have one done on you if you have a willing psychologist); they are fascinating and uncannily accurate.

### Nurse

Nurses play a more central role on a psychiatric unit than is the case on other wards, as they often know patients best and can therefore report on comments and behaviors that have been missed by the MDs (psychiatric patients are often very skilled at hiding their pathology during an interview but usually can't do so all day). As a result, nurses often speak first in rounds. Nurses may also have known the patient for a decade or more over repeated hospitalizations and can thus give you a great deal of insight into a given patient's longitudinal course, usual baseline presentation, home and family situation, etc. It's critical to develop a good rapport with the nurses.

## Social Worker

Social workers are expert on issues such as disposition, housing, finances, and transportation. Be nice to them, since they are very effective in mobilizing your patients.

## Psychiatry Assistant

Psychiatry assistants help the entire team with daily care tasks.

## Recreational Therapist ("RT")

When patient stays were longer (ie, months or even years), patients tended to have a lot of free time, which would principally be filled by "therapeutic" games, crafts, cooking, and other activities organized by an RT. However, RTs have now been phased out in many hospitals, and patients often watch TV instead.

## HOW IS THE DAY SET UP?

The day usually begins with a multidisciplinary-team meeting in which all the patients on the service are discussed. The team usually includes the attending, resident, nurse, and social worker together with the student. The nurse usually reports overnight events. If the student was on call, the previous evening's admission is presented by the student. During the discussion, plans are formulated for each patient.

    After the meeting, the student can complete as much work as he or she can before attending lectures and conferences; this includes checking labs and obtaining medical records. The student then has a chance to see the patient in the afternoon—a meeting that can vary in time and intensity depending on the specific circumstances. At the end of the workday, the student writes a progress note documenting both the overnight and day's events.

| 7:30–8:00 AM | Prerounds (optional) |
|---|---|
| 8:00–10:00 AM | Morning rounds/new-patient presentation |
| 10:00 AM–12:00 NOON | Conferences/lectures/grand rounds |
| 12:00 NOON–1:00 PM | Lunch |
| 1:00–4:00 PM | Clinic/floor work/scut time |
| 4:00–5:00 PM | Afternoon rounds |
| OR | |
| 1:00–5:00 PM | Consultation and liaison service |
| OR | |
| 1:00–5:00 PM | Emergency crisis intervention |

This is just a sample schedule; times and activities may vary depending on the structure of the rotation. In general, however, the afternoon on the inpatient psychiatry wards is generally scut time consisting of activities such as arranging medical, OB/GYN, and neurologic consultations on psychiatric patients, looking up articles on MEDLINE, and rounding up labs and x-rays (if necessary) for afternoon rounds.

## WHAT DO I DO DURING PREROUNDS?

On many psychiatry services, you will not be expected to preround on your patients. Instead, overnight events are reported during morning rounds. If you are expected to preround, look for hours of sleep the night before, percentage of meals eaten the day before, and the type and amount of PRN meds given. This information is often in the nursing notes. Definitely consider prerounding on patients with active nonpsychiatric diagnoses.

## HOW DO I DO WELL IN THIS ROTATION?

Emphasizing the biopsychosocial model, modern psychiatry incorporates biological, experiential, and sociocultural factors into a single paradigm. Doing well in psychiatry requires the development of interviewing skills, the study of psychopathology, and the acquisition of knowledge on psychopharmacology. Generally, psychiatry emphasizes the doctor–patient relationship in the healing process. Thus, the development of empathic skills and an ability to listen is critical to doing well in this rotation. The use of open-ended questions to acquire information about a patient's psychopathology is also a must.

**Good listening and observational skills are a must.**

Listening is an acquired skill that necessitates discipline and practice. Like a cardiologist who gathers much more information when listening to heart sounds than can a first-year medical student, a psychiatrist can distill a tremendous amount of information from an interview. What a patient tells a doctor extends beyond the content of his or her words; how the patient communicates and how the interviewer feels in response to that patient are just as important in assessing pathology.

In addition to developing interviewing skills, it is important to acquire a solid fund of psychiatric knowledge. Furthermore, observational skills need to be honed to monitor abnormalities in a patient's appearance, behavior, and affect. Specifically, this rotation provides an opportunity to learn the disorders of feeling, thinking, and behavior that interfere with the way a person functions and relates to others. You must also learn how to present a psychiatric history.

Often, the medical student has the most recent experience in medicine wards of any member of the team. You can thus be a real asset in helping the team manage medical problems in psychiatric patients.

**Some specific tips.** Many students find themselves initially disoriented by the unique organization and expectations of the psychiatry clerkship. Here are some tips from students and residents who've been there.

- Keep an open and inquiring mind. Psychiatric training benefits doctors in all fields.
- Be organized. Keep a card on every patient that includes a short history, a thorough medication list, and a checklist of things to do. Also

make a card with the generic and trade names, common dosages, and side effects of the most commonly used psychiatric drugs, as well as a card with an outline of the mental status exam.

- When interviewing a patient, obtain a very thorough medication history, including dates of use, effectiveness, and side effects.
- Get friendly with the support staff, especially the nurses! Psychiatry is highly multidisciplinary. Nurses know the patients well and often have great insight that can be shared with medical students.
- Remember—safety first. If you feel threatened, leave the room immediately and get help. You may witness a "take-down" in which the staff physically pins down a violently labile patient; this may look frightening and unpleasant, but it is often the safest and kindest option.
- Take the initiative. When discussing your patient, think ahead and consider issues such as housing, finances, social supports, time of discharge, cultural issues, and community services.
- Try to pick up on how your patient makes you feel (eg, depressed, anxious). You'll find that your patient often has similar feelings.
- Forget the white lab coat or any kind of uniform. Some institutions even ban ties and necklaces, as patients can use them to strangle the caretaker.
- Don't joke with your patients.
- Don't touch your patients. Touch is a very powerful and volatile tool that should be used only after you have gained more experience.
- Don't share details of your life with your patients.
- Before you interview a patient, discuss the goals of diagnosis and treatment with your resident or attending. Is it to gather information or to treat? How deep do you want to go? Are there any sensitive topics from which you should steer clear?
- You will often experience a mix of feelings when dealing with psychiatric patients. Be willing to explore these feelings comfortably with your team. Having such feelings is not seen as a sign of weakness, but failing to deal with them will not be viewed favorably.

Never let a labile patient get between you and the door.

## WHAT IS DSM-IV?

DSM-IV, or the *Diagnostic and Statistical Manual, Fourth Edition*, is published by the American Psychiatric Association. The DSM is the standard diagnostic classification system used by all U.S. mental health workers (clinicians and researchers) as well as by insurance companies and the federal government. It is revised about once a decade to incorporate new research findings and consists of long lists of the criteria that are required to assign specific psychiatric diagnoses to patients. At first glance, the DSM may appear lengthy, complex, and confusing. However, you do not need to know the details of all the criteria. The more important criteria will be found here under the appropriate headings.

It is important to note that despite its precise and detailed diagnostic criteria, the DSM is not meant to be used by nonpsychiatrists in a "check the appropriate boxes" or "cookbook" fashion. To the contrary, the DSM merely offers guidelines for trained psychiatrists to apply using their experience and clinical judgment and is intended to ensure better diagnostic agreement among clinicians and researchers.

DSM-IV uses a "multiaxial classification," which is just a fancy way of saying that information is broken down into five categories (which should be used for presenting patients in rounds, writeups, etc):

1. **Axis I:** The psychiatric disorders.
2. **Axis II:** Personality disorders and mental retardation.
3. **Axis III:** Physical and medical problems.
4. **Axis IV:** Social and environmental problems/stressors.
5. **Axis V:** The GAF (Global Assessment of Functioning), which rates a patient's overall level of social, occupational, and psychological functioning (current and best in the past year) on a scale of 1 (completely nonfunctional) to 100 (extremely high level of functioning in a wide number of areas).

## KEY NOTES

The psychiatric admit note is similar to its medicine counterpart except for the emphasis it gives to past psychiatric history and the patient's personal history. Large portions of a psychiatric history often need to be obtained from other sources. At a minimum, you must talk to a family member and to the patient's regular doctor and review any old charts.

**Chief complaint/reason for admission.** Psychiatric patients often do not have a chief complaint, or they may voice a complaint that is incoherent, obscene, or irrelevant, so it is often necessary to briefly state how and why the patient ended up in the hospital or ER.

**History of present illness.** This includes symptoms, precipitants, time course, any medication changes/noncompliance, effects on function at home and work, and current treatment.

**Past psychiatric history.** This includes age of onset of symptoms, first psychiatric contact, first psychiatric hospitalization, number of hospitalizations, the date and duration of the most recent hospitalization, suicide attempts (when, how, seriousness), substance abuse (what, how much, how often, how long, any withdrawal, shared needles), medications (what, how much, how long, what helped, side effects, why did patient stop taking them), legal history, and any history of violence or physical/sexual abuse.

**Past medical history.** Ask about history of seizures, CNS infections, endocrine difficulties (eg, thyroid), head trauma, and allergies.

**Social history.** In psychiatry, heavy emphasis is placed on the social/personal history, as the patient's health, lifestyle, and social interactions may heavily influence his or her current psychiatric illness. It is therefore important to flesh out the details of the patient's birth, childhood, school performance, marriage, education, religious and cultural beliefs, occupational history, family and social relations, sexual history, hobbies and special interests, community supports, and current living arrangements.

**Family history.** Ask about any psychiatric illnesses that run in the family. Get details on diagnoses, severity, outcomes, and what medications helped. Attention should also be paid to family structure and significant interpersonal dynamics (eg, divorced, adopted).

## KEY PROCEDURES

The mental status exam (MSE) is the single most important procedure medical students must learn. Like the physical exam, this exam provides a way to objectively document mental function and behavior. Although used most often in psychiatry, some form of mental status exam should be a part of all medical exams. In the same manner, ruling out organic causes of mental illness is crucial to psychiatry. It is therefore helpful to create a template of the mental status exam that can be filled in during the interview.

## WHAT DO I CARRY IN MY POCKETS?

You will want to carry a psychiatry handbook (see "Top-Rated Books" below) as well as your drug guide. You will rarely need a stethoscope. Female medical students may find themselves pocketless owing to the absence of a white coat.

**Memorize the mental status exam.**

# TOP-RATED BOOKS

## HANDBOOK/POCKETBOOK

**A**

### Current Clinical Strategies: Psychiatry
Hahn
Current Clinical Strategies, 1997, 129 pages, ISBN 1881528197, $12.75

A bare-bones, quick-reference pocketbook that is incredibly useful on the wards. Outline format with useful tables of drugs and side effects. Good value.

**A**

### Pocket Handbook of Clinical Psychiatry
Kaplan
Williams & Wilkins, 1996, 406 pages, ISBN 0683045830, $37.00

Pocket reference with brief summaries of psychiatric disorders in outline format. A bit long, but easily read. Includes DSM-IV diagnostic criteria, useful tables, a uniquely complete chapter on the MSE, and psychiatric pharmacotherapy.

**B+**

### Manual of Psychiatric Therapeutics
Shader
Little, Brown, 1994, 378 pages, ISBN 0316782238, $32.95

A pocketbook written in essay format, making it difficult to quickly retrieve information. Provides concise reviews of basic definitions, the MSE, and drug treatments for major psychiatric disorders. Excellent use of tables.

**B+**

### Practical Guide to Care of the Psychiatric Patient
Goldberg
Mosby, 1995, 258 pages, ISBN 081513648X, $26.95

Concise spiral-bound handbook geared toward medical students and primary-care residents. Contains basic information in outline format. Not comprehensive.

**B**

### Quick Reference to the Diagnostic Criteria from DSM-IV
APA
American Psychiatric Press, 1994, 358 pages, ISBN 0890420637, $21.00

A pocketbook that is a good distillation of DSM-IV. Best used as a guideline for clinical diagnostic criteria rather than for literal definitions of psychiatric disorders. Lacks coverage of drug dosages or etiologies and thus has only moderate clinical usefulness.

**B-**

### Psychiatry (House Officer Series)
Tomb
Williams & Wilkins, 1995, 292 pages, ISBN 0683088930, $24.95

A pocketbook written in essay format, making it less useful as a quick reference on the wards. A fair basic review book, but too incomplete to serve as a primary source.

### Psychiatry: Diagnosis and Therapy
Flaherty
Appleton & Lange, 1993, 544 pages, ISBN 0838512674, $28.95

Outdated pocket reference based on DSM-III-R criteria. Easily read and complete with many useful tables and appendices. Perhaps too detailed and lengthy for quick reference on the wards.

### Handbook of Psychiatry
Guze
Mosby, 1990, 727 pages, ISBN 0815136447, $34.00

An outdated clinically oriented pocketbook based on DSM-III. Rather cumbersome for a handbook, thus limiting its usefulness.

## REVIEW/MINI-REFERENCE

### Concise Textbook of Clinical Psychiatry
Kaplan
Williams & Wilkins, 1996, 669 pages, ISBN 0683300091, $39.95

Excellent, downsized version of Kaplan's *Synopsis* that retains all the clinical psychiatry you need to know minus the behavioral science. Tightly organized with practical chapters on psychopharmacology and laboratory tests. Good for the bookshelf of the non-psychiatry-bound.

### Psychiatry (BRS)
Shaner
Williams & Wilkins, 1997, 378 pages, ISBN 0683076744, $23.95

Concise, outline-format review book geared toward the USMLE Step 2. Covers a comprehensive number of subjects, stresses key points of disorders, and is an easy read. Quick learning in focused areas. End-of-chapter questions and a 100-question multiple-choice practice exam.

### DSM-IV Casebook
Spitzer
American Psychiatric Press, 1994, 576 pages, ISBN 0880486759, $37.95

Companion text for DSM-IV consisting of short cases followed by discussion of differential diagnosis, epidemiology, and follow-up. An easily read but somewhat long didactic tool for those interested in psychiatry, but not useful on the wards.

### Psychiatric Secrets
Jacobson
Mosby, 1996, 553 pages, ISBN 156053107X, $35.95

Q & A format typical of the *Secrets* series. Concise coverage of a wide range of subjects, including both clinically relevant and esoteric information. Not useful as a reference text. Good preparatory material for pimping sessions on rounds or for the student interested in psychiatry trivia.

**B+** **Review of General Psychiatry**
Goldman
Appleton & Lange, 1995, 535 pages, ISBN 0838584217, $35.00

A fact-based reference for students interested in psychiatry. Not clinically oriented, thus limiting its usefulness on the wards, although it does have some clinical vignettes.

**B** **Clinical Psychiatry for Medical Students**
Stoudemire
Lippincott, 1994, 717 pages, ISBN 0397513380, $39.95

Detailed review text for clinical psychiatry. Updated for DSM-IV. Major disorders logically arranged, but may be too long to be read straight through and too loosely organized to be a quick reference. Compare with Kaplan's *Concise Textbook of Clinical Psychiatry.*

**B** **NMS Psychiatry**
Scully
Williams & Wilkins, 1996, 318 pages, ISBN 0683062638, $30.00

Overly detailed and dense outline-format review book that is neither clinically oriented nor a quick reference. Has clinically useful questions with lengthy answers after each chapter. Could better serve as a good review for an end-of-rotation exam or for the boards.

**C** **Oklahoma Notes Psychiatry**
Shaffer
Springer-Verlag, 1996, 188 pages, ISBN 0387946330, $17.95

Outline-format review book geared toward the USMLE Step 2. Overly basic and incomplete; not useful for the wards.

## TEXTBOOK/REFERENCE

**A** **Kaplan & Sadock's Synopsis of Psychiatry**
Kaplan
Williams & Wilkins, 1994, 1257 pages, ISBN 068304530X, $64.00

Comprehensive reference text for those serious about psychiatry. Incredibly complete, yet readable. Interesting historical perspectives on psychiatric disease and treatment. Considered by most to be the "gold standard." Solid investment.

**B** **DSM-IV**
APA
American Psychiatric Press, 1994, 886 pages, ISBN 0890420610, $59.95

Comprehensive reference for psychiatric diagnostic criteria. Limited clinical usefulness for medical students, as it lacks discussion of treatment or etiologies. Not worth purchasing unless you are considering psychiatry as a career.

# HIGH-YIELD TOPICS

## ROTATION OBJECTIVES

Unlike other specialties, psychiatry has a more limited group of diagnoses. You should know the clinical characteristics, workup, and management of the following major psychiatric disorders. Disease entities and related issues discussed in this chapter are listed in italics.

- *Mental status exam*
- *Major depression*
- *Bipolar disorder*
- *Schizophrenia*
- *Dementia*
- *Delirium*
- *Attention-deficit hyperactivity disorder*
- *Suicidality*
- *Personality disorders*
- *Substance abuse/dependence*
- *Eating disorders*
- Anxiety disorders (posttraumatic stress disorders, phobias)
- Pathologic grief
- Sleep disturbances
- Mental retardation
- Issues regarding the dying patient

**Skills goals are as follows:**

- Gathering data using nonverbal and affective observations.
- Presenting the psychiatric history.
- Integrating information coherently, developing a differential diagnosis, and making a biopsychosocial formulation.
- Applying principles of intervention and treatment.

**Knowledge goals include:**

- Indications, interactions, and side effects of the major psychoactive drugs.
- Clinical characteristics of organic diseases presenting as psychiatric disorders.
- Neurobiological principles applied to emotions and behavior.

## MENTAL STATUS EXAM

Table 1 offers a brief outline of the key components of a mental status exam. You may want to use it as a guide in creating a template. One should, however, refer to a text or manual for a complete treatment of this subject.

## MAJOR DEPRESSION

Major depression is an affective (mood) disorder with a prevalence of approximately 5%. The lifetime risk of acquiring major depression is about 20%. Although it is thought that people with chronic stress may be predisposed to this condition, major depression is also commonly seen in caregivers of patients with chronic illness. Socioeconomic status does not corre-

| TABLE 1. Mental status exam | |
|---|---|
| **Component** | **Comments** |
| Appearance and behavior | Eye contact, grooming, kinetics, level of cooperation, posture, gait, facial expressions, mannerisms. |
| Speech | Rate, rhythm, tone, enunciation, volume, clarity, abnormalities. |
| Emotions | Mood: The patient's subjective and objective emotional state—depressed, euphoric, anxious, happy, sad, etc. <br> Affect: The observed emotional range of the patient—expansive, labile, normal, constricted, flat, inappropriate. |
| Thought | Rate: Decreased in depression, increased in mania. <br> Process: Organization of a patient's thoughts—circumstantial, tangential, linear, flight of ideas, "word salad," thought blocking/insertion/withdrawal/control. <br> Content: Content of a patient's thoughts—suicidality, homicidality, delusions, major themes, preoccupations. |
| Perception | Hallucinations, illusions. |
| Language | Testing to be done before memory testing. <br> Native language, fluency, naming, comprehension, repetition. |
| Cognition | Level of consciousness: Alert, drowsy, stuporous. <br> Orientation: Person, place, date. <br> Concentration: <br> 1. Spell "world" forward and backwards. <br> 2. Beginning with the number 100, serially subtract 7. <br> 3. Recite the months of the year backwards. <br> Memory: <br> 1. Immediate (registration): Instant recall of 3 objects, digit span. <br> 2. Short term: Recall of 3 objects at 5 minutes. <br> 3. Long term: Ask about a patient's history, corroborated by other sources. <br> General fund of knowledge: <br> 1. Name the last 4 presidents or 5 major cities. <br> 2. Ask about a current event. <br> Abstract thinking: Metaphors, analogies, meaning of aphorisms. <br> Visual-spatial: Have the patient copy a drawing. |
| Judgment | Based on patient observation, can patient formulate judgments? |
| Insight | How aware is the patient of his or her illness and need for treatment? |
| Impulse control | Based on observation, does patient have impulse control? Is the patient dangerous? |

late with the incidence of major depression. Major depression has a female-to-male ratio of 2:1, with the age of onset most commonly in the 20s–40s. Depression is a dangerous condition: up to 15% of all patients with major depression commit suicide. Depressed patients are also at greater risk for a wide spectrum of medical illnesses.

Numerous theories exist regarding the etiology and pathophysiology of major depression. Perhaps the most well-known theory (although it is now falling into disfavor) is the biogenic amine theory, which holds that depression is due to low levels of amine neurotransmitters (eg, norepinephrine, serotonin) in the synaptic cleft. Since antidepressants increase the functional amount of amine neurotransmitters in the CNS, they increase the amount of biogenic amine that can bind to the receptor on the postsynaptic neuron. Sleep changes (eg, decreased REM latency, early-morning awakening) are sometimes present in major depression as well.

## Signs and Symptoms

According to DSM-IV, the signs and symptoms of major depression include:

- Depressed mood by self-report or by observation.
- Anhedonia (marked decrease in interest/pleasure in activities most of the day).
- Weight changes (not due to dieting) or appetite changes.
- Sleep changes (insomnia or hypersomnia).
- Psychomotor agitation or retardation.
- Fatigue or loss of energy.
- Feelings of worthlessness or guilt.
- Decreased ability to concentrate or think.
- Recurrent thoughts of death or suicide.

The signs and symptoms of major depression sometimes exhibit a diurnal variation (ie, symptoms are worse in the early morning) and can be masked by somatic complaints (eg, headache, pain, and constipation).

> **Symptoms of depression— SIG E CAPS**
>
> **S**leep
>
> **I**nterest
>
> **G**uilt
>
> **E**nergy
>
> **C**oncentration
>
> **A**ppetite
>
> **P**sychomotor retardation
>
> **S**uicidal ideations

## Differential

**Psychiatric.** Mood disorder due to a general medical condition, substance-induced mood disorder, cocaine withdrawal, bereavement, dementia, bipolar disorder (depressed episode) or bipolar disorder (mixed episode) and adjustment disorder with depressed mood.

**Organic.** Hypothyroidism, AIDS, multiple sclerosis, Parkinson's disease, Addison's disease, Cushing's disease, anemia (especially pernicious anemia), infectious mononucleosis, neuroborreliosis, influenza, malnutrition, and malignancies (eg, pancreatic cancer).

**Drugs.** Oral contraceptives, cimetidine, and some beta blockers.

## Workup

According to DSM-IV, the criteria for the diagnosis of a major depressive episode include the presence of 5 or more of the symptoms listed above for a

Always ask about suicidal ideation.

2-week duration with a clinically significant impairment in level of functioning, including the symptoms of either depressed mood or anhedonia. These symptoms may not be accounted for by bereavement or substance abuse.

### Treatment

The treatment of major depression includes antidepressant medications (eg, SSRIs, tricyclic antidepressants, MAO inhibitors), psychotherapy, and electroconvulsive therapy (useful for psychotic depression, actively suicidal patients, and patients who are refractory to or who cannot tolerate antidepressant medications).

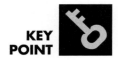

**KEY POINT**

---

## KEY ANTIDEPRESSANT MEDICATIONS

### Tricyclic antidepressants (TCAs)
Include amitriptyline (Elavil), imipramine (Tofranil), desipramine, clomipramine (Anafranil), and nortriptyline (Pamelor).

- **Side effects:** Anticholinergic (dry mouth, blurred vision, constipation, urinary retention, delirium, worsening glaucoma); cardiac arrhythmias (widened QRS, prolonged PR and QTc); orthostatic hypotension; seizures.
- **Pros:** Cheap, well studied, effective even in severe depression.
- **Cons:** Poor compliance due to side effects; lethal in overdose, have to titrate dose slowly.
- **Labs:** Check EKG before starting, after a few days, and at therapeutic dose; check blood levels if no response, excessive side effects, or suspected noncompliance.

### Selective serotonin reuptake inhibitors (SSRIs)
Include fluoxetine (Prozac), sertraline (Zoloft), paroxetine (Paxil), fluvoxamine (Luvox).

- **Side effects:** Agitation, anxiety, insomnia, sexual dysfunction, GI distress, anorexia, multiple drug interactions (always check in PDR).
- **Pros:** Relatively well tolerated, can usually start at therapeutic dose, safe in overdose.
- **Cons:** Expensive, less effective in severe depression, sexual dysfunction very common and often the cause of noncompliance.

### Monoamine oxidase inhibitors (MAOIs)
Include phenelzine (Nardil) and tranylcypromine (Parnate).

- **Side effects:** Hypertensive crises ("tyramine reaction" or "cheese reaction"; most foods are safe in moderation; main things to avoid are aged cheeses, cured/pickled foods, yeast extracts, and OTC sympathomimetic drugs); headache, dizziness, sleep abnormalities.
- **Pros:** Cheap, broad range of efficacy, best drugs for atypical depression.
- **Cons:** Dietary restrictions, should wear Medic Alert bracelet.

## Other medications

Include venlafaxine (Effexor), bupropion (Wellbutrin), trazodone (Desyrel), nefazodone (Serzone).

- **Comments:** Expensive, rarely first-line; venlafaxine associated with hypertension (follow BP), bupropion with seizures.

## Electroconvulsive therapy (ECT)

This is not like *One Flew Over the Cuckoo's Nest!* ECT is safe, simple, and one of the most effective treatments for depression. Usually need 6–12 treatments; can be done on an outpatient basis; can be life-saving for refractory or catatonic depression. Try to see it being performed.

- **Contraindications:** No absolute; relative contraindications include high anesthetic risk, intracranial mass lesions.
- **Side effects:** Postictal confusion, arrhythmias, retrograde amnesia, sore muscles.
- **Pre-ECT workup:** EKG, electrolytes, CBC, CXR; alert anesthesiology in advance.

## BIPOLAR DISORDER

Bipolar (manic-depressive) disorder is an affective (mood) disorder with a prevalence of about 1%. It is less common than major depression and affects males and females equally. Bipolar disorder has a strong genetic component, with a monozygotic-twin concordance rate of 40–90%. Commonly, the first manic episode occurs before age 30. Patients with bipolar disorder have an increased risk of committing suicide in comparison to both the general population and patients with major depression. Bipolar disorder is more commonly associated with substance abuse than are other psychiatric disorders.

Cyclothymia is a diagnosis that characterizes patients who have periods of hypomanic and depressive symptoms for at least two years and who do not meet the criteria for a major depressive episode. Cyclothymia differs from bipolar disorder in that the former is a more chronic disorder (at least 2 years in duration) with less severe depression and hypomania than is the case with bipolar disorder. Cyclothymia is not associated with hallucinations or delusions. In addition, the male-to-female ratio in bipolar disorder is 1:1, whereas that of cyclothymia is 1:2.

### Signs and Symptoms

According to DSM-IV, the signs and symptoms of a manic episode, which is characteristic of bipolar disorder, include the mnemonic "**DIG FAST.**"

The first presenting symptom in a bipolar patient is frequently depression. If an antidepressant medication is given to a depressed bipolar patient without the subsequent administration of lithium or some other type of mood stabilizer, a manic episode may result, a phenomenon known as "manic switch."

### Differential

**Psychiatric.** Schizophrenia, schizoaffective disorder, borderline personality disorder and ADHD.

> **Signs and symptoms of a manic episode— DIG FAST**
>
> **D**istractibility
>
> **I**nsomnia: Decreased need for sleep
>
> **G**randiosity: Inflated self-esteem
>
> **F**light of ideas
>
> Increase in goal-directed **A**ctivity/ psychomotor **A**gitation
>
> Pressured **S**peech
>
> **T**houghtlessness: Seeks pleasure without regard to consequences (eg, shopping sprees)

**Organic**. Medical conditions that can cause mania include brain tumors, CNS syphilis, encephalitis, metabolic derangements, hyperthyroidism, and multiple sclerosis.

**Drugs**. Cocaine, amphetamines, corticosteroids, anabolic steroids, phenyl-propanolamine, isoniazid, captopril, and antidepressants.

### Workup

According to DSM-IV, the criteria for the diagnosis of a manic episode include the presence of 3 or more of the signs and symptoms listed above lasting for a period of at least 1 week or less if hospitalization is necessary. These symptoms cannot be due to a preexisting medical condition or to a substance-related condition.

A hypomanic episode is like a manic episode except that the mood disturbance is not severe enough to cause marked impairment in social/occupational functioning or to necessitate hospitalization, and there are no psychotic features.

Six separate criteria sets exist for the diagnosis of bipolar I disorders with combinations of manic, hypomanic, and depressed episodes (see DSM-IV).

### Treatment

Treatment is divided into 3 parts: prophylaxis/maintenance, acute mania, and bipolar depression.

**Prophylaxis/maintenance.** The patient is normally given lifelong prophylaxis with a "mood stabilizer" after the second episode, or after the first episode if severe or life-threatening or if a strong family history exists.

- **Lithium**. Still the gold standard; aim for a level of 0.8–1.2 in acute mania and 0.6–1.0 for maintenance; start to see signs of toxicity at about 1.5 (coarse tremor, dysarthria, ataxia, nausea, diarrhea), seizures/coma around 2.5, death around 3–4.

  - **Side effects:** Fine tremor, nausea, acne, weight gain, benign leukocytosis, arrhythmias, hypothyroidism, nephrogenic diabetes insipidus, chronic renal failure.
  - **Pros:** Cheap, well studied in long-term use.
  - **Cons:** Regular lab work, narrow therapeutic index, long-term renal impairment common, have to titrate dose up due to side effects.
  - **Labs:** Before starting treatment: EKG, BUN/creatinine (maybe creatinine clearance), electrolytes, divalents, CBC, TFTs; first month— Li level weekly; every 3 months—Li level; every 6 months—chem 7; every year—TFTs, EKG (maybe creatinine clearance).

- **Valproic acid/divalproex** (Depakote). Probably as effective as lithium (better in mixed mania, substance abusers); alternative first-line agent or used with lithium; aim for a level of 75–125 in acute mania, 50–100 maintenance.

  - **Side effects:** GI distress, sedation, hepatotoxicity (extremely rare), thrombocytopenia.
  - **Pros:** Well tolerated, few blood draws once dose is established, high therapeutic index, can start at therapeutic dose.

- **Cons:** Extremely expensive, limited experience with long-term use in bipolar disorder.
- **Labs:** Before starting—LFTs, platelets; after a few days—level, LFTs; after a few weeks—level, LFTs, platelets; after a few months—LFTs, platelets (if all okay, no further labs needed).

- **Carbamazepine (Tegretol).** Probably less effective than others; not first-line agent. Main worries are aplastic anemia (very rare) and Stevens-Johnson syndrome (surprisingly common). Need CBC before starting, then monthly for 3–6 months, then every 3–6 months.

**Acute mania.** Treatment has three parts: control mood, resolve psychosis, and control manic/violent behavior until mood and psychosis are controlled. Mood is controlled with lithium or valproic acid (or ECT); psychosis is treated with antipsychotics (usually a fairly low dose); and behavior is managed with benzodiazepines—lots of benzodiazepines!

**Bipolar depression.** Bipolar depression is more difficult to treat than regular depression, as the depression is often more severe. In addition, there is a high risk of precipitating mania with antidepressants. Treatment includes lithium alone, lithium and a short course of an antidepressant, or ECT.

## SCHIZOPHRENIA

Schizophrenia has a lifetime prevalence of approximately 1%, with an incidence of 0.5 per 1000 persons per year. Like bipolar disorder, schizophrenia has a male-to-female ratio of 1:1. There is also an increased incidence of schizophrenia in lower socioeconomic groups, which has been explained by the theory that people with schizophrenia move into lower socioeconomic classes by virtue of their handicap (ie, poorly functional schizophrenic patients end up in unfavorable settings). This theory is known as the "downward drift of schizophrenia."

Although there are many theories that attempt to explain the pathophysiology of schizophrenia, the most well known is the dopamine hypothesis, which postulates that excessive dopamine activity in the CNS may be responsible for the pathogenesis of this disease. The dopamine hypothesis is supported by the fact that antipsychotic medications, which are dopamine receptor antagonists, help alleviate psychotic symptoms while dopamine agonists (such as cocaine and amphetamines) worsen them. Other hypotheses include the norepinephrine hypothesis (which states that schizophrenia may be due to excessive central norepinephrine activity in the limbic system), the GABA hypothesis (decreased central GABA activity in the limbic system), and the serotonin hypothesis (abnormal serotonin secretion in the CNS). Abnormalities seen in the brains of schizophrenic patients on CT/MRI scans and on autopsy include enlargement of the third ventricle and lateral ventricles, diffuse cortical atrophy, atrophy of the cerebellar vermis, a thickened corpus callosum, and a smaller left parahippocampal gyrus.

## Signs and Symptoms

According to DSM-IV, the signs and symptoms of schizophrenia during the active phase of the illness include:

- Delusions
- Hallucinations
- Disorganized, incoherent speech (eg, "word salad," clang associations)
- Disorganized/catatonic behavior
- Poor insight, concrete thinking
- Negative symptoms such as flat affect, thought blocking, low motivation, social withdrawal, and poor grooming

Acute schizophrenia usually presents with active psychosis, which may include hallucinations, delusions, loose associations, bizarre behavior, incongruent mood, and hyperverbal, incoherent speech. These are the "positive" symptoms of schizophrenia. Chronic schizophrenia is more frequently characterized by withdrawal, apathy, and blunting of affect (the "negative" symptoms).

## Differential

**Psychiatric.** It is important to differentiate schizophrenia from schizoaffective disorder, the major affective disorders such as bipolar disorder, and other psychotic disorders.

**Organic.** Early Huntington's chorea, early Wilson's disease, complex partial seizures (eg, temporal lobe epilepsy), frontal or temporal lobe tumors, early multiple sclerosis, early SLE, and acute intermittent porphyria.

**Drugs.** Substance abuse with amphetamine, cocaine, or PCP.

## Workup

According to DSM-IV, the criteria for the diagnosis of schizophrenia include the presence of 2 or more of the signs and symptoms listed above lasting for a period of at least 1 month, with continuous evidence of social and occupational dysfunction secondary to this psychiatric disturbance present for at least 6 months unless hospitalization is necessary. These symptoms cannot be due to a preexisting medical condition (eg, Wilson's disease) or to a substance-related condition (eg, amphetamine psychosis). Several subtypes of schizophrenia have been characterized (Table 2). Schizoaffective disorders, mood disorders, autism, and organic mental disorders must also be effectively ruled out.

**TABLE 2.** Types and characteristics of schizophrenia

| Schizophrenia Subtype | Characteristics |
|---|---|
| Disorganized | Disinhibited, disorganized, poor personal appearance, and inappropriate emotional responses<br>Worst prognosis |
| Catatonic | Stupor, bizarre posturing (waxy flexibility) |
| Paranoid | Delusions or hallucinations<br>Good self-care<br>Best prognosis |
| Undifferentiated | Has characteristics of more than one subtype |

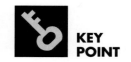 

## KEY ANTIPSYCHOTIC MEDICATIONS

Usually divided into "typical" and "atypical." Atypicals cause fewer extrapyramidal symptoms, don't increase prolactin levels, and may be more effective but are very expensive.

### Typical antipsychotics

Typical antipsychotics can be divided into high, medium, and low potency based mainly on doses needed; side effects are similar for all typical agents. Anticholinergic side effects occur more often with low-potency antipsychotics.

**High:** Haloperidol (Haldol), fluphenazine (Prolixin), thiothixene (Navane).

**Medium:** Trifluoperazine (Stelazine), perphenazine (Trilafon).

**Low:** Thioridazine (Mellaril), chlorpromazine (Thorazine).

Side effects:

1. Extrapyramidal symptoms (EPS) include the following:
   - **Acute dystonia:** Early, sudden onset of twisting of neck/rolling of eyes, mainly in young men; treat with intramuscular anticholinergics, eg, benztropine (Cogentin), trihexyphenidyl (Artane), or diphenhydramine (Benadryl).
   - **Akathisia:** Subjective sense of restlessness in legs; treat with beta blocker, eg, propranolol (Inderal) or benzodiazepine (Klonopin).
   - **Parkinsonism:** Tremor, rigidity, bradykinesia; treat with oral anticholinergics .
   - **Tardive dyskinesia:** Abnormal lip smacking, tongue protrusion, writhing movements of limbs; often irreversible. Occurs in 10–30% of long-term neuroleptic users, especially elderly, women, and patients with mood disorders; treat by withdrawing neuroleptic or change to clozapine.

2. **Neuroleptic malignant syndrome (NMS):** Fever, rigidity, autonomic instability, clouding of consciousness. Uncommon but life-threatening; treat by withdrawing neuroleptic, supportive measures, sometimes dantrolene/bromocriptine.

3. **Hyperprolactinemia:** Causes amenorrhea, gynecomastia. Must rule out pituitary tumor.

4. **Anticholinergic effects:** Dry mouth, urinary retention, constipation, orthostatic hypotension, etc.

5. Sedation.

6. Seizures.

7. EKG changes, arrhythmias.

### Atypical antipsychotics

The first atypical was clozapine (Clozaril); newer ones include risperidone (Risperdal), olanzapine (Zyprexa), sertindole, and quetiapine (Seroquel).

**Clozapine:** Highly effective for treatment-resistant schizophrenia; causes agranulocytosis in 0.5%, so requires weekly blood draws. Side effects include severe sedation, anticholinergic effects, drooling, weight gain, seizures, arrhythmias.

Other agents have fewer side effects (except more EPS) and don't cause agranulocytosis but are probably less effective in treatment-resistant patients (but at least as good as typical antipsychotics).

## Treatment

The treatment of schizophrenia consists primarily of antipsychotic (neuroleptic) medications as well as hospitalization and psychotherapy. Most neuroleptic medications work by blocking dopamine receptors. Psychosocial intervention includes supportive treatment to build a patient's ego and decrease his or her fears together with vocational rehabilitation and arranged social support in the community.

## DEMENTIA

Dementia, delirium, and depression — the 3 D's — can mimic each other.

Dementia is the development of multiple cognitive deficits—including memory impairment, aphasia, apraxia, agnosia, loss of abstract thought, behavioral/personality changes, and impaired judgment—that impair a person's level of social and/or occupational functioning. By definition, dementia has an organic etiology. Dementia has the highest prevalence in persons ages 85 and older. The most common etiologies of dementia include Alzheimer's disease (70–80%), vascular dementia (10%), head trauma, alcohol, Huntington's disease, and Parkinson's disease (each 1–5%). Only 10% of dementias are reversible.

Alzheimer's disease is the most common type of dementia in the elderly and is irreversible.

Theories of the etiology and pathophysiology of Alzheimer's disease include:

- Primary degeneration of cholinergic neurons in the nucleus basalis of Meynert, resulting in decreased levels primarily of acetylcholine but also of all other neurotransmitters.
- Accumulation of toxic amyloid precursors due to a mutation in the amyloid precursor protein gene on chromosome 21.
- Defect in the apolipoprotein E protein, which may serve a function in the prevention of β-amyloid deposition in the brain.

Pathologic findings in the brains of patients with Alzheimer's disease include:

- Involvement of the amygdala, hippocampus, frontal lobes, and basal forebrain.
- Senile plaques (degenerated nerve terminals with surrounding neurotoxic β-amyloid plaques).
- Neurofibrillary tangles (NFTs).
- Loss of cholinergic neurons in the nucleus basalis of Meynert.

Pathologic findings in patients with vascular dementia, the second most common type of dementia in the elderly, include multiple cerebral infarcts with diffuse cortical atrophy as seen on CT/MRI.

**4 A's of dementia**

**A**phasia

**A**praxia

**A**gnosia

Disturbances in **A**bstract thought

## Signs and Symptoms

According to DSM-IV, the signs and symptoms of both Alzheimer's and vascular dementia include:

- Memory impairment
- Aphasia

- Apraxia
- Agnosia
- Disturbances in abstract thought, planning, organizing, and sequencing

In a patient with Alzheimer's disease, one can expect to see a gradual and progressive worsening in cognitive abilities. The patient becomes less aware of his or her own surroundings and loses the ability to make rational decisions that are part of logical, everyday thinking. As a result, the patient may become frustrated and may deny that he has any loss of memory, accusing others of taking his money or his belongings. The patient also loses the ability to perform basic activities of daily living, such as eating, showering, and going to the bathroom.

Normal pressure hydrocephalus (NPH), which is a reversible form of dementia, is characterized by ataxia, urinary incontinence, progressive dementia, normal CSF pressure, and dilated cerebral ventricles.

## Differential

**Psychiatric.** Depression (pseudodementia), delirium, schizophrenia.

**Organic.** Normal aging can mimic dementia. Medical conditions that can cause dementia include hypothyroidism, malnutrition (vitamin $B_{12}$/folate deficiency), lead toxicity, Wilson's disease, Parkinson's disease, head trauma, brain tumors, Huntington's disease, HIV dementia, hypoxia, Creutzfeldt-Jakob disease, neurosyphilis, Down's syndrome, and multiple sclerosis.

**Drugs.** Alcohol.

Rule out reversible causes of dementia.

## Workup

According to DSM-IV, the criteria for the diagnosis of Alzheimer's and vascular dementia include the presence of memory impairment with 1 or more of symptoms 2–5 listed above, causing a clinically significant impairment in social and occupational functioning. Unlike Alzheimer's dementia, which is associated with a gradual decline in function, vascular dementia may be associated with a stepwise decline in cognitive function, becoming worse after each subsequent vascular insult. The signs and symptoms listed above cannot be due to a preexisting delirium, which must be ruled out, or to any other preexisting medical or substance-related condition.

The definitive diagnosis of Alzheimer's disease is made histopathologically at autopsy and is based on the findings of senile β-amyloid plaques and the presence of neurofibrillary tangles in the brain. A minimum workup to exclude reversible causes should include routine labs, TFTs, VDRL/RPR, $B_{12}$, folate, and a head CT or MRI scan.

## Treatment

Treat reversible causes. Rule out delirium (see Table 3). Tacrine (Cognex) is a relative acetylcholinesterase inhibitor that may help slow down the progression of Alzheimer's dementia but has shown little promise so far and is associated with hepatotoxicity. A newer acetylcholinesterase inhibitor,

| TABLE 3. Differentiating dementia, delirium, and depression | | | |
|---|---|---|---|
| | **Dementia** | **Delirium** | **Depression** |
| Hallmark feature | Memory loss | Fluctuating orientation | Depressed mood |
| Level of arousal | Normal | Stupor or agitation | Normal |
| Development | Slow and insidious | Rapid | Slow |
| Reversibility | Often irreversible | Frequently reversible | Fully reversible |
| Other comments | | Brain damage predisposes Most common in children and elderly Course fluctuates; duration brief | Neurovegetative signs |

donepezil (Aricept), is not hepatotoxic and may be more effective. Use supportive intervention (nutrition, physical activity, support for the family, etc). Provide environmental cues to help with orientation. Use low-dose, nonsedating antipsychotics with less anticholinergic activity (eg, haloperidol) for agitation, and avoid medications that can decrease cognition (eg, barbiturates, benzodiazepines).

Potentially treatable forms of dementia include:

- Multi-infarct dementia
- Normal pressure hydrocephalus
- Alcoholic dementia
- Hypothyroidism
- Brain trauma/tumors
- Infections
- Metabolic disorders of the heart, lung, liver, and kidney
- Vitamin $B_{12}$/folate deficiency
- CNS syphilis

> De**mem**tia = **Mem**ory impairment
>
> Deli**rium** = Change in senso**rium**

## DELIRIUM

Delirium is the acute development of disorientation, waxing and waning consciousness, decreased attention span and level of arousal, disorganized thinking, hallucinations, illusions, and disturbances in the sleep–wake cycle with associated cognitive dysfunction. By definition, delirium has an organic etiology. Like dementia, delirium most commonly occurs in the elderly population. Delirium is one of the most commonly seen complications on inpatient surgical and medical services.

### Signs and Symptoms

According to DSM-IV, the signs and symptoms of delirium include:

- Disturbance of consciousness with inability to maintain attention.
- Changes in cognition (eg, memory deficit).
- Disturbance that develops acutely (ie, hours to days) and tends to fluctuate.

## Differential

**Psychiatric.** The differential diagnosis of altered mental status includes delirium, dementia, schizophrenia, mania, psychotic depression, and acute functional psychosis.

**Organic.** Infections (eg, UTI, pneumonia, encephalitis, meningitis, AIDS, tertiary syphilis, disseminated tuberculosis), hypoxia, cerebrovascular accident, drug toxicity/side effects, illicit drug intoxication, heavy metal poisoning (lead, mercury, arsenic), endocrine abnormalities (eg, Cushing's disease, myxedema madness, hypothyroidism, Addison's disease, and hypo- or hyperparathyroidism), autoimmune diseases (eg, SLE), uremia, hepatic encephalopathy, Wilson's disease, and electrolyte abnormalities (eg, hyponatremia or hypercalcemia).

**Drugs.** Alcohol withdrawal, acyclovir, amphotericin B, antihistamines, anticholinergics (atropine), TCAs, phenytoin, corticosteroids, INH, rifampin, β blockers, digitalis, aminophylline, lithium, barbiturates, benzodiazepines, and many other drugs.

## Workup

According to DSM-IV, the criteria for the diagnosis of delirium due to a general medical condition include the presence of the symptoms listed above as well as clinical evidence that this disturbance is due to a general medical condition, causing a clinically significant impairment in social and occupational functioning. The signs and symptoms listed above cannot be due to a preexisting dementia, which must be ruled out.

Essential historical and medical information includes:

- Did the patient take any new medications?
- Did he or she overdose on any medications?
- Did the patient drink alcohol?
- Has this ever happened before?
- Does the patient have any medical problems?
- Has the patient had any symptoms of organ failure?
- How long have these episodes been going on?
- Any signs of UTI—dysuria, frequency, pruritis?

The medical workup for delirium includes:

- H&P
- Neurologic exam
- Vital signs
- Check of old labs and medical records
- Review of patient's current meds

**Labs.** The rationale for doing each lab test is to rule out specific diseases that are part of the differential diagnosis. Not all of these labs are indicated during the initial workup. Essential labs include:

- Electrolytes plus glucose plus Ca, BUN (rule out electrolyte abnormalities).
- CBC with differential (to rule out infection).
- ABG (rules out hypoxia).

> **Major causes of delirium— HIDE**
>
> **H**ypoxia
>
> **I**nfection (esp. UTI)
>
> **D**rugs (esp. anticholinergics)
>
> **E**lectrolyte disturbances

- EKG (rules out MI).
- CXR (rules out TB, CHF, etc).
- UA (rules out UTI).

Order additional studies based on clinical suspicion:

- Urine toxicology (rules out drug overdose, but misses many drugs).
- Liver profile (AST, ALT, alkaline phosphatase): Rules out liver damage causing hepatic encephalopathy.
- Total and direct bilirubin: Rules out hepatic encephalopathy due to liver failure/damage.
- Thyroid profile (TSH/TFTs): Rules out hypo- or hyperthyroidism.
- EEG (rules out seizure disorder).
- VDRL/RPR (rule out neurosyphilis).
- Lumbar puncture (rules out meningitis).
- Serum $B_{12}$ and folate (rules out vitamin deficiencies and malnutrition).

CT and MRI studies are performed if head trauma (fracture or hemorrhage) or CNS pathology (eg, brain tumor) is suspected and after lab work is done and has been noncontributory to a medical diagnosis. EEG shows diffuse slowing that is proportional to the severity of the delirium.

### Treatment

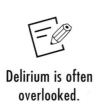

**Delirium is often overlooked.**

It is very important to treat the underlying disorder. Normalize fluid and electrolyte status. Provide an appropriate sensory environment. Nonsedating antipsychotics (eg, haloperidol) may be used for agitation but not in alcohol withdrawal. Benzodiazepines can also be used for agitation and insomnia. Because delirium has so many causes, the most important thing is to recognize that a patient is delirious. Look for a waxing and waning level of consciousness that develops rapidly.

### ATTENTION-DEFICIT HYPERACTIVITY DISORDER

Attention-deficit hyperactivity disorder (ADHD) is a disorder that affects approximately 3% of all children and occurs more commonly in boys than in girls. A genetic predisposition exists for this condition; thus, it is important to obtain a good family history when considering this diagnosis. ADHD most commonly occurs in boys aged 3–13 years and is typically manifested by poor performance in school. About one-third of patients will continue to have symptoms and require treatment as adults.

### Signs and Symptoms

According to DSM-IV, the signs and symptoms of ADHD include:

**Inattention:**

- Manifests inability to pay close attention to detail, making careless mistakes.
- Has difficulty maintaining attention in schoolwork or play.
- Does not listen when spoken to directly.
- Has inability to follow through with instructions or tasks or fails to complete schoolwork.

- Has difficulty organizing tasks/activities.
- Avoids or dislikes tasks requiring concentration or sustained mental effort.
- Loses items necessary for completion of school tasks (eg, pencils, paper, books).
- Is easily distracted by external stimuli.
- Is forgetful in daily activities.

**Hyperactivity/impulsivity:**

- Fidgety (eg, squirms in seat).
- Unexpectedly leaves desk in classroom.
- Runs about excessively in inappropriate situations.
- Has difficulty playing quietly.
- Is often "on the go" or often acts as if "driven by a motor."
- Talks excessively.
- Blurts out answers before questions have been completed.
- Has difficulty awaiting his turn.
- Often interrupts or intrudes on others.

## Differential

The differential diagnosis of ADHD includes certain medications (eg, sedatives such as sleeping pills may exhibit a paradoxic stimulant effect in children), head trauma, learning disability, major depression, bipolar disorder, cyclothymic disorder, anxiety disorders, intermittent explosive disorder, and, of course, a normal active child.

## Workup

According to DSM-IV, the criteria for the diagnosis of ADHD include having 6 or more of the above symptoms of inattention and/or 6 or more of the above symptoms of hyperactivity/impulsivity that were present before 7 years of age and that cause clinically significant impairment in social and academic functioning. The signs and symptoms must have been present for at least 6 months and cannot be accounted for by another axis I disorder.

## Treatment

The treatment of ADHD includes psychostimulants like methylphenidate (Ritalin), dextroamphetamine (Dexedrine), and pemoline (Cylert), some antidepressants (eg, nortriptyline, imipramine, bupropion), and $\alpha_2$-agonists (clonidine, guanfacine) along with behavior modification. Initial treatment should be conservative and nonpharmacologic, with stimulant medication initiated when conservative therapy fails. Adverse effects of stimulant medication include stunted growth, tics, insomnia, irritability, and decreased appetite. Methylphenidate is a schedule 2 controlled substance with a significant potential for abuse, particularly by teenagers. Avoid desipramine, as it has been associated with arrhythmias. $\alpha_2$-agonists can cause hypotension. Restricting a child's caffeine intake may also help control hyperactive symptoms. Note that sugar and food additives are not etiologic factors in ADHD despite the attention they have received in the popular press.

## SUICIDALITY

Suicide is the eighth leading cause of death in the U.S. and is the second leading cause of death in people aged 15–24, behind accidents. The incidence of suicide in the U.S. is increasing. In general, woman are more likely to *attempt* suicide than men, but men are more likely to *commit* suicide. Men are also more likely to commit suicide by violent means (eg, firearms). Women are more likely to commit suicide by drug ingestion. Suicide rates increase with age; elderly people account for approximately one-quarter of all suicide cases.

### Signs and Symptoms

There are no signs or symptoms of suicide except for the act itself. However, risk factors for suicide that you should be aware of include:

- Depression (approximately half of all suicidal patients are depressed; depressed patients are 30 times more likely to commit suicide).
- Other major psychiatric disorders (eg, schizophrenia). A greater percentage of schizophrenic patients commit suicide than depressed patients.
- Past history of suicide attempts.
- Alcoholism and substance abuse.
- Elderly individuals.
- A recent severe stressor (eg, bereavement, job loss, examinations).
- Single, divorced, or widowed individuals (marriage is associated with a decreased risk of suicide) or anyone without good social support.
- Divorced parents.
- Positive family history of suicide.
- Caucasians, especially Caucasian males (whites commit suicide more frequently than do blacks).
- Patients recovering from a suicidal depression (since they have regained the energy to kill themselves) or a first schizophrenic episode (since they have developed insight).
- Policemen and doctors (and medical students) have an increased suicide risk in comparison to the general population.
- Individuals with a chronic medical condition (eg, terminal cancer, AIDS).

### Workup

The identification of patients at high risk for suicide is key (see risk factors listed above in "Signs and Symptoms"). Pertinent information includes:

- Patient has expressed to someone a desire to kill himself (ie, has given others warning).
- Patient has made out a plan to kill himself.
- Patient has a positive family history for suicide.
- Patient has tried to commit suicide before.
- Patient is ambivalent about death.

To obtain the above information, do the following:

- Ask the patient directly for suicidal ideation, intent, and plan.
- Look for available means of committing suicide.
- Assess suicide risk in every mental status examination.

**Asking the patient about suicide will not plant the idea in the patient's head.**

## Treatment

Treat the underlying disorder. This frequently requires intensive psychotherapy and inpatient hospitalization as well as antidepressant and antipsychotic medications. Electroconvulsive therapy may be used as a second-line agent in the treatment of an actively suicidal patient who is refractory to medications and psychotherapy. The actively suicidal patient needs intensive monitoring, close contact, and ongoing assessment for hospitalization. Two- or four-point soft leather restraints may also be necessary in the acute phase to protect the patient from himself. Often, severely depressed patients with suicidal ideations are at greatest risk for suicide in the first 1–2 weeks after antidepressant medication has started, since they have regained the energy to kill themselves. Actively suicidal patients who have formulated a plan may need to be emergently hospitalized, sometimes against their will.

Actively suicidal patients should be kept hospitalized under close observation.

## PERSONALITY DISORDERS

A personality trait is an enduring pattern of perceiving, relating to, and thinking about the environment and oneself that is exhibited in a wide range of important social and personal contexts. A personality disorder exists when these personality traits become inflexible and maladaptive enough to cause significant impairment in social or occupational functioning or to cause subjective distress. Personality disorders are axis II psychiatric disorders that can be seen in all medical contexts. Personality disorders are, in addition, pervasive, persistent, maladaptive patterns of behavior that are deeply ingrained and are not attributable to axis I disorders.

Personality disorders typically begin in childhood, crystallizing by late adolescence and affecting all facets of the personality (eg, cognition, mood, behavior, and interpersonal style). Behaviors secondary to personality disorders are constant, not situational. The coping strategies outlined under the different clusters are meant to aid any clinician with these difficult patients. Personality disorders (axis II disorders) often coexist with and have an impact on the treatment of acute psychiatric illnesses (axis I disorders).

### Signs and Symptoms

Table 4 outlines the signs and symptoms of personality disorders.

### Differential

The differential diagnosis of personality disorders includes normal variants of an individual's personality, axis I psychiatric disorders (eg, schizophrenia, major depression, bipolar disorder, anxiety disorders), environmental stressors, and substance abuse.

### Diagnosis

The diagnosis of personality disorders is made through the identification of persistent signs and symptoms as listed above as well as through the presence of significant impairment in social or occupational functioning or subjective distress. The diagnosis cannot be made in a person under 18 years of age. In addition, it is difficult to make in the face of an active axis I disorder.

| TABLE 4. Signs and symptoms of personality disorders | | | | |
|---|---|---|---|---|
| Cluster | Examples | Characteristics | Clinical Dilemma | Coping Strategy |
| Cluster A | Paranoid Schizoid Schizotypal | Eccentric, strange, fearful of social relationships, paranoid, suspicious, social isolation, odd beliefs, shy, withdrawn, impoverished personal relationships | Patient is suspicious of doctor and does not trust doctor. | Use clear, honest attitude, noncontrolling, nondefensive, no humor; keep distance. |
| Cluster B | Borderline Histrionic Narcissistic Antisocial | Emotional, dramatic, erratic, self-indulgent, hostile, aggressive, exploitive relationships, attention seeking | Patient will change rules on doctor. Clingy and demands attention. Feels that he or she is special. Will manipulate doctor and staff ("splitting"). | Firm: Stick to treatment plan and don't waffle. Fair: Don't be punitive or derogatory. Consistent: Don't change the rules on them. |
| Cluster C | Obsessive-compulsive Avoidant Dependent Passive-aggressive | Fearful, anxious, adheres to rules and regulations, anxiety, repressed, unable to express affect | Patient may subtly sabotage his or her own treatment. Very controlling. | Avoid power struggles. Passive wins over active. Give clear treatment recommendations, but do not push the patient into a decision. |

## Treatment

Psychotherapy is usually the treatment of choice for personality disorders. Behavioral therapy and pharmacotherapy have also been successful in specific contexts. Addressing the underlying personality disorder will assist in treating the major psychiatric (axis I) disorders.

## SUBSTANCE ABUSE/DEPENDENCE

Substance abuse has a 13% lifetime prevalence in the U.S., with alcohol being the most common substance abused (not counting tobacco and caffeine). Alcohol abuse/dependence has a lifetime prevalence of 6% in the general U.S. population with a male-to-female ratio of 3.5:1, but the incidence of alcoholism in women is increasing. In the U.S., approximately 10% of the drinking population consumes 50% of all alcohol, while approximately 70% of all Americans use alcohol. The highest prevalence of alcoholism occurs in males between the ages of 21 and 34 years. Substance abusers are at increased risk for accidental and traumatic injuries, especially motor vehicle accidents. Intravenous drug abusers are at increased risk for acquiring HIV, hepatitis B, endocarditis, cellulitis (especially among "skin poppers"), and STDs. Substance abusers are often exceptionally destructive, both to themselves and to their families. Some—particularly opioid and crack addicts—will do almost anything to get money for drugs, including dealing, stealing, and prostituting themselves (and even their children). Always ask about the care of their children (you may need to contact child protection agencies) and where they get their drug money (this may give you clues to other potential medical and legal problems).

Substance abuse will teach you about the real (or unreal) world.

Ask them where they get their money and who is caring for their children.

## Signs and Symptoms/Workup

According to DSM-IV, substance dependence is characterized by the presence of 3 or more of the following signs and symptoms that last for at least 1 year:

- Tolerance.
- Withdrawal.
- Substance taken in larger amounts than intended.
- Persistent desire or attempts to cut down.
- Considerable time and energy spent trying to obtain substance.
- Important social, occupational, or recreational activities given up or reduced because of substance use.
- Continued use despite awareness of the problems that it causes.

According to DSM-IV, substance abuse is a maladaptive pattern of substance use leading to clinically significant impairment or distress; symptoms have not met the criteria for substance dependence. DSM-IV criteria for substance abuse are met when 1 or more of the following symptoms are present for at least 1 year:

- Recurrent use resulting in failure to fulfill major obligations at work, school, or home.
- Recurrent use in physically hazardous situations.
- Recurrent substance-related legal problems.
- Continued use despite persistent problems caused by use.

Alcohol withdrawal syndromes consist of the following:

- **Uncomplicated withdrawal:** Occurs within the first 12–18 hours after cessation of drinking and is characterized by tremulousness, hypervigilance, hyperreflexia, weakness, tinnitus, blurred vision, paresthesias, and numbness.
- **Alcohol hallucinosis:** Occurs in the first 3–6 days after cessation of drinking and is characterized by striking auditory hallucinations, some withdrawal symptoms, and clear sensorium (no delirium).
- **Delirium tremens (DTs):** Occur approximately 2–8 days after cessation of drinking; can be life-threatening (untreated mortality of 15–20%). DTs are characterized by disorientation, fever, agitation/tremor, delusions, seizures, memory deficits, visual and tactile hallucinations, and autonomic instability.

Table 5 outlines drug-specific signs and symptoms of substance abuse.

## Differential

The differential diagnosis of substance abuse includes axis I psychiatric disorders (eg, schizophrenia, major depression, bipolar depression, anxiety disorders) and delirium.

## Workup

The diagnosis of alcohol intoxication can be confirmed with a Breathalyzer test and serum alcohol level. Get CBC, electrolytes, and LFTs. An elevated gamma-glutamyl transpeptidase and MCV suggest chronic alcohol abuse. If other substances are suspected, check a urine tox screen. Always offer HIV

> **Screening questions for alcoholism— CAGE**
>
> 1. Have you have felt the need to **C**ut down on your drinking?
> 2. Have you ever felt **A**nnoyed by criticism of your drinking?
> 3. Have you ever felt **G**uilty about drinking?
> 4. Have you ever had to take a morning **E**ye opener?
>
> More than one "yes" answer makes alcoholism likely.

Substance abuse is a huge risk factor for HIV. Try to get them tested.

| TABLE 5. Signs and symptoms of substance abuse | | |
|---|---|---|
| Drug | Intoxication | Withdrawal |
| Alcohol | Disinhibition, emotional lability, incoordination, slurred speech, ataxia, coma, blackouts (retrograde amnesia) | Tremor, tachycardia, hypertension, malaise, nausea, seizures, delirium tremens (DTs), tremulousness, agitation, hallucinations |
| Opioids | CNS depression, nausea and vomiting, constipation, pupillary constriction, seizures, respiratory depression (overdose is life-threatening) | Anxiety, insomnia, anorexia, sweating, fever, rhinorrhea, piloerection, nausea, stomach cramps, diarrhea |
| Amphetamines | Psychomotor agitation, impaired judgment, pupillary dilation, hypertension, tachycardia, euphoria, prolonged wakefulness and attention, cardiac arrhythmias, delusions, hallucinations, fever | Post-use "crash," including anxiety, lethargy, headache, stomach cramps, hunger, severe depression, dysphoric mood, fatigue, insomnia/hypersomnia |
| Cocaine | Euphoria, psychomotor agitation, impaired judgment, tachycardia, pupillary dilation, hypertension, hallucinations (including tactile), paranoid ideations, and angina and sudden cardiac death | Hypersomnolence, fatigue, depression, malaise, severe craving, suicidality |
| PCP | Belligerence, impulsiveness, fever, psychomotor agitation, vertical and horizontal nystagmus, tachycardia, ataxia, homicidality, psychosis, delirium | Recurrence of symptoms due to reabsorption in GI tract; sudden onset of severe, random, homicidal violence |
| LSD | Marked anxiety or depression, delusions, visual hallucinations, flashbacks | |
| Marijuana | Euphoria, anxiety, paranoid delusion, slowed time, impaired judgment, social withdrawal, increased appetite, dry mouth, persecutory delusions, hallucinations, amotivational syndrome | |
| Barbiturates | Low safety margin, respiratory depression | Anxiety, seizures, delirium, life-threatening cardiovascular collapse |
| Benzodiazepines | Alcohol interactions, amnesia, ataxia, sleep, minor respiratory depression | Rebound anxiety, seizures, tremor, insomnia |
| Caffeine | Restlessness, insomnia, diuresis, muscle twitching, cardiac arrhythmia | Headache, lethargy, depression, weight gain |
| Nicotine | Restlessness, insomnia, anxiety, arrhythmias | Irritability, headache, anxiety, weight gain, craving, tachycardia |

testing to substance abusers, even those who don't use needles. They often engage in high-risk behaviors for money or while intoxicated.

### Treatment

Treatment depends on the substance abused and the context in which it was used (see Table 6). The first goal is usually abstinence; then treatment tar-

| TABLE 6. Management of substance intoxication | | |
|---|---|---|
| Drug | Symptoms of Acute Intoxication | Management |
| Hallucinogens (eg, LSD) | Maladaptive behavior changes, changes in perception, pupillary dilation, tachycardia, palpitations, sweating, anxiety | If severe, diazepam (Valium) PO; otherwise provide reassurance. |
| Cocaine/crack | Diaphoresis, chills, tachycardia, pupillary dilation, nausea and vomiting, hypertension, tremor, visual and tactile hallucinations ("cocaine bugs") | Severe agitation is treated with haloperidol and lorazepam. |
| PCP | Belligerent, assaultive behavior; agitated, impulsive patient with hypertension and unpredictability | If severe, diazepam (Valium) PO; otherwise provide reassurance. |
| Amphetamines | Same symptoms as cocaine, with fever, arrhythmias, and convulsions. | Same as with cocaine/crack. |

gets the patient's physical, psychological, and social well-being. In other words, detoxification followed by rehabilitation is the model used to treat substance abuse. Treatment modalities vary widely because of the great variety in addictive substances.

Treatment of alcohol withdrawal includes:

1. Rule out any medical complications (eg, hepatic dysfunction, Wernicke's encephalopathy) by physical exam, laboratory tests, etc.
2. Give chlordiazepoxide (Librium) 50–100 mg PO every 4 hours. Give lorazepam (Ativan) or oxazepam (Serax) if patient has liver dysfunction.
3. Give thiamine (before glucose), folate, and multivitamins as well as electrolytes (if low).
4. Check vital signs and give fluid replacement if necessary.
5. If history of seizures, add carbamazepine and avoid neuroleptics, since they decrease seizure threshold.

## EATING DISORDERS

Eating disorders, which include anorexia nervosa, bulimia nervosa, and disorders not otherwise specified, are generally characterized by disturbed eating behaviors with an intense fear of gaining weight.

Approximately 5–10% of the population suffers from eating disorders, with 90% of all cases occurring in females. Nearly 1% of all females in late adolescence and early adulthood are diagnosed with anorexia nervosa, while 3–5% of females in the same age group are diagnosed with bulimia nervosa. The long-term mortality rate for anorexia nervosa is greater than 10%; the bulimia mortality rate is unknown. The etiology of eating disorders is thought to be partially neurochemical and partially environmental.

Anorexia nervosa is characterized by the refusal to maintain a body weight greater than or equal to 85% of the ideal body weight. Two subgroups of anorexia nervosa have been defined: restricting type and binge-eating/purging type. Restricting types will maintain their low weight by fasting, dieting, or exercise, while binge-eating/purging types may or may not binge eat but will purge whatever food they have consumed. Anorexics are afraid of gaining weight even when they are excessively thin. This fear does not resolve with weight loss; in fact, it may get worse. Their body image is distorted in that their self-esteem is intimately related to their weight and body image. Their weight loss and ability to stay thin are, to them, representative of self-control, while body fat and weight gain are signs of failure. Their denial of the medical consequences of their low body weight is often overwhelming. These patients often abuse diet pills such as Dexatrim. Females who suffer from anorexia nervosa are amenorrheic owing to the low levels of estrogen, LH, and FSH circulating in their bodies.

Bulimia nervosa is characterized by binge eating, which is defined as eating more food than what most people would eat in a certain period of time, with the feeling of being out of control during the eating period. Bulimics then engage in behaviors to prevent weight gain, which can include vomiting, laxative abuse, diuretics, enemas, fasting, or excessive exercise. This binge–purge activity must occur twice a week for at least 3 months to be diagnosed as bulimia nervosa. Patients also have a distorted body image, as in anorexia nervosa; however, they are usually not as thin as anorexics, tending to be close to their ideal body weight or even slightly overweight. Bulimia nervosa is also divided into two subgroups: purging and nonpurging. In the purging type, patients will engage in vomiting, laxatives, enemas, or diuretics to control their weight. In the nonpurging type, patients will engage in excessive fasting or exercise to control their weight. Unlike anorexics, bulimics are usually ashamed of their eating behaviors and generally keep them a secret.

## Signs and Symptoms

Anorexia is characterized by amenorrhea, lanugo, cold intolerance, lethargy, excess energy, emaciation, hypotension, hypothermia, dryness of skin, bradycardia, and hypercarotenemia. Bulimia is characterized by dental enamel erosion (from vomiting), enlarged parotid glands, scars on the dorsal surfaces of the hands, menstrual irregularities, and laxative dependence in chronic users. Both groups often have electrolyte abnormalities, including hypokalemia.

## Differential

The differential includes gastrointestinal disease, occult malignancy, hypothalamic tumor, AIDS, thyroid disorders, diabetes, superior mesenteric artery syndrome, depression, affective disorders, schizophrenia, and substance abuse. These disorders may have physical symptoms similar to those of eating disorders; however, the associated fear of weight gain is what differentiates the eating disorders.

## Workup

DSM-IV defines anorexia nervosa and bulimia nervosa according to the following criteria:

**Anorexia nervosa:**

- Refusal to maintain body weight at or above 85% of the ideal body weight.
- Intense fear of becoming fat.
- Disturbance in body image, with a heightened influence of body weight on self-esteem.
- Amenorrhea or the absence of 3 consecutive menstrual periods.

**Bulimia nervosa:**

- Recurrent episodes of binge eating.
- Recurrent inappropriate compensatory behaviors to prevent weight gain (vomiting, laxatives, diuretics, enemas, fasting, exercise).
- Both of the above occurring at least twice weekly for 3 months.
- Self-evaluation is overly dependent on body weight.
- Does not occur exclusively during episodes of anorexia nervosa.

Don't forget baseline CBC, electrolytes, TFTs, amylase (for parotitis), and EKG.

## Treatment

Patients are usually brought in by family members and loved ones, rarely coming in on their own. Often, they are still in denial with regard to their disorder. Early treatment is centered on weight gain for the emaciated patient. Both individual and family psychotherapy is used to help motivate the patient to gain weight; group therapy is also a popular mode of treatment. Psychopharmacology is of no benefit in anorexia. SSRIs do reduce binging/purging behaviors in some bulimic patients.

# Notes

# Abbreviations

| Abbreviation | Meaning |
|---|---|
| A&O × 3 | alert and oriented to person, place, and date |
| A&O × 4 | alert and oriented to person, place, time, and date |
| AAA | abdominal aortic aneurysm |
| Ab | antibody |
| ABCs | airway, breathing, circulation |
| ABD | abdomen |
| ABG | arterial blood gases |
| ABX | antibiotics |
| ACE | angiotensin-converting enzyme |
| ACLS | advanced cardiac life support |
| ADA | American Diabetic Association |
| ADH | antidiuretic hormone |
| ADHD | attention-deficit hyperactivity disorder |
| AFB | acid-fast bacillus |
| AIDS | acquired immunodeficiency syndrome |
| Alk phos | alkaline phosphatase |
| ALT | alanine transaminase |
| AMS | altered mental status |
| ANA | antinuclear antibody |
| A/P | assessment and plan |
| ARDS | acute respiratory distress syndrome |
| AST | aspartate transaminase |
| AT | atraumatic |
| ATS | American Thoracic Society |
| AV | atrioventricular |
| AVM | arteriovenous malformation |
| AZT | azidothymidine |
| β-HCG | β-human chorionic gonadotropin |
| BP | blood pressure |
| bpm | beats per minute |
| BR | bathroom |
| BRBPR | bright red blood per rectum |
| BS | breath sounds, bowel sounds |
| BUN | blood urea nitrogen |
| c̄ | with |
| C&S | culture and sensitivity |
| Ca | calcium |
| CA | cancer |
| CABG | coronary artery bypass grafting |
| CAD | coronary artery disease |
| cal | calorie |
| CBC | complete blood count |
| CBD | common bile duct |
| cc | cubic centimeter |
| CC | chief complaint |
| C/C/E | clubbing, cyanosis, edema |
| C/D/I | clean, dry, intact |
| CEA | carcinoembryonic antigen |
| CFTR | cystic fibrosis transmembrane regulation |
| chem 7 | lab tests for sodium, potassium, chloride, carbon dioxide, bicarbonate, blood urea nitrogen, and glucose |
| CHF | congestive heart failure |
| CK | creatine phosphokinase |
| CK-MB | creatine phosphokinase, MB isoenzyme |
| CL | contralateral |
| CMT | cervical motion tenderness |

| Abbreviation | Meaning |
|---|---|
| CMV | cytomegalovirus |
| CN | cranial nerve |
| CNS | central nervous system |
| c/o | complains of |
| CO | cardiac output, carbon monoxide |
| $CO_2$ | carbon dioxide |
| COPD | chronic obstructive pulmonary disease |
| CPR | cardiopulmonary resuscitation |
| Cr | creatinine |
| CRNA | certified registered nurse anesthetist |
| CSF | cerebrospinal fluid |
| CT | computed tomography |
| CTA | clear to auscultation |
| CTAB | clear to auscultation bilaterally |
| CTD | connective tissue disease |
| CV | cardiovascular |
| CVP | central venous pressure |
| CVS | chorionic villi sampling |
| CW | compared with |
| CX | culture |
| CXR | chest x-ray |
| D&C | dilation and curettage |
| D5 | dextrose 5% |
| DC | direct current |
| D/C | discontinue |
| DEF | drugs/fluids, EKG, fibrillation |
| DES | diethylstilbestrol |
| DIC | disseminated intravascular coagulation |
| Dispo | disposition |
| DKA | diabetic ketoacidosis |
| dL | deciliter |
| DLCO | diffusion capacity for carbon monoxide |
| DM | diabetes mellitus |
| DNR | do not resuscitate |
| DRE | digital rectal exam |
| DSM | *Diagnostic and Statistical Manual* |
| DT | delirium tremens |
| DTP | diphtheria, tetanus toxoids, pertussis (vaccine) |
| DTR | deep tendon reflex |
| DUB | dysfunctional uterine bleeding |
| DVT | deep venous thrombosis |
| dx | diagnosis |
| EBL | estimated blood loss |
| ECT | electroconvulsive therapy |
| EDD | estimated date of delivery |
| EEG | electroencephalogram |
| EGD | esophagogastroduodenoscopy |
| EKG | electrocardiogram |
| ELISA | enzyme-linked immunosorbent assay |
| EMG | electromyogram |
| EOM | extraocular movement |
| EOMI | extraocular movements intact |
| EPS | extrapyramidal symptoms |
| ER | emergency room |
| ERCP | endoscopic retrograde cholangiopancreatography |
| ERRLA | equal, round, responsive to light and accommodation |
| ESR | erythrocyte sedimentation rate |
| EtOH | ethanol |
| exp lap | exploratory laparotomy |

| Abbreviation | Meaning | Abbreviation | Meaning |
|---|---|---|---|
| EXT | extremities | ID | identification |
| FB | finger breadth | IDDM | insulin-dependent diabetes mellitus |
| F/C/S | fever, chills, sweating | IgA | immunoglobulin A |
| $FEF_{25-75}$ | forced expiratory flow, mid-expiratory phase | IHSS | idiopathic hypertrophic subaortic stenosis |
| $FE_{Na}$ | excreted fraction of filtered sodium | IM | intramuscular |
| $FEV_1$ | forced expiratory volume in 1 second | INH | isoniazid |
| FFM | fast finger movements | INR | International Normalized Ratio |
| FH | family history | I/O | intake/output |
| FHT | fetal heart tone | IOC | intraoperative cholangiogram |
| FNA | fine needle aspiration | ITP | idiopathic thrombocytopenic purpura |
| FSH | follicle-stimulating hormone | IUD | intrauterine device |
| FTA/ABS | fluorescent treponemal antibody absorption (test) | IUGR | intrauterine growth retardation |
| | | IU/L | International Units per liter |
| FTN | finger to nose | IV | intravenous |
| FUO | fever of unknown origin | IVC | inferior vena cava |
| FVC | forced vital capacity | J | joules |
| G-tube | gastrostomy tube | J-tube | jejunostomy tube |
| GABA | gamma-aminobutyric acid | JP | Jackson-Pratt |
| GAF | Global Assessment of Functioning | JPS | joint position sense |
| GB | gallbladder | JVD | jugular venous distention |
| GCS | Glasgow Coma Scale | JVP | jugular venous pressure |
| GE | gastroesophageal | K | potassium |
| GEN | general | KCl | potassium chloride |
| GERD | gastroesophageal reflux disease | KUB | kidney, ureter, bladder |
| GFR | glomerular filtration rate | KVO | keep vein open |
| GGT | gamma-glutamyl-transferase | L&D | labor and delivery |
| GI | gastrointestinal | L4–5 | fourth and fifth lumbar vertebrae |
| Glu | glucose | LDH | lactate dehydrogenase |
| GNR | gram-negative rod | LEEP | loop electrosurgical excision procedure |
| GnRH | gonadotropin-releasing hormone | | |
| GU | genitourinary | LES | lower esophageal sphincter |
| GUSTO | Global Utilization of Streptokinase and Tissue Plasminogen Activator for Occluded Arteries | LFT | liver function test |
| | | LGI | lower gastrointestinal |
| | | LGIB | lower gastrointestinal bleeding |
| H&P | history and physical | LH | luteinizing hormone |
| HA | headache | Li | lithium |
| Hb | hemoglobin | LLE | left lower extremity |
| HBV | hepatitis B virus | LLQ | left lower quadrant |
| HCT | hematocrit | LMN | lower motor neuron |
| HCV | hepatitis C virus | LMP | last menstrual period |
| HD | hospital day | LOC | laxative of choice, loss of consciousness |
| HEENT | head, eyes, ears, nose, and throat | | |
| HELLP | hemolysis, elevated liver (enzymes), low platelets | LP | lumbar puncture |
| | | LR | Ringer's lactate |
| hep | heparin | LT | light touch |
| Hgb | hemoglobin | LUE | left upper extremity |
| HIB | *Haemophilus influenzae* type B (vaccine) | LUQ | left upper quadrant |
| | | LV | left ventricle, left ventricular |
| HIDA | hepato-iminodiacetic acid | LVEF | left ventricular ejection fraction |
| HIS | hospital information system | MAE | moves all extremities |
| HIV | human immunodeficiency virus | MAI | *Mycobacterium avium-intracellulare* |
| HLA | human leukocyte antigen | MAO | monoamine oxidase |
| HMO | health maintenance organization | MAOI | monoamine oxidase inhibitor |
| h/o | history of | MCA | middle cerebral artery |
| HP | human papillomavirus | MCV | mean corpuscular volume |
| HPF | high-power field | mEq/L | milliequivalents per liter |
| HPI | history of present illness | mg | milligram |
| HR | heart rate | Mg | magnesium |
| HRT | hormone replacement therapy | MHA-TP | microhemagglutination assay— *Treponema pallidum* |
| HSM | hepatosplenomegaly | | |
| HSV | herpes simplex virus | MI | myocardial infarction |
| HTN | hypertension | mmHG | millimeter of mercury |
| HTS | heel to shin | MMR | measles, mumps, rubella (vaccine) |
| I&D | incision and drainage | MPH | master's in public health |
| IBD | inflammatory bowel disease | M/R/G | murmurs, rubs, gallops |
| ICA | internal carotid artery | MRI | magnetic resonance imaging |
| ICP | intracranial pressure | MS | multiple sclerosis |
| ICU | intensive care unit | MS-I, II, etc | medical student |

| Abbreviation | Meaning |
|---|---|
| MSE | mental status examination |
| Na | sodium |
| NABS | normal active bowel sounds |
| NC | nasal cannula, normocephalic |
| ND | nondistended |
| NDDG | National Diabetes Data Group |
| NEURO | neurologic |
| NFT | neurofibrillary tangles |
| NG | nasogastric |
| NIDDM | non-insulin-dependent diabetes mellitus |
| NKDA | no known drug allergies |
| nl | normal |
| NMS | neuroleptic malignant syndrome |
| NP | nurse practitioner |
| NPH | normal pressure hydrocephalus |
| NPO | nil per os (nothing by mouth) |
| NQWMI | non-Q-wave myocardial infarction |
| NS | normal saline |
| NSAID | nonsteroidal anti-inflammatory drugs |
| NSVD | normal spontaneous vaginal delivery |
| NT | nontender |
| N/V | nausea, vomiting |
| $O_2$ sat | oxygen saturation |
| OB/GYN | obstetrics and gynecology |
| OCP | oral contraceptive pill |
| OGTT | oral glucose tolerance test |
| OI | opportunistic infection |
| OOB | out of bed |
| O/P | oropharynx |
| OR | operating room |
| OTC | over the counter |
| O/W | otherwise |
| P | pulse |
| PA | posteroanterior |
| $PaCO_2$ | partial pressure of carbon dioxide in arterial blood |
| PCA | posterior cerebral artery, patient-controlled analgesia |
| PCO | polycystic ovary |
| $pCO_2$ | partial pressure of carbon dioxide |
| PCP | phencyclidine ("angel dust"), *Pneumocystis carinii* pneumonia |
| $P_{Cr}$ | plasma creatinine |
| PDA | personal digital assistant |
| PDR | *Physician's Desk Reference* |
| PDS | polydioxanone sutures |
| PE | physical examination, pulmonary embolism |
| PEFR | peak expiratory flow rate |
| PERRL | pupils equal, round, responsive to light |
| PFT | pulmonary function test |
| PGY | postgraduate year |
| PID | pelvic inflammatory disease |
| PIH | pregnancy-induced hypertension |
| Plts | platelets |
| PMH | past medical history |
| PMN | polymorphonuclear (leukocytes) |
| PN | progress note |
| $P_{Na}$ | plasma sodium |
| $pO_2$ | partial pressure of oxygen |
| POD | postoperative day |
| PP | pin prick |
| ppd | pack per day |
| PPD | purified protein derivative (of tuberculin) |
| PR | per rectum |

| Abbreviation | Meaning |
|---|---|
| PRBC | packed red blood cells |
| prn | pro re nata (as required) |
| Pt | patient |
| PT | prothrombin time |
| PTC | percutaneous transhepatic cholangiography |
| PTCA | percutaneous transluminal coronary angioplasty |
| PTT | partial thromboplastin time |
| PUD | peptic ulcer disease |
| q4h | every four hours |
| qd | every day |
| qhs | every night |
| qod | every other day |
| R | respiration |
| RA | room air, rheumatoid arthritis |
| RBC | red blood cell |
| REM | random eye movement |
| Rh | Rhesus (factor) |
| RHM | rapid hand movements |
| RIND | reversible ischemic neurologic deficit |
| RLQ | right lower quadrant |
| ROM | rupture of membranes |
| ROS | review of symptoms |
| RPGN | rapidly progressive glomerulonephritis |
| RPR | rapid plasma reagin (test) |
| RR | rate regular, respiratory rate |
| RT | recreation therapy, recreational therapist |
| RUL | right upper lobe |
| RUQ | right upper quadrant |
| RV | residual volume, right ventricle, right ventricular |
| SA | sinoatrial |
| SAB | spontaneous abortion |
| SAH | subarachnoid hemorrhage |
| SBO | small bowel obstruction |
| SBP | systolic blood pressure |
| SCM | sternocleidomastoid |
| SGOT | serum glutamic oxaloacetic transaminase |
| SH | social history |
| sl | slightly |
| SLE | systemic lupus erythematosus |
| SMX | sulfamethoxazole |
| SOAP | subjective (data), objective (data), assessment, and plan |
| SOB | shortness of breath |
| s/p | status post(operatively) |
| SQ | subcutaneous |
| SSRI | selective serotonin uptake inhibitor |
| STD | sexually transmitted disease |
| T | temperature |
| T. bili | total bilirubin |
| T&P | tongue and palate |
| TAB | therapeutic abortion |
| TB | tuberculosis |
| Tc | technetium |
| $T_c$ | current temperature |
| TCA | tricyclic antidepressant |
| TFT | thyroid function test |
| TID | three times a day |
| TIPS | transjugular intrahepatic portosystemic shunt |
| TLC | total lung capacity |
| TM | tympanic membrane |
| $T_M$ | maximum temperature |
| TMP | trimethoprim |
| TOA | tubo-ovarian abscess |

| Abbreviation | Meaning | Abbreviation | Meaning |
|---|---|---|---|
| ToRCHeS | toxoplasmosis, rubella, cytomegalovirus, herpes simplex, syphilis | U/S | ultrasound |
| | | USMLE | United States Medical Licensing Examination |
| tPA | tissue-type plasminogen activator | UTI | urinary tract infection |
| TPN | total parenteral nutrition | VA | Veterans Administration |
| TSH | thyroid-stimulating hormone | VC | vital capacity |
| TTP | thrombotic thrombocytopenic purpura | VCUG | voiding cystourethrogram |
| TyCo | Tylenol and codeine | VDRL | Venereal Disease Research Laboratory (test) |
| UA | urinalysis | | |
| $U_{Cr}$ | urinary concentration of creatinine | VFFTC | visual fields full to confrontation |
| UGI | upper gastrointestinal | V-fib | ventricular fibrillation |
| UGIB | upper gastrointestinal bleeding | V-Q | ventilation-perfusion |
| UMN | upper motor neuron | VS | vital signs |
| $U_{Na}$ | urinary concentration of sodium | V-tach | ventricular tachycardia |
| UO | urine output | WBC | white blood cell, white blood (cell) count |
| UP | universal precautions | | |
| URI | upper respiratory infection | WHO | World Health Organization |

# Index

TSH/prolactin levels, 248
T-tube, 99
Tuberculosis, pulmonary (TB), 81
Tubes and drains, 99–100
Tubo-ovarian abscess (TOA), 238
Typical medical day, 5–7
 afternoon work, 8
 attending rounds, 6
 communicating with patients/family members, 19
 consults, 20–21
 internal medicine, 46
 labs and studies, checking, 21
 neurology, 174–175
 noon conference, 6
 OB/GYN, 211
 pediatrics, 146
 prerounds, 5
 procedures, 19–20
 psychiatry, 255–256
 reading up on your patient's problems, 21–22
 signing out, 7
 surgery, 7, 94–95
 work rounds, 6
 work time, 6
 writing notes, 17
 writing orders, 17–18

## U

Ulcerative colitis, 79, 80, 128
Ultrasound, 69, 116, 227, 227
Umbilical hernia, 134
Unconjugated hyperbilirubinemia, 163–164
Understanding Electrocardiography (Conover), 42
Universal precautions, 32
University hospitals, 24
Upper gastrointestinal bleeding (UGIB)
 differential diagnosis, 129
 signs and symptoms, 129
 treatment, 130
 workup, 130
Upper GI series, 124
Upper motor neuron (UMN), 206
Urinary tract infection (UTI)
 differential diagnosis, 162–163
 pathogens, common, 162

signs and symptoms, 162, 163
 treatment, 163
Urine and renal failure, 84–85
Uterine bleeding, abnormal
 etiology, 248–249
 treatment, 250
 workup, 249

## V

Vaginal examinations and ultrasound, 228
Vaginitis
 causes of, 243
 defining, 243
 differential diagnosis, 243
 signs and symptoms, 243
 treatment, 244
 workup, 243
Vagus and cranial nerve exam, 184
Valproate, 171, 195
Valproic acid, 268–269
Vascular dementia, 272
Vasopressin, 130
VA system, 23–24
Venereal warts. See Condylomata acuminata
Venlafaxine, 267
Ventricular systolic function, left/right, 61–63
Ventriculitis, 159
Vertigo, central vs. peripheral, 205
Vesicoureteral reflux, 162
Vestibulocochlear and cranial nerve exam, 184
Vestibulotoxic drugs, 205–206
Violent patients, 35
Viral meningitis, 158
Virchow's triad, 69
Vital signs, 95, 149
V-Q scans, 69, 70

## W

Wards experience, understanding the. See also various subject headings
 admission, the, 8–14
 advantages, your, 37–38
 books, top-rated, 39–43
 call nights, surviving, 28
 daily ward activities, 17–22
 difficult situations, 31–38

evaluations, 30–31
 mental/physical health, strategies for, 28
 oral presentation, 15–17
 organizational aids, 26–28
 preparatory measures for getting off to good start, 29–30
 rotation sites, choosing, 23–25
 scheduling rotations, 22
 team, medical, 1–5
 time and patient management, 25–26
 typical medical day, 5–7
Washington Manual of Medical Therapeutics, 21
Washington Manual of Surgery (Doherty), 106
Water and electrolyte balance, 159
Water brash, 123
Weakness
 anatomic localization, 207
 causes of, 206
 clinical localization, 207
 investigation of patient with, 208
 lesions in the motor pathways, 207
Wellbutrin, 267
Western blot test, 82
Wheezing, 123
White blood cell counts
 asthma, 165
 croup, viral, 169
 epiglottitis, 170
 febrile seizures, 171
 meningitis, 158
 pneumonia, 161
Williams Obstetrics (Cunningham), 218
Withdrawal, alcohol, 282
Work rounds, 6
Writing notes/orders, 17–18. See also Records, medical
Written evaluations, 30

## X

Xanthines, 72

## Z

Zebra decision making, 24
Zollinger-Ellison syndrome, 77, 78
Zoloft, 266
Zyprexa, 271

# Notes

# Notes

# Notes

# Notes

# Notes

# Notes

# Notes

# Notes

# Notes

**NEW from the authors of *First Aid for the USMLE Step 1*
and *First Aid for the Wards* comes...**

# First Aid for the Match

*Le, Bhushan, & Amin*

*First Aid for the Match* helps medical students effectively and efficiently navigate the residency application process. This book allows students to make the most of their limited time, money, and energy. The book draws on the advice and experiences of successful student applicants as well as residency directors. Features application and interview tips tailored to each specialty, successful personal statements and CVs with analyses, current trends, and common interview questions with suggested strategies for responding. Available in bookstores. ISBN 0-8385-2596-2.

---

# About the Authors

**Tao Le, MD,** earned his medical degree from the University of California at San Francisco in 1996. He has been involved in major writing and editing projects over the past six years. As a medical student he was editor-in-chief of *Synapse,* a campus-wide student-run newspaper with a weekly circulation of 5000. His continuing interest in medical student education led to the development of *First Aid for the Match* and *First Aid for the Wards*. He is currently a resident in internal medicine at Yale-New Haven Hospital. He is married and lives in New Haven with his wife, Thao, a resident in pediatrics. Tao can be reached at taotle@aol.com.

**Vikas Bhushan, MD,** completed residency training in diagnostic radiology at the University of California at Los Angeles. He is currently working part-time *locum tenens* in radiology while taking time off to travel and write. His work in medical education led to the development and publication of the original *First Aid for the USMLE Step 1* in 1992. He is active in medical informatics and digital radiology. Vikas earned his MD with Thesis from the University of California at San Francisco. Vikas is single and resides in the Beverly Glen area of Los Angeles. He can be reached at vbhushan@aol.com.

**Chirag Amin, MD,** graduated from medical school at the University of Miami and is now training in orthopedic surgery at Orlando Regional Medical Center. Chirag has been involved extensively in teaching and in writing books. He recently led the completion of *Jump Start MCAT* (Williams & Wilkins), a preparation guide for the MCAT. Chirag is single and lives in Orlando, Florida. He can be reached at chiragamin@aol.com.

**Ross Berkeley, MD,** recently finished his medical degree form the University of California at San Francisco and is now a resident in emergency medicine at the University of Pittsburgh. He helped coordinate *First Aid for the Wards* and was a contributing author for the 1996 revision of *First Aid for the USMLE Step 1*. Ross is single and lives in Pittsburgh. He enjoys the outdoors and Belgian beers. He can be reached at emergdoc@aol.com.

**For the latest on the Boards, Wards, and Match, tune into**
# http://www.s2smed.com